Standard Operating Procedures
and Regulatory Guidelines
BLOOD BANKING

GW01057421

Standard Operating Procedures
and Regulatory Guidelines
BLOOD BANKING

Second Edition

GP Saluja MBBS MD (Pathology)
Senior Consultant
Blood Center
Alchemist Hospitals Ltd
Panchkula, Haryana, India

GL Singal M. Pharm. Ph.D. LLB
Former State Drugs Controller
Food and Drug Administration
Ministry of Health and Family Welfare
Government of Haryana
Panchkula, Haryana, India

Forewords
Ratti Ram Sharma
Manmohan Taneja
Ravneet Kaur
Arvind Kukrety

JAYPEE

JAYPEE BROTHERS MEDICAL PUBLISHERS
The Health Sciences Publisher
New Delhi | London

Jaypee Brothers Medical Publishers (P) Ltd

Headquarters

EMCA House
23/23-B, Ansari Road, Daryaganj
New Delhi 110 002, India
Landline: +91-11-23272143, +91-11-23272703
+91-11-23282021, +91-11-23245672
E-mail: jaypee@jaypeebrothers.com

Corporate Office

Jaypee Brothers Medical Publishers (P) Ltd.
4838/24, Ansari Road, Daryaganj
New Delhi 110 002, India
Phone: +91-11-43574357
Fax: +91-11-43574314
E-mail: jaypee@jaypeebrothers.com

Overseas Office

JP Medical Ltd.
83, Victoria Street, London
SW1H 0HW (UK)
Phone: +44-20 3170 8910
Fax: +44(0)20 3008 6180
E-mail: info@jpmedpub.com

Website: www.jaypeebrothers.com
Website: www.jaypeedigital.com

Inquiries for bulk sales may be solicited at: jaypee@jaypeebrothers.com

Standard Operating Procedures and Regulatory Guidelines—Blood Banking / GP Saluja, GL Singal

First Edition: 2014

Second Edition: **2024**

ISBN: 978-93-5696-188-3

Printed at Rajkamal Electric Press, Kundli, Haryana.

Dedicated to

Our families
and
our dear parents
whose inspiration, motivation, blessings
and moral support continue to contribute
a great deal to our academic endeavors
&
Everybody striving to contribute
to the blood safety

Foreword

स्नातकोत्तर चिकित्सा शिक्षा एवं अनुसंधान संस्थान, चंडीगढ़–160012 (भारत)

Postgraduate Institute of Medical Education & Research,
Chandigarh - 160012

रक्ताधान औषधि विभाग
Department of Transfusion Medicine

डा. रत्ती राम शर्मा
प्राध्यापक एवं अध्यक्ष

Dr Ratti Ram Sharma
Professor & Head

संख्या/No. DTM/ ....
दिनांक/Dated ....

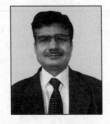

Blood and its components are treated as drugs and its collection storage and supply is regulated under the Drugs and Cosmetics Act and Rules framed thereunder. The regulations are amended from time to time to address new challenges and incorporate new developments and advancements in the related field. The entire statutory framework focuses on safety starting from donor selection, screening, handling, testing, storage, preservation, transportation, etc. Lapse at any stage may adversely impact the final product.

To do things right, each time, it is necessary to standardize procedures, methods, and systems being followed by the blood centers. To keep pace with the ever-changing environment, all stakeholders need regularly update oneself on law, its understanding and technical advancements. This void needs to be managed by each blood center by providing training and latest material on the subject to their team.

Dr GL Singal, Ex Drugs Controller, Haryana a known expert in the regulatory field and Dr GP Saluja a renowned expert in the field of transfusion medicines have been working in this area for many years. The duo has through this Second Edition of their book made an excellent effort to share the updates on the subject. This manual covers all the technical aspects on blood center operations, right from blood collection, processing, preparation of components, basics of blood serology, transfusion transmitted infections, and current regulatory guidelines. This will certainly help the blood center officers, technicians, regulatory officials, and student in understanding the technical and regulatory aspects of the subject.

Dr Ratti Ram Sharma

दूरसंचार
Grams POSTGRADMED

दूरभाष/Phone: Off: 0172-2756481
M/fax: 0172-2744401, 2744450, 2745078
{ई-मेल/Email:rrsdoc@hotmail.com}

Foreword

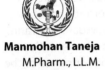

State Drugs Controller-cum-Licensing Authority
Food & Drugs Administration
Haryana

Manmohan Taneja
M.Pharm., L.L.M.

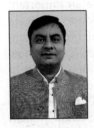

I am extremely happy to know that Dr GP Saluja and Dr GL Singal have taken an initiative for revision of their book titled "*Standard Operating Procedures and Regulatory Guidelines—Blood Banking*" which was published in 2014. I am writing this foreword because Dr GP Saluja, on account of being nominated expert by Government of India and Dr GL Singal, former State Drugs Controller, Haryana, have vast experience in joint inspections for grant of license of blood centers and their subsequent renewal, training to blood center medical officers and regulators and there cannot be more appropriate experts in revision of their book in view of amendments in Drugs and Cosmetics Act, 1940 and Rules thereunder and recently released "National Standards for Blood Centres and Blood Transfusion Services (2nd Edition)" by the National Blood Transfusion Council (NBTC).

Blood transfusion services are integral part of healthcare delivery system and save considerable number of lives. Blood transfusions are needed for a wide range of health conditions including anemia, complications during pregnancy and childbirth, severe trauma due to accidents and surgical procedures. They are also regularly used for patients with conditions such as sickle cell disease and thalassemia and for the products to treat hemophilia.

Blood transfusions are generally considered safe, but there is some risk of complications and, hence the need of provisions for safe blood arises. Safe blood can only be ensured by implementing Quality management in blood centers. Quality management can be achieved by adopting *Good Manufacturing Practice, Good Laboratory Practice and Good Clinical Practice* through establishing a comprehensive and coordinated approach of the total quality management. All those who are involved in blood transfusion related activity must be aware of the importance of quality management for its successful implementation. Good record-keeping and documentation, use of Standard Operating Procedures and laboratory worksheets, and implementation of safety guidelines will further improve the quality performance of the services. Standard Operating Procedures constitute an important parameter for quality control; these are specific procedures which are written by the incharge of the blood center and shall be consistent with either DGHS (Directorate General of Health Services) manual or other organization/individual blood center's manuals subject to the approval of *Licensing Authority*. The use of Standard Operating Procedures is compulsory every time an activity is performed in the blood center. Standard procedures must ensure that whole human blood or blood component is issued only after performing all mandatory tests.

Besides, those involved in blood transfusion service, must also be aware of the statutory provisions, guidelines and ethical practices to carry out safe blood transfusion.

I hope that the Second Edition of this book would be of immense help to all those involved in blood transfusion services for understanding the importance of Standard Operating Procedures, documentation and statutory requirements pertaining to the provisions of safe blood to the community.

Warm regards,

Manmohan Taneja

Department of Food & Drug Administration, Haryana
SCO-94, Sector-5, Panchkula-134108

Website: www.fdaharyana.gov.in   E-mail ID: haryanafda@gmail.com

Foreword

**GOVERNMENT MEDICAL COLLEGE AND HOSPITAL
SECTOR-32, CHANDIGARH
DEPARTMENT OF TRANSFUSION MEDICINE**

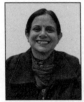

Dr Ravneet Kaur MD MAMS
Professor & Head

It gives me immense pleasure to know that Dr GP Saluja and Dr GL Singal have spearheaded the Second Edition of their book titled "*Standard Operating Procedures and Regulatory Guidelines—Blood Banking*". The first edition was published long back in 2014 and since then, with the amendments in the Drugs and Cosmetics Act in March 2020, the issuance of National Standards for Blood Centres and Blood Transfusion Services by Ministry of Health and Family Welfare (MoHFW), Govt of India in August 2022, and changes in technologies, there is need to update the book.

I commend the efforts of Dr GP Saluja and Dr GL Singal for giving their valuable contributions and efforts in the publication of the Second Edition. I am sure that all the technical developments in the field, regulatory changes in the transfusion medicine as well as guidelines of Govt of India have been adequately incorporated in the book.

I am confident that this book will be of immense benefit to one and all working in this field and will help them in achieving the objective of providing adequate, safe, and quality blood/blood components by updating and following the standard operating procedures.

Ravneet Kaur

Dr Ravneet Kaur

Foreword

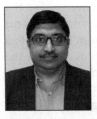

Arvind Kukrety
Deputy Drugs Controller (India) Central Drugs Standard
Control Organisation (CDSCO)
Ministry of Health and Family Welfare
New Delhi

त्दिवशुध्म हि रुधिरं ब्ल्वर्नसुख्युषा।
युन्क्ति प्रवीनम प्राणः शोणितं हस्नुवर्त्ते।।

Living creatures are endowed with:
- **Bala:** Strength and immunity
- **Varna:** Skin complexion
- **Sukha:** Happiness comfort
- **Ayusha:** Longevity due to pure blood

Blood plays a vital role in the sustenance of vital force of life.

"Blood is Life" as can be seen from the quote above from Charaka Samhita. Offering blood to save someone's life is the biggest service one can offer toward humanity. But this can also be fatal if contaminated. There have been constant and consorted efforts by the Governments, Medical Fraternity, Researchers, and Members of the Society, Private Players, NGOs, etc., to ensure its adequacy, availability, accessibility, quality, and safety. As such having a well-organized and a strong framework for Blood Transfusion Service which is an essential component of healthcare system, has become need of the hour. Blood and its components are treated as drugs and its collection storage and supply is regulated under the Drugs and Cosmetics Act and Rules framed thereunder. The regulations are amended from time to time to address new challenges and incorporate new developments and advancements in the related field. The entire statutory framework focuses on safety starting from donor selection, screening, handling, testing, storage, preservation, transportation, etc. Lapse at any stage may adversely impact the final product.

Dr GL Singal, former State Drugs Controller, Haryana, a known expert in the regulatory field and Dr GP Saluja a renowned expert in the field of transfusion medicine have been working in this area for many years. The duo has through this Second Edition of their book made an excellent effort to share the updates on the areas. They besides reflecting on the need of changes in the regulatory frameworks and standard operating procedures, have shared the updates, new developments, and crucial judicial pronouncements in the related field. The inputs being provided through the chapters on technical aspects on blood center operations covering all the aspects right from collection, processing, preparation of components, immunohematology, transfusion transmitted infections, regulatory guidelines, etc., shall immensely add value to quality output and performances of the centers and shall also help the associated persons like the blood center officers, technicians, regulatory officials, and student in understanding legal and regulatory aspects of the subject.

Arvind Kukrety

Preface to the Second Edition

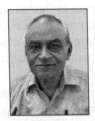

GP Saluja

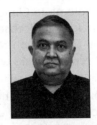

GL Singal

Blood transfusion services have become an integral part of the healthcare system. It is an essential function of the health services to provide quality safe blood to all those who need it in an efficient, coordinated and cost-effective manner. The developments in the blood transfusion services with emergence of newer technologies, digital platforms, and current knowledge in immunohematology, have been able to make safe blood and blood components available for the patients.

Having been associated with blood transfusion services since last many decades, we have witnessed gigantic changes in blood banking starting from the era when blood center licensing was not mandatory and glass bottles were being used for collection of blood units after preparing and sterilizing anticoagulant solution by autoclave. It was after the Supreme Court verdict in *Common Cause vs. Union of India and others*", delivered on 4th January 1996, licensing of blood centers was made mandatory, elimination of professional donors and the National Blood Transfusion Council (NBTC) and State Blood Transfusion Councils (SBTCs), were set up. The Drugs and Cosmetics Rules, 1945 were also amended to maintain and follow "Standard Operating Procedures" (SOP) by all blood centers, including methodology to be followed in the collection, processing, compatibility testing, storage and supply or distribution of blood, and preparation of blood components. The Standards for Blood Centers and Blood Transfusion Services published by the NBTC recommended quality assurance system as per international standards. Recent amendment in Drugs and Cosmetics Act 1940 and

Rules 1945 requiring 3 months experience in licensed blood center for MD (Pathology) or DNB (Pathology) and MBBS with Diploma in Transfusion Medicine or Diploma in Immunohematology or Blood Transfusion; 6 months experience in licensed blood center for MBBS with Diploma in Clinical Pathology or Diploma in Pathology and Bacteriology in licensed blood center and no experience for MD or DNB (Transfusion Medicine), for whole-time medical officer in blood center, speaks about the evolution in the field of transfusion medicine.

While auditing functioning of blood centers during statutory inspections of blood centers under the provisions of Drugs and Cosmetics Act 1940 and Rules 1945 for grant/renewal of blood center license, we realize the importance and dire necessity of appropriate SOPs to streamline their functioning for ensuring safe and quality blood. Therefore, feeling the need to provide adequate knowledge to the technical personnel working in the field of blood banking, the first edition of book titled "Standard Operating Procedures and Regulatory Guidelines—Blood Banking" was authored in 2014.

Keeping in view the mammoth advancement in the technology, changes by way of amendments after the year 2014 in the Drugs and Cosmetics Act 1940 and Rules 1945 as well as revision of "National Standards for Blood Centers and Blood Transfusion Services (2nd Edition)" in August 2022, it was need of the hour to update the readers on SOPs, regulatory guidelines and judicial pronouncements. The importance of SOPs and quality control of blood and blood components has also been highlighted. This book is suitable for medical graduate and postgraduate students, blood center officers, and medical laboratory technicians, and even for drug regulatory officers.

We are thankful to Ortho Clinical Diagnostics India, Terumo Penpol Private Limited and Mylab Discovery Solutions Pvt Ltd for their help and support in designing equipment specific SOPs.

We are thankful to our colleagues and friends for their never ending inspiration and support. We are grateful to our families who have always stood beside us in thick and thin and encouraging us in authoring edition/publication of this book.

Preface to the First Edition

This book *"Standard Operating Procedures and Regulatory Guidelines–Blood Banking"* has been designed to provide blood bank technicians, students undergoing various courses in medical technology, blood bank specialists and residents with a concise and thorough practical and simple procedural guide to all the procedures to check the quality and safety of the blood donated for transfusion.

The first section of the book focuses on routine blood bank practices including donor selection, phlebotomy procedure, sample collection, component preparation, blood grouping—both routine and gel technology, screening for the transfusion transmitted infections (TTIs), compatibility testing, storage of blood/blood components, apheresis, labeling, issue and transport of blood units, transfusion of the right blood to the right patient, quality control/ assurance, equipment maintenance and bio-waste disposal.

The second section deals with the regulatory guidelines including the Drugs and Cosmetics Act, 1940 and Rules, 1945, NACO guidelines for the safety of blood/blood components and procedural details as well as various documents required for processing of application for grant of license under the said Act to operate the blood banks.

Some of the judicial pronouncements related to the blood safety have also been included so as to create awareness amongst the blood bank fraternity regarding the various legal issues involved in blood transfusion.

The book is a culmination of the tremendous efforts of the dedicated professionals because they care about the blood bank profession, and it also aims at fostering improved patient care by providing the readers with a basic understanding of the various blood bank procedures and legal issues. We express our gratitude to all those associated including Dr Gautam Wankhede, Director, Medical Affairs, Alliance Transfusion (Pvt) Ltd, for contributing valuable inputs in compiling this publication.

GP Saluja
GL Singal

Acknowledgments

First and foremost, praises and thanks to the God, the Almighty, for His showers of blessings throughout the period of updating and completing this book.

We owe an enormous debt of gratitude to blood transfusion professionals who gave us detailed and constructive comments for the first edition and pushed us to clarify concepts in this edition.

Our sincere thanks go to Dr Anchal Mahajan, Consultant Microbiology; Alchemist Hospitals Ltd; Panchkula for her expert advice on chapter of sterility testing.

Our thanks are extended to M/s Jaypee Brothers Medical Publishers (P) Ltd, New Delhi, India, and their dedicated staff for professionally designing and printing this book.

We would like to thank Mr Ashok Kumar, data entry operator, who has helped in typing this manuscript.

Additionally, our special thanks to Mr Ved Prakash, senior technical supervisor, Alchemist Hospitals Ltd Panchkula for his help in designing the various formats for registers and other documents.

This book would not have been possible without the concrete suggestions of our colleagues—seniors and juniors that allowed us to prepare this manuscript.

Last but not the least, we thank our families and friends as any attempt at any level cannot be completed without their support.

Contents

Component Section

Immunohematology

Transfusion Transmitted Infections (TTIs)

Quality Control

Biomedical Waste

Section 3: Regulatory Guidelines

PLATE 1

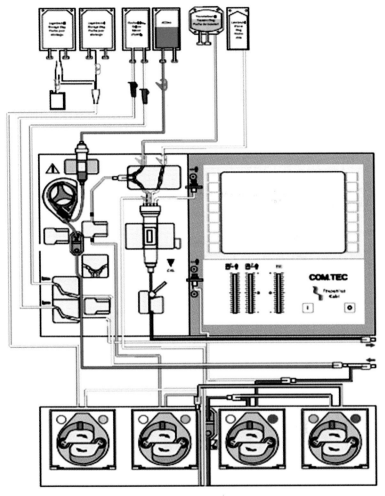

FIG. 6: Checks after apheresis set and separation chamber installation. (*Chapter 14*)

PLATE 2

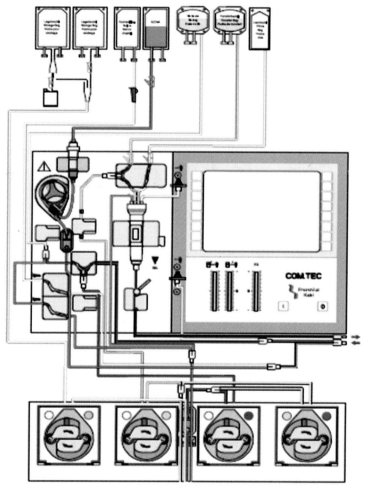

FIG. 6: Checks after apheresis set and separation chamber installation.
(*Chapter 15*)

PLATE 3

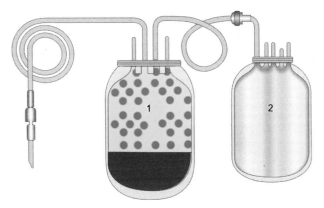

FIG. 2: Blood bag no. 1 contains red blood cell (RBC) at the bottom and platelet-rich plasma (PRP) on the top. **(*Chapter 20*)**

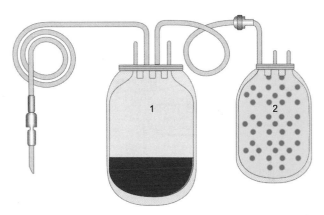

FIG. 3: Packed red blood cells (RBCs) in bag no. 1 and platelet-rich plasma in bag no. 2. **(*Chapter 20*)**

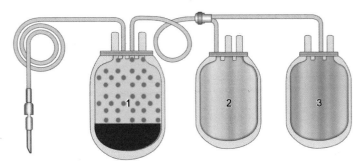

FIG. 2: Triple bag after centrifugation. **(*Chapter 21*)**

PLATE 4

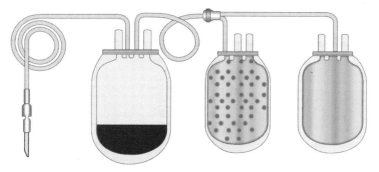

FIG. 3: Platelet-rich plasma (PRP) transferred to bag no. 2. (*Chapter 21*)

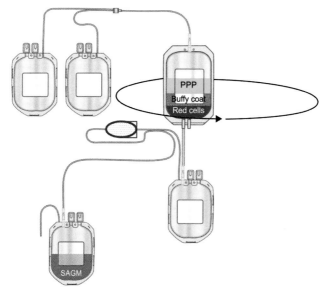

FIG. 4: Centrifuging whole blood with hard spin (first spin). (*Chapter 22*)
(PPP: platelet poor plasma; SAGM: saline-adenine-glucose-mannitol)

PLATE 5

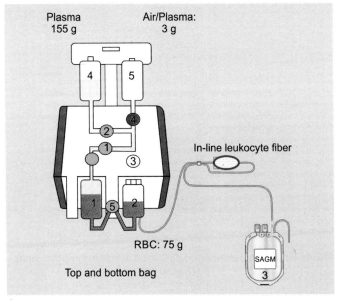

FIG. 5: Graphical placement of top and bottom penta blood bags. **(*Chapter 22*)**

(RBC: red blood cell; SAGM: saline-adenine-glucose-mannitol)

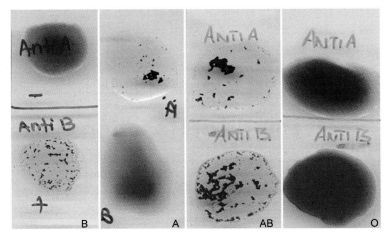

FIG. 1: Slide method for blood grouping. **(*Chapter 28*)**

PLATE 6

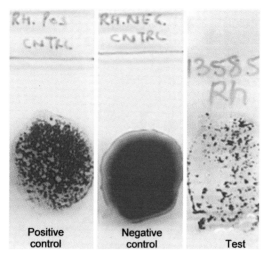

FIG. 1: Rh grouping showing agglutination in test and positive control. (*Chapter 29*)

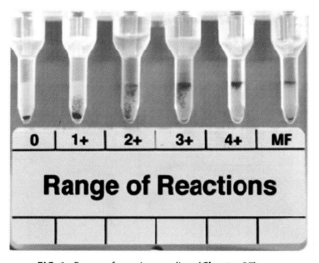

FIG. 1: Range of reaction grading. (*Chapter 37*)

PLATE 7

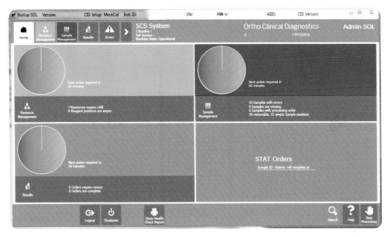

FIG. 3: Screen status for any error (red color) and review status (yellow color).
(*Chapter 37*)

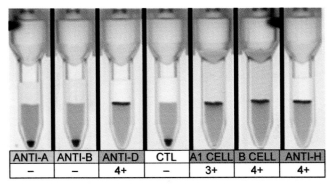

ANTI-A	ANTI-B	ANTI-D	CTL	A1 CELL	B CELL	ANTI-H
–	–	4+	–	3+	4+	4+

Annexure 38.1: Blood grouping with reverse grouping "O" Rh positive.
(*Chapter 38*)

PLATE 8

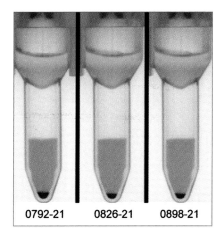

0792-21   0826-21   0898-21

Annexure 39.1: Negative reaction in polyspecific crossmatch showing compatible unit. *(Chapter 39)*

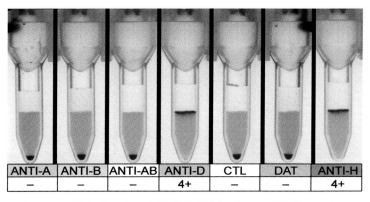

ANTI-A	ANTI-B	ANTI-AB	ANTI-D	CTL	DAT	ANTI-H
–	–	–	4+	–	–	4+

Annexure 40.1: New born ABO/Rh/DAT (Blood group O DAT negative). *(Chapter 40)*

PLATE 9

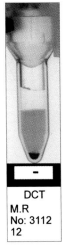

DCT
M.R
No: 3112
12

Annexure 43.1: DAT negative
(*Chapter 43*)

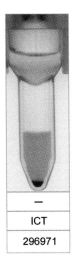

ICT

296971

Annexure 43.2: IAT negative
(*Chapter 43*)

Purple Top	
Additive	EDTA
Mode of action	Forms calcium salts to remove calcium
Uses	Hematology (CBC) and Blood Center (Crossmatch); requires *full draw*—invert eight times to prevent clotting and platelet clumping

FIG. 1: Purple top vacutainer. (*Chapter 46*)
(CBC: complete blood count; EDTA: ethylenediaminetetraacetic acid)

Red top	
Additive	None
Mode of action	Blood clots, and the serum is separated by centrifugation
Uses	Blood chemistries, immunology and serology, Blood Center (crossmatch)

FIG. 2: Red top vacutainer. (*Chapter 46*)

PLATE 10

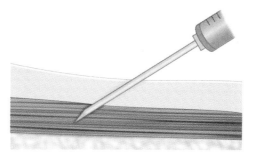

FIG. 3: Needle angle. *(Chapter 46)*

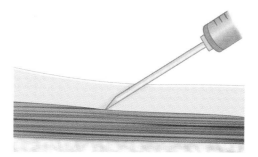

FIG. 4: Needle not in the lumen of the vein. *(Chapter 46)*

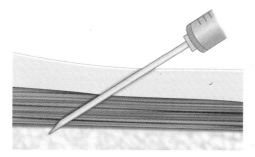

FIG. 5: Needle penetrated too far. *(Chapter 46)*

PLATE 11

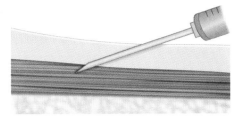

FIG. 6: Bevel touching the vein wall. **(Chapter 46)**

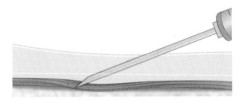

FIG. 7: Collapsed vein. **(Chapter 46)**

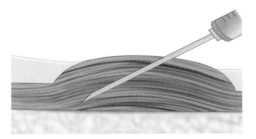

FIG. 8: Hematoma under the skin. **(Chapter 46)**

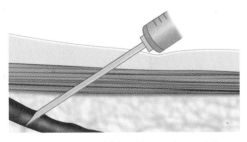

FIG. 9: Bright red (arterial) blood being drawn. **(Chapter 46)**

PLATE 12

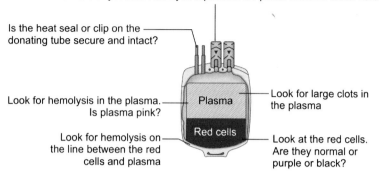

FIG. 1: Various signs of deterioration to be looked for. (**Chapter 47**)

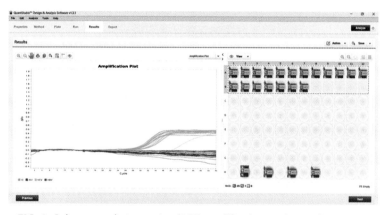

FIG. 6: Polymerase chain reaction (PCR) amplification result in real-time PCR. (**Chapter 56**)

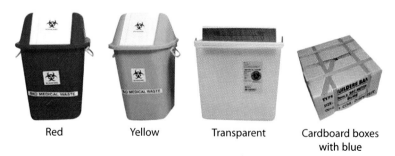

| Red | Yellow | Transparent | Cardboard boxes with blue |

Category of Bins used for segregation of biomedical waste as given in **Table 1**. (**Chapter 72**)

SECTION 1

General

CHAPTER 1

Procedure for Creating Standard Operating Procedures

INTRODUCTION

A standard operating procedure (SOP) is a set of written instructions that describes a step-by-step process put together by an organization to enable technicians and workers to properly perform their day-to-day activities within the organization. The SOPs should be followed in the same way every time to ensure that the organization remains consistent and adheres to mandatory regulations and standards. SOP aims to achieve efficiency, quality output, and performance consistency while reducing misunderstandings and regulatory violations. SOPs provide policies and processes, and the organization needs to be successful. It provides a platform by reducing errors, increasing efficiency and profitability, creating a safe working environment, and providing policies to solve problems and overcome obstacles.

PURPOSE

A blood center SOP is essential to ensure the smooth, efficient, and legal operation/operation of a blood center; achieve efficiency, quality performance, and consistency in performance; and reduce misunderstandings and regulatory violations. These SOPs are numerous within a particular blood center, each defining its role and function, but there are also some SOPs common to all blood centers with common procedures, equipment, e.g., SOP for donor selection, blood collection, pre- and postdonation counseling, blood grouping and blood crossmatching, issuing procedures, and testing for adverse transfusion reactions, etc. These SOPs must contain the following:
- Guidelines for rational use of blood and blood components
- Availability time frames of whole blood and its components
- Rapid assessment of reported transfusion reactions and other adverse events

- Release of uncrossmatched blood in emergency, which should include compatibility testing performed after release

Standard operating procedures are an important part of quality system and ensure that procedures are performed in a standardized manner and produce consistent results.

Each blood center is an independent distinct entity holding specific drug license under the Drugs and Cosmetics Act 1940 and Rules 1945. Schedule "F" of the Drugs and Cosmetics Rules 1945 provides that written SOPs must be maintained and used for collection, processing, compatibility testing, storage, and sale or distribution of blood and/or preparation of components for homologous transfusion, autologous transfusion, and further manufacturing purposes. These SOPs must be available to the personnel for use in the concerned areas to ensure that all procedures are performed at the blood center under the license. Therefore, each blood center should develop its own blood center-specific SOPs based on available infrastructure, laboratory procedures to be followed, and reagent availability. The SOPs described here will assist licensees in creating their own blood center-specific SOPs, which will be approved by the State Licensing Authority (SLA) and Central License Approving Authority (CLAA).

BENEFITS

- Indicate compliance to Drugs and Cosmetics Act 1940 and Rules 1945
- Minimize deviation and improve quality by consistently enforcing processes or procedures within the organization
- Minimize opportunities for misunderstandings and help address safety concerns
- Used as a checklist for inspectors to audit procedures
- Improved operational efficiency

STANDARD OPERATING PROCEDURE TEMPLATE OVERVIEW

An SOP template is a preformatted document that an organization uses as a starting point to create its own SOPs. Like other templates, it also serves as a basic structural guideline for creating operating procedures. The template determines what information the document contains and how each topic is laid out in SOP. This is important to ensure consistency from one SOP to another SOP so that users can easily find the information they need. The first step in creating a template is deciding on the style and layout. Create a framework that builds on each other's SOPs, from fonts to line spacing to sections, ensuring a consistent flow of information in each SOP. To ensure that blood center staff have the information they need, the various sections of the template are divided into two categories from the blood center's perspective.

1. Technical
2. General

Technical

The technical part provides guidelines to the user for performing various analytical methods in the laboratory. The technical content of the SOP should include the following:

- *Scope and application*: Description of the purpose of the process or procedure, regulatory requirements, and restrictions on the use of the procedure
- *Responsibility*: The responsibility of the person performing the procedure
- Materials required to perform the procedure
- Step-by-step details of procedures to be performed
- Interpretation of results
- Performing quality assurance of reagents/chemicals
- Documentation

General

The SOP header should contain:

- *Title of SOP*: Each procedure or activity should be assigned a unique title
- Number of SOP
- Issue date of SOP
- Effective date of SOP
- Page number and total number of pages of each SOP
- Revision date and revision number (SOP should be reviewed/ updated as per blood center policy)

The header specimen is given below:

Name and Address of Blood Center: .... Drug License No.: .... Valid up to	SOP No.
	Version No./Date of issue
	Effective Date
	Review Date
	Page No. Page ___ of ___

The footer contains the signatures of the authorized person(s) who has prepared it and the person from the management approving the SOP.

The footer specimen is given below:

Prepared and Issued By	Approved By

Each SOP should be validated. This includes establishing criteria for accepting the results generated by the SOPs, reporting workshops to develop protocols, conducting tests using the SOPs, and predefining observed results and whether they match the statement that the SOP has been validated.

USE OF STANDARD OPERATING PROCEDURES

- The SOPs, once developed and approved, becomes a roadmap for blood center operations.
- SOPs related to conduct and areas of responsibility must be accessible to all staff.
- Blood centers must follow and maintain SOPs as approved. Any changes required to the SOPs should only be made by authorized individuals following appropriate procedures.
- Deviations from SOPs must be documented and approved by an authorized person.
- All SOPs, including old ones, will be retained by the blood center for a period of time as per blood center policy.
- All blood center staff are required to use SOPs in all blood center activities.
- The approval and accreditation process also mandates the use of SOPs.
- SOPs are also used to establish quality control capabilities for blood transfusion services. The focus is on ensuring consistency in the implementation of various activities to ensure blood safety and quality.
- Outdated procedural documents and forms must be retained and accessible for at least 5 years. Start and end dates are recorded.

STANDARD OPERATING PROCEDURE VALIDATION AND APPROVAL

One or more individuals with appropriate training and experience in writing SOPs should review the SOPs. This is especially useful when someone other than the 'SOP's original writer cross checks or reviews the draft before actually completing the SOP. The SOP must be finally approved by management. Approved means that the SOP has been reviewed and approved by management.

REVISION AND REVIEW FREQUENCY

The SOP should be updated regularly and reapproved as necessary. If necessary, change only the relevant parts of the SOP and note the change/revision date along with the revision number in the table of contents and document control notes. In addition, SOPs should be periodically and systematically reviewed every 1–2 years to ensure that policies and procedures are current and appropriate or to determine whether SOPs are required. Each reviewed SOP must include a review date. Obsolete SOPs should be removed from the current file and archived. The frequency of reviews should be determined by management in the organization's quality control plan, which identifies the person responsible for ensuring that the SOPs are up to date.

DOCUMENT CONTROL

All organizations should develop a numbering system to systematically identify and number SOPs and incorporate document control into quality control plans. In general, each SOP page should have a formal description, as shown in **Box 1**. A short title and identification number (ID) can be used as a reference.

This type of document description is usually found in the upper right corner of each document page after the title page.

TRACK AND ARCHIVE DOCUMENTS

A master list of all SOPs, including historical information such as SOP number, version number, publication date, title, author, status, organizational unit, industry, section, and previous versions if any, must be maintained by all blood centers. The quality assurance (QA) manager (or officer) is usually responsible for maintaining record of all currently used SOPs for quality within the organization. The quality control plan should identify the person responsible for ensuring that only the latest versions are used. The plan should also indicate where and how obsolete versions are stored or archived to prevent future use and to be available for review of historical data.

Box 1:	Formal description on each page of standard operating procedure (SOP).

Short title/ID #

Rev. #:

Date:

Page 1 of

SECTION 2

Blood Center Operation

CHAPTER

2

Predonation Counseling and Donor Registration

SCOPE AND APPLICATION

This standard operating procedure (SOP) covers the methods for blood donor reception, counseling, and collection of information from donors to determine their initial eligibility, registering blood donors for further reference to the medical officer for donor selection and donation. Donor identification and registration ensures that returning donors are correctly linked to existing records, first-time donors are correctly registered, and future donors are easily identified. This process also ensures that each blood donation is matched to the correct donor for traceability of blood components.

Predonation counseling is usually provided to potential donors at the same time when the donor is asked to answer the set of questions given in blood donor questionnaire and health checkup form/blood donor questionnaire and health checkup (Apheresis) form during the donor registration process.

RESPONSIBILITY

A blood center counselor/staff nurse in the blood donation area assigned to the registration of donors at both fixed and mobile donation sites is responsible for all the activities described in this SOP to ensure that all donors are accurately identified and registered.

MATERIALS REQUIRED

- Blood donor questionnaire and health checkup form **(Annexure 2.1)**
- Blood donor questionnaire and health checkup (Apheresis) form **(Annexure 2.2)**
- Pen
- General information in pamphlet format about donating blood

PROCEDURE

Predonation counseling is part of the donor selection process, in which each individual's suitability to donate blood is carefully assessed at each donation time based on the set of donor selection criteria. It also gives donors an opportunity to ask questions and understand the reasons behind deferred donations.

The steps for donor selection include:
1. Predonation information
2. Predonation counseling
3. Donor questionnaire and health checkup

A. *Predonation Information:*
   It is intended for the following purposes:
   - Raise the awareness of blood transfusion donors
   - Increase donor confidence in transfusion services
   - Encourage individuals to self-defer:
     1. Confidentiality must be maintained at all times during this process.
     2. Whenever potential donors come to a blood center, they must be greeted warmly, acknowledged that they have come to donate blood, and asked to sit comfortably.
     3. He/she should be offered a glass of water and asked to relax.
     4. If there is any likelihood of any inadvertent delay in blood donation, inform the donor of the waiting period.
     5. Ask blood donors to review the donation information leaflet which should include:
        a. The nature and uses of blood and its components
        b. Eligibility to donate blood
        c. Reason for donor questionnaire and predonation health assessment
     6. Option for the donor to withdraw or self-defer at any time before or during the donation.
     7. The blood donation process and likely adverse donor reactions.
     8. General information about transfusion transmitted infection (TTI), transmission mode, and window period.
     9. Basic information about tests performed on the donated blood.
     10. Possible consequences for donors and donated blood in the case of abnormal TTI test results.
   After the donor has read this pamphlet, make sure that they understand the information provided and answer any questions the donor may have.

B. *Predonation Counseling*:
Blood donor counseling is a confidential dialogue between a blood donor and a counselor regarding issues relating to the donor's health and blood transfusion. This is donor-focused and preferably one-on-one.

The goals of this counseling are to:
- Be able to understand blood donor questionnaire and health checkup form to enable correct answers
- Confirm the understanding of TTI test and disclosure of results
- Clarify misconceptions about donor selection, blood donation, and blood screening
- Describe self-deferral (self-deferral is the process by which a person identifies that he/she may be at high risk for transfusion)
- Describe temporary and permanent deferral
- Inform donors about the blood donation process
- Obtain donor-informed consent

C. *Donor questionnaire and health checkup form:*
11. Donors will receive a blood donor questionnaire and health checkup form/blood donor questionnaire and health checkup (Apheresis) form and will be asked to complete them. If the form is difficult to complete, the donor should be assisted in completing the form:
    a. After the form is completed and duly signed by the donor, retrieve his/her donation record from the database if the donor has donated before.
    b. Check the following:
       - The donor has not been previously deferred.
       - The donor is due for donation.
       - There is no reason for not drawing blood from a donor.
       - If you are unable to draw blood from your donor, you will need counseling to complete the registration process.
12. To prevent donor reactions, identify the following high-risk donors:
    a. First-time donor
    b. Donor who has not slept
    c. Anxious donors
    d. Donor with previous history of reaction during donation
13. The apheresis procedure donor will be briefed about the apheresis process and asked to complete the platelet apheresis donor selection, registration form, and informed consent form.
14. Donors are informed and given the opportunity to ask questions about all blood tests that are required for recipient safety. Informed consent is obtained in writing if the donor gives verbal consent and determines the initial eligibility of the donor.

15. Blood center medical officer will then conduct a physical examination of the donor and declare that he/she is eligible for blood donation/apheresis procedures.

PRECAUTION

Important information, i.e., full name, father's name, and date of birth of donor, should be verified at all stages of the donor registration process to ensure and guard against any possible mix-up of donor records.

RECORD

Blood donor questionnaire and health checkup form/blood donor questionnaire and health checkup (Apheresis) form, on which complete information is recorded, is required to be preserved as a permanent record in compliance with provisions under Drugs and Cosmetic Rules 1945.

ANNEXURE 2.1

| Logo of Institution | **Blood Donor Questionnaire and Health Checkup Form** |

Blood Center: _____   License No: _____

Blood Unit and Segment No.: _____	Donor's Name: _____
Type of Blood Bag Used: _____	Father's Name: _____
	Age/DOB: _____

Blood Donor Questionnaire
(Confidential)

(√) Tick wherever applicable

Please answer the following questions correctly. This will help to protect you and the patient who receives your blood.

Occupation: _____   Address: _____   Pin Code: _____
Tel. No.: _____   Mobile No.: _____
E-mail: _____

Your blood group: _____ Time of last meal: _____

Type of donor: ☐ **Voluntary** ☐ **Replacement, if replacement patient name:**
_____ **MR No.:** _____

Would you like us to call you on your mobile for emergency voluntary donation?
☐ Yes   ☐ No

Have you donated previously?   ☐ Yes   ☐ No If yes, on how many occasions?
_____ When   Last _____

Did you experience any ailment, difficulty or discomfort during previous
donation?   ☐ Yes   ☐ No

What was the difficulty? _____

Have you ever been advised not to donate the blood? ☐ Yes ☐ No

After donating blood do you have to engage in heavy works, driving heavy vehicle or work at heights? ☐ Yes ☐ No

Tick (√) the appropriate answer

1. Do you feel well today?
   ☐ Yes ☐ No
2. Did you have something to eat in the last 4 hours?
   ☐ Yes ☐ No
3. Did you sleep well last night? (Minimum 6–8 hours)
   ☐ Yes ☐ No
4. Have you any reason to believe that you may be infected by Hepatitis, Malaria, HIV/AIDS, and/or Venereal disease?
   ☐ Yes ☐ No
5. In the last 6 months have you had any history (signs and symptoms of AIDS) of the following?
   ☐ Unexplained weight loss
   ☐ Persistent diarrhea
   ☐ Swollen glands
   ☐ Night sweats
   ☐ Continuous low-grade fever
   ☐ Sexually transmissible diseases
6. In the last 6 months have you had any?
   ☐ Tattooing
   ☐ Ear piercing
   ☐ Dental procedure
   ☐ Foreign travel
   ☐ Minor surgery
7. Are you taking or have taken any of these in the past 72 hours?
   ☐ Antibiotics ☐ Ticlopidine
   ☐ Clopidogrel ☐ Piroxicam
   ☐ Aspirin ☐ Dutasteride
   ☐ Finasteride ☐ Steroids
   ☐ Alcohol ☐ Ketoconazole
   ☐ Vaccination
   ☐ Any medication of unknown nature
   ☐ Dog bite/antirabies vaccine
8. Is there any history of surgery or blood transfusion in the past 12 months?
   ☐ Major surgery
   ☐ Endoscopy
   ☐ Blood transfusion
9. Do you suffer from or have suffered from any of the following diseases?
   ☐ Heart disease
   ☐ Leprosy
   ☐ Diabetes
   ☐ Thyroid disorders
   ☐ Other endocrine disorders
   ☐ Acute infection of bladder (cystitis)/UTI
   ☐ Chronic nephritis
   ☐ Cancer/Malignant disease
   ☐ Tuberculosis
   ☐ Abnormal bleeding tendency
   ☐ Measles, Mumps, Chickenpox, Dengue
   ☐ Zika virus
   ☐ Conjunctivitis
   ☐ Osteomyelitis
   ☐ Acid peptic disease

☐ Hepatitis B/C

☐ Asthma

☐ Liver disease

☐ Autoimmune disorders like SLE, Scleroderma, Dermatomyositis, Ankylosing spondylitis, or Severe Rheumatoid arthritis

☐ Bleeding disorders

☐ Any history of organ/Stem cell/Tissue transplant?

☐ Any history of unexplained/delayed faint or delayed faint with injury or consecutive faints following a blood donation?

☐ Polycythemia vera

☐ Malaria (within 6 months)

☐ Typhoid (within 1 year)

☐ Epilepsy

☐ Fainting attacks

☐ Schizophrenia

10. For women donors:

  a. Are you menstruating?

    ☐ Yes ☐ No

  b. Are you pregnant?

    ☐ Yes ☐ No

  c. Have you had an abortion in the last 6 months?

    ☐ Yes ☐ No

  d. Do you have a child less than one year old/Are you breastfeeding?

    ☐ Yes ☐ No

11. Would you like to be informed about any abnormal test results done on your donated blood at the address furnished by you?

  ☐ Yes ☐ No

Consent for Blood Donation

I understand that:

i. Blood donation is a totally voluntary act, and no inducement or remuneration has been offered.

ii. Donation of blood/components is a medical procedure, and that by donating voluntarily, I accept the risk associated with this procedure.

iii. I confirm that I have answered all questions truthfully and accurately without hiding any facts willfully. I also understand that any willful misinterpretation of the facts could endanger the life of the patient who receives my blood/components.

iv. My donated blood and plasma recovered from my donated blood may be sent for plasma fractionation for the preparation of plasma-derived medicines, which may be used for the larger patient population and not just this Blood Center.

v. My blood will be tested for Hepatitis B, Hepatitis C, Malaria parasite, HIV/AIDS and Syphilis, in addition to any other screening tests required to ensure blood safety.

vi. I would like to be informed about any abnormal test results done on my donated blood: Yes/No

vii. I understand that screening tests are not diagnostic and may yield false-positive results, which may need further confirmatory tests.

viii. I confirm that my age is more than 18 years and not beyond 65 years.

ix. My donated blood/blood components may be utilized in this Blood Center or beyond this Blood Center for any patient in need.

x. My donated blood/blood components may be used for the purpose of preparation of panels, indigenous manufacture and scientific research.

Date and Time: _____   **Donor's Sign:** _____

General Physical Examination

1. **History Checklist**

   Feeling well: ☐ Yes   ☐ No

   Adequate sleep: ☐ Yes   ☐ No

   Ever hospitalized: ☐ Yes   ☐ No

   Current illness or medication: ☐ Yes   ☐ No

2. **Examination Checklist**

   Look unhealthy/Pallor/Icterus/Alcohol smell: ☐ Yes   ☐ No

   Weight: _____kg_____Height: _____cms

   Hb: _____g/dL

   Temp: _____ °F_____Pulse: _____ per minute

   BP: _____mm Hg

   Heart: _____   Lungs: _____

Outcome:	Donor Accepted/Temporary Deferral/ Permanent Deferral

Signature of the Medical Officer: _____   **Date:** _____

3. **COUNSELING:**
   a. **Predonation Counseling**
      - Understanding of donor questionnaire to enable correct responses
      - Reiterate understanding of TTI testing and the disclosure of results
      - Clarify any misunderstanding about donor selection, blood donation and blood screening
      - Explain self-deferral
      - Explain temporary and permanent deferral
      - Familiarize donor to the process of blood donation
      - Obtain donor's informed consent
   b. **Counseling during donation**
      - Ensure that the donor feels comfortable
      - Provide gentle reassurance to relax the donor
      - Reduce his/her anxiety and minimize the risk of any adverse reactions.
   c. **Post-donation Counseling:**
      Do's and Don'ts immediately after blood donation
      - Remove the wrap bandage after 1 hour and clean the wrap area with soap and water.
      - Take more fluids for next 24 hours.
      - Avoid heavy workout for next 24 hours.
      - Avoid driving for next 30 minutes
      - Do not smoke for next 30 minutes.
      - Do not take alcohol for next 24 hours.
      - In case of bleeding from phlebotomy site, raise the arm and apply pressure.
      - If there is feeling of faintness or dizziness, lie down with legs slightly raised above the head level. If the condition does not improve, contact the nearest Doctor or contact the Blood Center.
      - In case of emergency, contact at _____
      - *Need for follow-up for TTI purposes*: Donors who have consented to be contacted by the Blood Center in case of an abnormal test result shall be recalled to the Blood Center so as to inform them about the sero-reactive result of transfusion-transmitted infection (TTI) and shall be provided post-donation counseling prior to referring to appropriate medical services for confirmation of diagnosis, follow-up and treatment whenever necessary.

Phlebotomy site: Right/Left antecubital fossa: _____
Starting time of phlebotomy: _____
Ending time of phlebotomy: _____
Duration of phlebotomy: _____
Blood collection: _____mL
Weight of blood unit: _____ g
Name of the phlebotomist: _____
Signature _____

Complications:

Fainting: ☐ Yes ☐ No   Fits: ☐ Yes ☐ No

Hematoma: ☐ Yes ☐ No

Double prick: ☐ Yes ☐ No   Sweating: ☐ Yes ☐ No

BP: _____mm Hg

Pulse: _____ per minute   Loss of consciousness: ☐ Yes ☐ No

Others (Please specify): _____

_____

Management: _____

_____

_____

_____

_____

Blood safety begins with a Healthy Donor
रक्त सुरक्षा की शुरूआत स्वस्थ रक्तदाता से होती है

ANNEXURE 2.2

Logo of Institution	**Blood Donor Questionnaire and Health Checkup Form (Apheresis)**

Blood Center: _____   License No: _____

Blood unit and Segment No.: _____ _____ Type of Blood Bag Used: _____ _____	Donor's Name: _____ _____ Father's Name: _____ _____ Age/DOB: _____ Sex: _____

Blood Donor Questionnaire
(Confidential)

(√) Tick wherever applicable

Please answer the following questions correctly. This will help to protect you and the patient who receives your blood.

Occupation: _____ Address: _____ Pin Code: _____
Tel. No.: _____ Mobile No.: _____
E-mail: _____

Your blood group: _____ Time of last meal: _____

Type of donor: ☐ **Voluntary** ☐ **Replacement, if replacement patient name:**
_____ **MR No.:** _____

Would you like us to call you on your mobile for emergency voluntary donation?
☐ Yes   ☐No

Have you donated previously?   ☐ Yes   ☐ No   If yes, on how many occasions?
_____ When   Last _____

Did you experience any ailment, difficulty or discomfort during previous donation?   ☐ Yes   ☐ No

What was the difficulty? _____

Have you ever been advised not to donate the blood?   ☐ Yes   ☐ No

After donating blood do you have to engage in heavy works, driving heavy vehicle or work at heights?   ☐ Yes   ☐ No

---

Tick (√) the appropriate answer

1. Do you feel well today?
   ☐ Yes   ☐ No

2. Did you have something to eat in the last 4 hours?
   ☐ Yes   ☐ No

3. Did you sleep well last night? (Minimum 6–8 hours)
   ☐ Yes   ☐ No

4. Have you any reason to believe that you may be infected by Hepatitis, Malaria, HIV/AIDS, and/or Venereal disease?
   ☐ Yes   ☐ No

5. In the last 6 months have you had any history (signs and symptoms of AIDS) of the following?
   ☐ Unexplained weight loss
   ☐ Persistent diarrhea
   ☐ Swollen glands
   ☐ Night sweats
   ☐ Continuous low-grade fever
   ☐ Sexually transmissible diseases

6. In the last 6 months have you had any?
   ☐ Tattooing
   ☐ Ear piercing
   ☐ Dental procedure
   ☐ Foreign travel
   ☐ Minor surgery

7. Are you taking or have taken any of these in the past 72 hours?
   ☐ Antibiotics   ☐ Ticlopidine
   ☐ Clopidogrel   ☐ Piroxicam
   ☐ Aspirin   ☐ Dutasteride
   ☐ Finasteride   ☐ Steroids
   ☐ Alcohol   ☐ Ketoconazole
   ☐ Vaccination
   ☐ Any medication of unknown nature
   ☐ Dog bite/antirabies vaccine

8. Is there any history of surgery or blood transfusion in the past 12 months?
   ☐ Major surgery
   ☐ Endoscopy
   ☐ Blood transfusion

9. Do you suffer from or have suffered from any of the following diseases?
   ☐ Heart disease
   ☐ Leprosy
   ☐ Diabetes
   ☐ Thyroid disorders
   ☐ Other endocrine disorders
   ☐ Acute infection of bladder (cystitis)/UTI
   ☐ Chronic nephritis
   ☐ Cancer/Malignant disease

☐ Tuberculosis

☐ Abnormal bleeding tendency

☐ Measles, Mumps, Chickenpox, Dengue

☐ Zika virus

☐ Conjunctivitis

☐ Osteomyelitis

☐ Acid peptic disease

☐ Hepatitis B/C

☐ Asthma

☐ Liver disease

☐ Autoimmune disorders like SLE, Scleroderma, Dermatomyositis, Ankylosing spondylitis, or Severe rheumatoid arthritis

☐ Bleeding disorders

☐ Any history of organ/Stem cell/ Tissue transplant?

☐ Any history of unexplained/ delayed faint or delayed faint with injury or consecutive faints following a blood donation?

☐ Polycythemia vera

☐ Malaria (within 6 months)

☐ Typhoid (within 1 year)

☐ Epilepsy

☐ Fainting attacks

☐ Schizophrenia

10. For women donors:

a. Are you menstruating?

☐ Yes ☐ No

b. Are you pregnant?

☐ Yes ☐ No

c. Have you had an abortion in the last 6 months?

☐ Yes ☐ No

d. Do you have a child less than one year old/Are you breastfeeding?

☐ Yes ☐ No

11. Would you like to be informed about any abnormal test results done on your donated blood at the address furnished by you?

☐ Yes ☐ No

Consent for Blood Donation

I understand that:

i. Blood donation is a totally voluntary act, and no inducement or remuneration has been offered.

ii. Donation of blood/components is a medical procedure, and that by donating voluntarily, I accept the risk associated with this procedure.

iii. During apheresis, blood is withdrawn through a needle and mixed with an anticoagulant as it is drawn. The blood is pumped through the cell separator and the desired components are collected in a sterile plastic container. Most of the blood in the cell separator is then returned to the donor. All equipment used is commercially available, and all materials coming in contact with the donor's blood are sterile, only used once and then disposed as biomedical waste.

iv. Apheresis is a medical procedure and that by undergoing the procedure voluntarily, I accept the risks associated with this procedure which is safe and most people tolerate very well.

v. I confirm that I have answered all questions truthfully and accurately without hiding any facts willfully. I also understand that any willful misinterpretation of the facts could endanger the life of the patient who receives my blood/components.

vi. My donated plasma may be sent for plasma fractionation for the preparation of plasma-derived medicines, which may be used for the larger patient population and not just this blood center.

vii. My blood will be tested for Hepatitis B, Hepatitis C, Malaria parasite, HIV/AIDS and Syphilis, in addition to any other screening tests required to ensure blood safety.

viii. I would like to be informed about any abnormal test results done on my blood: Yes/No

ix. I understand that screening tests are not diagnostic and may yield false-positive results, which may need further confirmatory tests.

x. I confirm that my age is more than 18 years and not beyond 65 years.

xi. My donated blood components may be utilized in this Blood Center or beyond this Blood Center for any patient in need.

xii. My donated blood components may be used for the purpose of preparation of panels, indigenous manufacture and scientific research.

xiii. I hereby voluntarily consent to one of the following procedures checked below:

☐ Platelet apheresis   ☐ Plasma apheresis

I hereby authorize blood center services personnel to perform the withdrawal of my blood by either a continuous or intermittent flow cell separator; the extraction of the appropriate blood component; the reinfusion of my own anticoagulated blood and replacement fluids.

The procedure and risks have been explained to me. I have been given ample opportunity to ask questions about the procedures and about the risks, hazards and possible complications involved. All questions have been answered to my satisfaction. In the event of a reaction or complication, the medical staff will provide immediate emergency medical care as per protocol.

Date and Time: _____   **Donor's Sign:** _____

I (attendant name)_____Related to (patient's name) _____ have been explained that my patient needs an urgent transfusion of _____ (Blood component) which has to be prepared from one of my known directed donor Mr./Mrs. (Donor Name) _____

I understand that since this component is needed for my patient's treatment urgently, it has to be tested for infectious diseases like HIV, HCV, VDRL, MP, by Rapid method which have slightly lower sensitivity and may miss such infection, if present in the donor even after testing. Keeping in view of the urgency, I am willing to take the risk.

I also give my consent that in case the procedure is aborted or unsuccessful for any reason, the cost of the kit and consumables shall be borne by me as per the hospital/blood center policy.

Signature of the patient's guardian: _____

Date: _____

Date and Time: _____

Donor's Sign: _____

General Physical Examination

1. **History Checklist**

Feeling well:	☐ Yes	☐ No
Adequate sleep:	☐ Yes	☐ No
Ever hospitalized:	☐ Yes	☐ No
Current illness or medication:	☐ Yes	☐ No

2. **Examination Checklist**

   Look unhealthy/Pallor/Icterus/Alcohol smell: ☐ Yes   ☐ No

   Weight: _____kg_____Height: _____cm

   Hb: _____g/dL

   Temp: _____°F_____Pulse: _____ per minute

   BP: _____mm Hg

   Heart: _____   Lungs: _____

Screening for TTI				
Test	**Method**	**Result**	**Date/Time**	**Signatures**
HIV I and II				
HBsAg				
HCV				
VDRL				
MP				
ABS				

Outcome: ☐ Donor accepted   ☐ Rejected   ☐ Defferred

_____

_____

Signature of the Medical Officer: _____ **Date:** _____

Apheresis Procedure Detail

Name of the patient: _____ MR No.: _____

IPD No.: _____   Age: _____

Sex: _____ Ward /Bed No.: _____

Consultant in charge: _____

Clinical diagnosis: _____

Blood group: _____ Platelet count: _____

Yield: _____

Set used: _____ Batch used: _____

Batch No. and Expiry (ACD): _____

Venipuncture performed by (Name): _____

Date and time of commencement of apheresis: _____

Total volume of blood processed: _____

PLT. Conc. volume collected: _____mL

Total volume of ACD used in platelet concentrate: _____ mL
and to donor_____mL

Total volume of replacement fluid used: _____

Date and time of completion of apheresis procedure: _____

_____

Expiry date of component: _____

Any complaint by the donor during the procedure: _____

Any medicine given during the procedure: _____

Remarks: _____

_____

Signature of blood center officer: _____

Space for pasting sticker of the kit used	Space for pasting sticker of the kit used

Bill No. and Date: _____

Spillovers No.	Blood process volume	Time

Donor Screening for Hemoglobin (Copper Sulfate Solution Method)

SCOPE AND APPLICATION

This standard operating procedure (SOP) describes donor screening for hemoglobin status based on the principle of blood relative density (or specific gravity) to ensure donor safety and blood/blood component quality. This method is fast and reasonably reliable. This method is only meant for screening of donors at outdoor blood donation camps.

RESPONSIBILITY

It is the responsibility of the medical officer/technician to perform the screening of hemoglobin of the donor.

MATERIALS REQUIRED

- *Equipment*:
  - Urinometer
- *Reagents*:
  - Copper sulfate solution
  - Distilled water
  - Ethylenediaminetetraacetic acid (EDTA) blood samples of known hemoglobin concentration
- *Glassware*:
  - Coplin jar
  - Test tubes
- *Miscellaneous*:
  - Tissue paper
  - Weighing scale
  - Crystalline $CuSO_4 \cdot 5H_2O$
  - Copper sulfate record book
  - Test tube stand

PROCEDURE

Principle

This method is based on the specific gravity values of blood and copper sulfate solution. A copper sulfate solution with a specific gravity of 1.053 corresponds to 12.5 g/dL of blood hemoglobin. Normal blood has a specific gravity between 1.052 and 1.063, averaging 1.057 in men and 1.053 in women. The specific gravity of blood depends on the amount of hemoglobin present in red blood cells and plasma protein levels. A drop of blood is collected from a finger prick and dropped into the solution. Each drop of blood that enters the copper sulfate solution is encapsulated in a copper protein bag and remains as a separate drop with unchanged specific gravity for 15–20 seconds. Therefore, drop behavior is considered during these 15–20 seconds. If the specific gravity of the blood is less than the specific gravity of the solution, the blood will rise for a few seconds and then fall. If the specific gravity is the same, it will stay still for that period of time before falling. If the drop of blood is heavy, it will continue to drip during this interval.

Method

1. Dissolve 170 g of crystalline $CuSO_4 \cdot 5H_2O$ in 1,000 mL of distilled water.
2. Dilute 51 mL of stock solution with distilled water to make it 100 mL. Label it as "working solution."
3. Check the specific gravity of the working solution using a urinometer and adjust to 1.053 by adding stock solution or distilled water. Check the copper sulfate solution to make sure that a single drop of blood with a specific hemoglobin level reacts (sinks/floats) as expected.
4. Transfer 30 mL of copper sulfate working solution to a Coplin jar.
5. Clean your fingertips thoroughly with an alcohol swab. Let it dry.
6. Transfer 30 mL of copper sulfate working solution to a Coplin jar.
7. Puncture the fingertip with a sterile disposable lancet to ensure good free flow of blood. Do not squeeze the finger repeatedly to avoid dilution of blood with excess tissue fluid.
8. Wipe away the first drop of blood. Allow the second drop of blood to fall gently from the finger from a height of about 1 cm above the surface of the copper sulfate solution into the Coplin jar.
9. Watch the movement of the drop for approximately 15 seconds.

Note:
- The working solution is prepared fresh each morning and changed after every 25 tests.
- The Coplin jar is kept covered when not in use.
- The lancet and capillaries are discarded in a container with 1% sodium hypochlorite solution.

INTERPRETATION

- If the drop of blood sinks within 15 seconds, this indicates that the donor's hemoglobin level exceeds 12.5 g/dL as per this procedure, and the donor is eligible to donate blood.
- However, if the blood drop floats for >15 seconds or sinks in the middle, it indicates that the donor's hemoglobin is <12.5 g/dL following this procedure. It will be either postponed or retested in a quantitative testing system.
- After >15 seconds, the drop of blood in CuSO$_4$ solution will sink even if the hemoglobin level is very low. This must NOT be taken as an indication for bleeding of donor. If so, test donor hemoglobin using Sahli's method.
- Test the hemoglobin of the donor using Sahli's method in case the drop sinks slowly, hesitates, and then goes to the bottom of the jar. The donors having hemoglobin ≥12.5 g/dL are accepted for blood donation.

RECORD

The results are entered in the **Blood Donor Questionnaire and Health Checkup Form**/Donor Register.

CHAPTER 4

Estimation of Hemoglobin of Donor (Sahli's Method)

SCOPE AND APPLICATION

This standard operating procedure (SOP) describes how to measure a donor's hemoglobin prior to donation using Sahli's hemoglobin meter. This method is used to reassess the hemoglobin status of donors who fail the copper sulfate solution method.

RESPONSIBILITY

It is the responsibility of the medical officer/technician working in the donor area.

MATERIALS REQUIRED

- Sahli's hemoglobin meter
- 0.1 N hydrochloric acid (HCl)
- Distilled water
- Pasteur pipettes
- Lancet
- Sterile cotton swabs

PROCEDURE

Principle

Mixing the blood with 0.1 HCl converts the hemoglobin into a brown, acidic hematin. Dilute the solution until its color matches the amber glass in the comparison box. The hemoglobin measurement tube reading represents the donor's hemoglobin level as a percentage.

Method

1. Fill the graduated tube with 0.1 N HCl to the 20 mark with a Pasteur pipette.
2. Thoroughly clean the fingertip with an alcohol swab. Let it dry.
3. Puncture the fingertip with a sterile disposable lancet to ensure good free blood flow. Do not squeeze the finger repeatedly to avoid diluting the blood with excess tissue fluid.
4. Draw blood up to 20 µL mark with a hemoglobin pipette. Adjust the column carefully and make sure that there are no air bubbles. Wipe off excess blood from the side of the dropper with a dry cotton ball.
5. Transfer blood to the graduated tube containing 0.1 N HCl. Aspirate and dispense HCl two to three times to wash out the contents of the pipette. Mix the contents well.
6. Allow the mixture to stand undisturbed for 10 minutes.
7. Place the hemoglobin meter tube in the comparator and add distilled water drop by drop to the solution and stir with a glass rod until the color matches the color of the comparator glass.
8. Remove the glass rod and take the reading directly by noting the lower meniscus of the diluted acid hematin and express in g/dL.

INTERPRETATION

The donors having hemoglobin 12.5 g/dL and more are accepted for blood donation.

RECORD

Enter the hemoglobin values in **Blood Donor Questionnaire and Health Checkup Form**/Donor Register.

Estimation of Hemoglobin (HemoCue Method)

SCOPE AND APPLICATION

This standard operating procedure (SOP) describes the method to determine a donor's hemoglobin status for safety and product quality assurance.

RESPONSIBILITY

It is the responsibility of the medical officer/technician working in the donor area.

MATERIALS REQUIRED

- HemoCue Analyzer
- Mains adapter for HemoCue
- 4 × AA batteries
- Gloves
- Lancets
- HemoCue microcuvettes

PROCEDURE

Principle

The HemoCue Analyzer is used to measure total hemoglobin in finger-prick whole blood. The system consists of an analyzer with specially designed cuvettes containing dry reagents in ug/g; < 300 sodium azide, < 300 sodium nitrite, and < 350 nonreactive ingredients. Cuvettes serve as pipettes, reaction vessels, and measuring cuvettes. No dilution is required. Hemoglobin measurements are performed on a factory calibrated analyzer using the international standard hemiglobincyanide (HiCN) method. Sodium deoxycholate hemolyzes red blood cells, releasing hemoglobin. Sodium nitrite converts hemoglobin to methemoglobin and forms hemiglobinazide with sodium azide. Absorbance is measured at two wavelengths (570 and 880 nm) to correct for sample turbidity.

Sample Type and Additives

Whole blood from:
- Capillaries
- Veins
- Suitable anticoagulants, such as ethylenediaminetetraacetic acid (EDTA) or heparin, can be used in their solid form to avoid dilution effects.

Method

Start-up Procedure

1. If AC power is available, connect the adapter to the socket on the back of the analyzer. If mains power is not available, insert 4 × AA batteries into the battery compartment.
2. Pull out the cuvette holder out to the loading position.
3. Press and hold the left button until the display becomes active (all symbols appear on display).
4. The display will show the version number of the program followed by an hourglass and an Hb icon.
5. After 10 seconds, the display will show three flashing dashes and the HemoCue symbol. It is now ready for use.

Measuring Capillary Blood

1. Remove the cuvette from the container and immediately close it again. Hold the cuvette by the straight edge.
2. Make sure the donor's hands are warm and relaxed. Use middle or ring finger to sample; avoid fingers with rings.
3. Clean the finger and dry it with a lint-free cloth.
4. Use your thumb to gently press the finger from the top of the knuckle toward the tip. This stimulates blood flow to the sampling site.
5. For the best blood flow and minimal pain, the sample is taken from the side of the fingertip rather than the middle.
6. Apply slight pressure toward the fingertip; prick the finger with the lancet.
7. Wipe off the first two drops of blood with a lint-free cloth.
8. Gently press toward the fingertip until another drop of blood appears. When the drop of blood is large enough, fill the cuvette

with blood in one continuous process to avoid air bubbles. DO NOT refill. Before inserting the cuvette into the cuvette holder, wipe it on three sides and then gently slide it into the measuring position. An hourglass appears on the display during the measurement.

9. After 15–60 seconds, the sample hemoglobin value will be displayed. The results remain on the display as long as the cuvette holder is in the measuring position.

10. All results must be recorded in the donors' notes, signed and dated by the technician using a HemoCue.

11. Open the cuvette holder and discard the cuvette in red biowaste bin.

12. To turn-off HemoCue, press and hold the left button until the display reads OFF and goes blank.

13. Slide the cuvette holder into the measuring position.

14. Make sure that the meter is clean and tidy.

INTERPRETATION

The donors having hemoglobin 12.5 g/dL and more are accepted for blood donation.

RECORD

The results are entered in the **Blood Donor Questionnaire and Health Checkup Form**/Donor Register.

Calibration

The system is factory calibrated to the HiCN method, the international standard method for determining hemoglobin concentration in blood.

INTERNAL QUALITY CONTROL

Self-test

The HemoCue Hb 201 analyzer has an internal electronic "self-test." The performance of the analyzer's optronics unit is automatically checked each time the analyzer is turned on. If the self-test passes, the display will show its HemoCue icon and three flashing dashes, indicating that the analyzer is ready to run the test.

Donor Health Checkup

SCOPE AND APPLICATION

This standard operating procedure (SOP) describes the conduct of a blood donor physical examination to confirm compliance with legal standards for blood donations, thereby ensuring donor and recipient safety and blood and blood component quality.

RESPONSIBILITY

It is the responsibility of the blood center medical officer to determine if a donor is suitable for donating blood according to donor selection criteria after evaluating the information of Donor Questionnaire and health checkup form, the donor physical examination, and the results of the predonation screening tests.

ACTIVITIES

The screening process of the donor comprises three major activities:
1. Donor registration
2. Medical history
3. Physical examination
   Donor is declared fit for donation only after completion of above three interrelated activities.

The donor screening process has one of the three outcomes for the prospective donors:
1. Acceptance
2. Temporary deferral
3. Permanent deferral
The *accepted donors* continue on to donation process.

Temporary deferred donors are advised on how long they must wait before visiting the blood center again for donation. They are also advised as to what should be done to increase their chances of acceptance for blood donation after the waiting period is over. For example, if a donor's hemoglobin is too low to qualify as a donor, he or she is advised to increase his/her hemoglobin level through diet/medication.

Permanent deferral is given to those donors who are not accepted as donors under any circumstances.

A medical history and physical examination must be undertaken on the actual day of donor registration/donation.

The donor screening process begins with obtaining complete and accurate demographic information of the donor at the time of donor registration. The information must fully identify the donor and entered in the existing donor record. This information must be captured/recorded for each donation.

Unique characteristics of the donor: Separate records should be kept for all donors of known Rh-negative blood group/Bombay phenotype.

MATERIALS REQUIRED

- Weighing and height-measuring scale
- Sphygmomanometer
- Stethoscope
- Thermometer
- Complete the Donor Questionnaire and health checkup form
- Clinical thermometer

PROCEDURE

Each potential donor undergoes a health check based on the information provided in the Donor Questionnaire and health checkup form and undergoes a physical examination by the blood center physician.

Selection Criteria of Blood Donors

- *Only voluntary/replacement nonremunerated blood donors are accepted for blood donation if the following criteria are fulfilled*: The donor must be healthy, mentally alert, physically fit, and shall not be in prison or any other confinement. Blood donors who have communication difficulties and are visually impaired may donate blood if clear and confidential communication is established by fully understanding the blood donation process and providing valid consent. Donors must meet the following requirements:
    - *Age*: The donor must be in the age group of 18–65 years. First-time donors must not be older than 60 years, and for repeat donors, the upper limit is 65 years.

- *Weight*: Donor weight must be at least 45 kg for 350 mL of blood collection and 55 kg for 450 mL of blood collection.
- *Blood donation interval*: Whole blood donation is once every 3 months (90 days) for men and once every 4 months (120 days) for women. If reinfusion of the red cell mass was complete in the last platelet apheresis donation, the apheresis donor is not accepted for whole blood donation until 28 days after the last platelet donation. Donors were not accepted within 90 days if the reinfusion of the red cell mass was incomplete.
- *Donor mouth temperature*: Afebrile; 37°C/98.4°F
- *Blood pressure*: 100–140 mm Hg systolic and 60–90 mm Hg diastolic with or without medications History and physical examination should be free of findings suggestive of end-organ injury or secondary complications (cardiac, renal, ocular, or vascular) or dizziness or syncope. No change in medication or dosage in the past 28 days.
- *Pulse*: 60–100/min and regular
- *Respiration*: The donor must not have acute respiratory illness.
- *Hemoglobin*: Should not be <12.5 g/dL. Thalassemia trait may be accepted, provided hemoglobin is acceptable.
- *Meal*: No fasting before the blood donation or fasting during the period of blood donation and last meal must be at least 4 hours prior to donating blood. Donors must not have consumed alcohol prior to donating blood and must not show signs of intoxication. The donor should not be someone who regularly consumes large amounts of alcohol.
- *Donor skin*: Donors must not have any skin disease at the site of phlebotomy. Donor arms and forearms should be free of skin punctures and wounds that indicate addiction to professional blood donors or self-injecting narcotics.
- *Occupation*: Aircrew, long-distance vehicle drivers at sea or below sea level, emergency medical services, or donors working where strenuous work is required should not donate blood at least 24 hours prior to their next duty shift. Donors must not be night shift workers who do not get enough sleep.
- *Risk behavior*: Donors must not have any transfusion communicable disease established by medical history and physical examination. The donor should not be considered at risk for human immunodeficiency virus (HIV) and hepatitis B or C infections (transgender, men who have sex with men, female sex workers, injecting drug users, persons with multiple sexual partners, or any other high risk as determined by the medical officer who determines their eligibility to donate blood).

- – *Travel and residence*: The donor should not be a person with history of residence or travel in a geographical area that is endemic for diseases that can be transmitted by blood transfusion and for which screening is not mandated or there is no guidance in India.
- *Criteria for blood donation*: The donors shall be accepted/deferred for phlebotomy according to the amended criteria for blood donation notified by Ministry of Health and Family Welfare, Govt. of India, vide G.S.R. 166(E) dated 11th March, 2020 **(Annexure 6.1)**.
- *Private interview*: Detailed sexual history must be taken. Positive history should be recorded on confidential notebook by the blood center counselor to exclude any risky behavior.
- *Informed consent*: If the donor is declared fit on his/her history and medical examination, informed consent providing following information must be obtained before blood donation.
  - – Need for blood donation
  - – Necessity of voluntary blood donation
  - – Transfusion transmissible infections
  - – Need for questionnaire and honest answers
  - – Blood donation safety
  - – Blood processing and use of donor blood
  - – Tests performed on donor blood
  - – Blood/blood components used by the blood centers according to government blood safety guidelines, including the use of donor blood for plasma fractionation and derivation of essential plasma-derived medicines

Note: The donors are requested to sign the **Blood Donor Questionnaire and Health Checkup Form** (Annexure 2.1/2.2), indicating that he/she is donating blood voluntarily. This will give the donor an opportunity to give his/her consent if they feel themselves as safe donors.

RECORD

- Information obtained from donors on the registration form and physical examination entered in donor record register.
- Deferred donors and reasons for their deferral should be recorded in the register.
- Record of adverse donor reaction and its management.

ANNEXURE 6.1

Criteria for Selection of Blood Donors

S. No.	Condition	Criteria
1.	Well being	• The donor shall be in good health, mentally alert and physically fit and shall not be inmates of jail or any other confinement • Differently abled or donor with communication and sight difficulties can donate blood provided that clear and confidential communication can be established and he/she fully understands the donation process and gives a valid consent
2.	Age	• Minimum age 18 years • Maximum age 65 years • First time donor shall not be over 60 years of age, for repeat donor upper limit is 65 years • For apheresis donors 18–60 years
3.	Whole Blood Volume Collected and weight of donor	• 350 mL – 45 kg • 450 mL – >55 kg • Apheresis – 50 kg
4.	Donation Interval	• For whole blood donation, once in three months (90 days) for males and four months (120 days) for females • For apheresis, at least 48 hours interval after platelet/plasmapheresis shall be kept (not >2 times a week, limited to 24 in one year) • After whole blood donation a plateletpheresis donor shall not be accepted before 28 days • Apheresis platelet donor shall not be accepted for whole blood donation before 28 days from the last platelet donation provided reinfusion of red cell was complete in the last plateletpheresis donation. If the reinfusion of red cells was not complete then the donor shall not be accepted within 90 days • A donor shall not donate any type of donation within 12 months after a bone marrow harvest, within 6 months after a peripheral stem cell harvest

Continued

Continued

5.	Blood Pressure	• 100–140 mm Hg systolic 60–90 mm Hg diastolic with or without medications • There shall be no findings suggestive of end organ damage or secondary complication (cardiac, renal, eye or vascular) or history of feeling giddiness, fainting made out during history and examination. Neither the drug nor its dosage should have been altered in the last 28 days
6.	Pulse	60–100 Regular
7.	Temperature	Afebrile; 37°C/98.4°F
8.	Respiration	The donor shall be free from acute respiratory disease
9.	Hemoglobin	≥12.5 g/dL Thalassemia trait may be accepted, provided hemoglobin is acceptable
10.	Meal	• The donor shall not be fasting before the blood donation or observing fast during the period of blood donation and last meal should have been taken at least 4 hours prior to donation • Donor shall not have consumed alcohol and show signs of intoxication before the blood donation. The donor shall not be a person having regular heavy alcohol intake
11.	Occupation	The donor who works as air crew member, long distance vehicle driver, either above sea level or below sea level or in emergency services or where strenuous work is required, shall not donate blood at least 24 hours prior to their next duty shift. The donor shall not be a night shift workers without adequate sleep
12.	Risk behaviour	• The donor shall be free from any disease transmissible by blood transfusion, as far as can be determined by history and examination • The donor shall not be a person considered at risk for HIV, Hepatitis B or C infections (Transgender, Men who have sex with men, Female sex workers, Injecting drug users, persons with multiple sexual partners or any other high risk as determined by the medical officer deciding fitness to donate blood)

Continued

Continued

13.	Travel and residence	The donor shall not be a person with history of residence or travel in a geographical area which is endemic for diseases that can be transmitted by blood transfusion and for which screening is not mandated or there is no guidance in India
14.	Donor Skin	The donor shall be free from any skin diseases at the site of phlebotomy. The arms and forearms of the donor shall be free of skin punctures of scars indicative of professional blood donors or addiction of self-injected narcotics
Physiological Status for Women		
15.	Pregnancy or recently delivered	Defer for 12 Months after delivery
16.	Abortion	Defer for 6 months after abortion
17.	Breast feeding	Defer for total period of lactation
18.	Menstruation	Defer for the period of menstruation
Nonspecific Illness		
19.	Minor nonspecific symptoms including but not limited to general malaise, pain, headache	Defer until all symptoms subside and donor is afebrile
Respiratory (Lung) Diseases		
20.	Cold, flu, cough, sore throat or acute sinusitis	Defer until all symptoms subside and donor is afebrile
21.	Chronic sinusitis	Accept unless on antibiotics
22.	Asthmatic attack	Permanently Defer
23.	Asthmatics on steroids	Permanently Defer
Surgical Procedures		
24.	Major surgery	Defer for 12 months after recovery. [Major surgery being defined as that requiring hospitalization, anesthesia (general/spinal) had Blood Transfusion and/or had significant Blood loss]
25.	Minor surgery	Defer for 6 months after recovery
26.	Received Blood Transfusion	Defer for 12 months

Continued

27.	Open heart surgery Including Bypass surgery	Permanently defer
28.	Cancer surgery	Permanently defer
29.	Tooth extraction	Defer for 6 months after tooth extraction
30.	Dental surgery under anesthesia	Defer for 6 months after recovery
Cardiovascular Diseases (Heart Disease)		
31.	Has any active symptom (Chest Pain, Shortness of breath, swelling of feet)	Permanently defer
32.	Myocardial infarction (Heart Attack)	Permanently defer
33.	Cardiac medication (digitalis, nitroglycerin)	Permanently defer
34.	Hypertensive heart disease	Permanently defer
35.	Coronary artery disease	Permanently defer
36.	Angina pectoris	Permanently defer
37.	Rheumatic heart disease with residual damage	Permanently defer
Central Nervous System/Psychiatric Diseases		
38.	Migraine	Accept if not severe and occurs at a frequency of less than once a week
39.	Convulsions and Epilepsy	Permanently defer
40.	Schizophrenia	Permanently defer
41.	Anxiety and mood disorders	Accept person having anxiety and mood (affective) disorders like depression or bipolar disorder, but is stable and feeling well on the day regardless of medication

Continued

Continued

		Endocrine Disorders	
42.	Diabetes	• Accept person with Diabetes Mellitus well controlled by diet or oral hypoglycemic medication, with no history of orthostatic hypotension and no evidence of infection, neuropathy or vascular disease (in particular peripheral ulceration) • Permanently defer person requiring insulin and/or complications of Diabetes with multi-organ involvement • Defer if oral hypoglycemic medication has been altered/dosage adjusted in last 4 weeks	

43.	Thyroid disorders	• Accept donations from individuals with Benign Thyroid Disorders if euthyroid (Asymptomatic Goiter, History of Viral Thyroiditis, Autoimmune Hypothyroidism)
		• Defer if under investigation for Thyroid Disease or thyroid status is not known
		• Permanently defer if:
		  1) Thyrotoxicosis due to Graves' Disease
		  2) Hyper/Hypothyroid
		  3) History of malignant thyroid tumors	

44.	Other endocrine disorders	Permanently defer	
		Liver Diseases and Hepatitis Infection	
45.	Hepatitis	• Known Hepatitis B, C—Permanently defer • Unknown Hepatitis—Permanently defer • Known Hepatitis A or E—Defer for 12 months	
46.	Spouse/partner/close contact of individual suffering with hepatitis	Defer for 12 months	
47.	At risk for hepatitis by tattoos, acupuncture or body piercing, scarification and any other invasive cosmetic procedure by self or spouse/partner	Defer for 12 months	

Continued

Continued

48.	Spouse/partner of individual receiving transfusion of blood/components	Defer for 12 months
49.	Jaundice	Accept donor with history of jaundice that was attributed to gall stones, Rh disease, mononucleosis or in neonatal period
50.	Chronic Liver disease/Liver Failure	Permanently defer
HIV Infection/AIDS		
51.	At risk for HIV infection (Transgender, Men who have Sex with Men, Female Sex Workers, Injecting drug users, persons with multiple sex partners)	Permanently defer
52.	Known HIV positive person or spouse/partner of PLHA (person living with HIV/AIDS)	Permanently defer
53.	Persons having symptoms suggestive of AIDS	Permanently defer person having lymphadenopathy, prolonged and repeated fever, prolonged and repeated diarrhea irrespective of HIV risk or status
Sexually Transmitted Infections		
54.	Syphilis (Genital sore, or generalized skin rashes)	Permanently defer
55.	Gonorrhea	Permanently defer
Other Infectious Diseases		
56.	History of Measles, Mumps, Chickenpox	Defer for 2 weeks following full recovery
57.	Malaria	Defer for 3 months following full recovery
58.	Typhoid	Defer for 12 Months following full recovery

Continued

Continued

59.	Dengue/ Chikungunya	• In case of history of Dengue/Chikungunya: Defer for 6 Months following full recovery • Following visit to Dengue/Chikungunya endemic area: 4 weeks following return from visit to dengue endemic area if no febrile illness is noted
60.	Zika Virus/ West Nile Virus	• In case of Zika infection: Defer for 4 months following recovery • In case of history of travel to West Nile Virus endemic area or Zika virus outbreak zone: Defer for 4 months
61.	Tuberculosis	Defer for 2 years following confirmation of cure
62.	Leishmaniasis	Permanently defer
63.	Leprosy	Permanently defer
Other Infections		
64.	Conjunctivitis	Defer for the period of illness and continuation of local medication
65.	Osteomyelitis	Defer for 2 years following completion of treatment and cure
Kidney Disease		
66.	Acute infection of kidney (pyelonephritis)	Defer for 6 months after complete recovery and last dose of medication
67.	Acute infection of bladder (cystitis)/ UTI	Defer for 2 weeks after complete recovery and last dose of medication
68.	Chronic infection of kidney/kidney disease/renal failure	Permanently defer
Digestive System		
69.	Diarrhea	Person having history of diarrhea in preceding week particularly if associated with fever: Defer for 2 weeks after complete recovery and last dose of medication
70.	GI endoscopy	Defer for 12 months

Continued

Continued

71.	Acid Peptic disease	• Accept person with acid reflux, mild gastroesophageal reflux, mild hiatus hernia, gastroesophageal reflux disorder (GERD), hiatus hernia • Permanently defer person with stomach ulcer with symptoms or with recurrent bleeding
	Other Diseases/Disorders	
72.	Autoimmune disorders like Systemic lupus erythematosus, scleroderma, dermatomyositis, ankylosing spondylitis or severe rheumatoid arthritis	Permanently defer
73.	Polycythemia vera	Permanently defer
74.	Bleeding disorders and unexplained bleeding tendency	Permanently defer
75.	Malignancy	Permanently defer
76.	Severe allergic disorders	Permanently defer
77.	Hemoglobinopathies and red cell enzyme deficiencies with known history of hemolysis	Permanently defer
	Vaccination and Inoculation	
78.	**Non live vaccines and Toxoid:** Typhoid, Cholera, Papillomavirus, Influenza, Meningococcal, Pertussis, Pneumococcal, Polio injectable, Diphtheria, Tetanus, Plague	Defer for 14 days

Continued

Continued

79.	**Live attenuated vaccines**: Polio oral, Measles (Rubella) Mumps, Yellow fever, Japanese encephalitis, influenza, Typhoid, Cholera, Hepatitis A	Defer for 28 days
80.	Anti-tetanus serum, Antivenom serum, Antidiphtheria serum, and Antigas gangrene serum	Defer for 28 days
81.	Antirabies vaccination following animal bite, Hepatitis B Immunoglobulin, Immunoglobulins	Defer for 1 year
82.	Swine Flu	Defer for 15 days
Medications taken by Prospective Blood Donor		
83.	Oral contraceptive	Accept
84.	Analgesics	Accept
85.	Vitamins	Accept
86.	Mild sedative and tranquilizers	Accept
87.	Allopurinol	Accept
88.	Cholesterol lowering medication	Accept
89.	Salicylates (aspirin), other NSAIDs	Defer for 3 days if blood is to be used for Platelet preparation
90.	Ketoconazole, Antihelminthic drugs including mebendazole	Defer for 7 days after last dose if donor is well
91.	Antibiotics	Defer for 2 Weeks after last dose if donor is well
92.	Ticlopidine, clopidogrel	Defer for 2 Weeks after last dose
93.	Piroxicam, dipyridamole	Defer for 2 Weeks after last dose

Continued

Continued

94.	Etretinate, Acitretin or Isotretinoin. (Used for acne)	Defer for 1 month after the last dose
95.	Finasteride used to treat benign prostatatic hyperplasia	Defer for 1 month after the last dose
96.	Radioactive contrast material	8 weeks deferral
97.	Dutasteride used to treat benign prostatatic hyperplasia	Defer for 6 months after the last dose
98.	Any medication of unknown nature	Defer till details are available
99.	Oral antidiabetic drugs	Accept if there is no alteration in dose within last 4 weeks
100.	Insulin	Permanently defer
101.	Antiarrhythmic, Anticonvulsant, Anticoagulant, Antithyroid drugs, Cytotoxic drugs, Cardiac Failure Drugs (Digitalis)	Permanently defer
Other Conditions Requiring Permanent Deferral		
102.	• Recipients of organ, stem cell and tissue transplants • Donors who have had an unexplained delayed faint or delayed faint with injury or two consecutive faints following a blood donation	Permanently defer
Residents of Other Countries		
103.	Residents of other countries	Accept only after stay in India for three continuous years

Selection of Blood Bags for Blood Collection and Preparation of Components

SCOPE AND APPLICATION

This standard operating procedure (SOP) describes the type of blood bag to be selected for blood collection and preparation of blood components.

RESPONSIBILITY

The blood center medical officer/laboratory technician determines the type of blood bag to use to optimize the availability of blood and its components.

MATERIALS REQUIRED

- Different types of blood bags
- Marker pen
- Identification labels

PROCEDURE

1. If the final product is whole human blood, a single blood bag with Citrate-phosphate-dextrose solution with adenine CPDA-1 solution should be used to collect the blood units.
2. Select the type of blood bag to be used for blood component preparation according to **Table 1**.

Note:
- Visually inspect the blood bag prior to blood collection.
- Do not use in case of puncture or discoloration or suspended particulate matter in the bag.
- Check the expiry date on the blood bag.

Table 1: Selection of blood bags for blood collection and preparation of blood components.				
Donor		**Components**	**Blood bags**	
Weight (kg)	**Aspirin intake**	**Required**	**Type**	**Quantity of Blood (mL)**
>45	–	Whole blood	Single	350
>55	No	PRBC + FFP + PLT	Triple or quadruple	450
>55	Yes	PRBC + FFP PRBC + FFP + CRYO	Double/triple	450
45–55	No	PRBC + FFP + PLT	Triple	350
45–55	Yes	PRBC + FFP PRBC + FFP + CRYO	Double/triple	350

(CRYO: cryoprecipitate; FFP: fresh frozen plasma; PLT: platelets; PRBC: packed red blood cells)

3. Assign a unique identification (UID) number to the donor. Label the primary/satellite bag/pilot tube with this UID. Record her/his UID number in the donor's record to ensure accountability/traceability and unique identifier of blood units/components, e.g., voluntary/exchange/autologous.

Note:
- Blood centers using automated component extractors must use blood bags compatible with those extractors.
- The blood bag also has diversion bags to divert the initial blood flow, thereby reducing the bacterial load entering the blood bag.
- The Luer adapter with holder (LAH) allows blood to be collected for sampling in multiple tubes by a closed technique for screening of transfusion transmitted infections (TTIs) and blood grouping.
- LAH also ensures safe handling and collection of blood and prevents needle stick injuries and blood spills.
- The blood bag is equipped with a needle injury protector (NIP) that locks the needle inside NIP after phlebotomy, reducing the accidental needle stick injury during and after phlebotomy.

RECORD

Record UID, type, and segment number of blood bags in the donor register.

CHAPTER 8

Labeling of Blood Bag

SCOPE AND APPLICATION

This standard operating procedure (SOP) covers the assignment of unique identification (UID) numbers to donors and the accurate labeling of blood units and pilot tubes after donor screening. This is essential for complete traceability or tracking of blood from donor to blood components and to recipient.

RESPONSIBILITY

It is the responsibility of the phlebotomist (under supervision of medical officer) performing the blood collection to ensure that the blood bags and sample tubes are properly labeled with the UID number. The UID number must also be provided on the donor registration form.

MATERIALS REQUIRED

- Robust sticker label with preprinted serial number
- Blood bag with a preprinted unique segment number on its tubing
- **Blood Donor Questionnaire and Health Checkup Form**

PROCEDURE

1. After selecting the type of blood bag for whole blood collection, perform a visual inspection for any signs of deterioration, particulate matter, or damage (in case of puncture, particulate matter, or discoloration, do not use it).
2. Affix a sticker label with UID number to identify the donor on top of the manufacturer's label of the primary collection bag and the satellite bags in case of multiple bags.

3. Record the date of blood collection on the manufacturer's label on the primary blood collection bag.
4. Affix a sticker label with the same UID number on the vacutainer to take blood samples for testing purposes.
5. Check the tube segment number of the primary collection bag and record in the donor register and Donor Questionnaire and health checkup form.
6. Verify the donor's identity using the Donor Questionnaire and health checkup form. Affix the UID number on it.
7. Cross-check UID number on the blood unit, pilot tubes, and Donor Questionnaire and health checkup form to ensure donor identity. Record it in the donor register using the same UID number. Transcribe this UID number on all records henceforth (storage, testing, issue, and transfusion records).
8. At this point, the blood bag is ready for blood collection.
9. After donating blood, fill in the blood collection start time, date, blood collection end time, and duration for blood collection on the **Blood Donor Questionnaire and Health Checkup Form**.
10. Samples collected in the vacutainer are used for blood grouping and transfusion transmitted infection (TTI) screening.

DOCUMENTATION

Make sure that the sticker with the same UID number is on the primary and satellite bags and vacutainers and there are no transcription errors, as this UID number will trace any blood/blood component to the donor of the blood and vice versa in case of requirement.

CHAPTER 9

Preparation of Phlebotomy Site

SCOPE AND APPLICATION

This standard operating procedure (SOP) describes the skin preparation at the phlebotomy site prior to venipuncture to ensure aseptic collection of blood.

RESPONSIBILITY

The phlebotomist who collects the blood unit from the donor is responsible for preparing the phlebotomy site.

MATERIALS REQUIRED

- Sterilization tray
- Methylated spirit
- 70% ethyl alcohol/alcohol swabs
- Povidone-iodine solution 5%
- Sterile cotton/gauze/swabs
- Artery forceps
- Blood pressure (BP) apparatus

PROCEDURE

1. Make the donor lie down with a pillow under his/her head or recline in a comfortable donor chair. Loosen tight clothes.
2. Select an antecubital venipuncture site on the arm.
3. Apply a BP cuff, inflate to 50–60 mm Hg, and select a large and good caliber vein in an area free of skin lesion.
4. Deflate the BP cuff and thoroughly cleanse the selected venipuncture site with methylated spirit, povidone-iodine solution, and finally a methylated spirit (70% ethyl alcohol or denatured alcohol) swab. Begin by disinfecting a 5 cm diameter area of skin in circular motions from the center to the periphery.

5. Rub the povidone-iodine swab vigorously for at least 30 seconds or till froth is formed.
6. Do not touch, the site prepared for venipuncture. Should the skin be touched away from the point of insertion of needle? If the puncture site is touched, repeat skin preparation procedure as previously.
7. Inspect each swab used. If it is physically observed soiled, take a new swab and repeat the skin preparation procedure as detailed above.
8. Discard the used swab in a biohazard waste container.
9. Allow the skin to air dry. Do not wipe the area with cotton wool, fan, or blow on it.

Note: If the donor is allergic to spirit/iodine, savlon antiseptic solution should be used for preparation of the phlebotomy site.

CHAPTER 10

Blood Collection and Counseling during Blood Donation

SCOPE AND APPLICATION

This standard operating procedure (SOP) provides instructions for aseptic blood collection from donors and guidelines for counseling during blood donation to achieve the following objectives:

- Make the donor comfortable during the blood donation process, including venipuncture.
- Reduce donor anxiety and minimize the risk of adverse donor reactions (ADRs), such as fainting.
- Postdonation counseling, including venipuncture site care
- Ensuring donors' cooperation in the exclusion of confidential entities or postdonation information processes
- Increase donor confidence in donor retention

RESPONSIBILITY

The phlebotomist is responsible for confirming donor screening details, verifying the assigned unique identification (UID) number, preparing the blood collection site, and then drawing blood from the donor. The phlebotomist is also responsible for counseling during the donation process.

MATERIALS REQUIRED

- Sterile cotton/gauze swabs
- Artery forceps
- Sterile disposable syringes (2 mL)
- Sterile disposable hypodermic needles (26 gauge)
- *Pilot tubes*: Plain and ethylenediaminetetraacetic acid (EDTA)
- Oxygen cylinder with accessories
- First aid kit

- Tube sealer
- Needle destroyer
- Citrate-phosphate-dextrose solution with adenine (CPDA) bag for blood collection
- Scissors
- Adhesive tapes
- Blood collection monitor
- Donor couch

PROCEDURE

1. Make the donor recline on a comfortable donor couch. Loosen tight clothes.
2. Identify the donor by name. Enter the bag and segment numbers into the Donor Questionnaire and informed consent form.
3. Ask the donor if he/she is comfortable. Give a hand roller/squeezer in hand to the donor.
4. Select the appropriate blood bag for blood collection.
5. Clean the venipuncture site.
6. Set the blood collection monitor to the desired blood collection volume (350/450 mL) and place the blood bag on it. Route the tube through the clamp.
7. Apply the blood pressure (BP) cuff to the donor arm.
8. Clamp the bleed line of the blood bag using artery forceps to prevent air from entering the tube or bag when the needle cover is removed.
9. Hold the needle with the bevel of the needle facing upward and hold the shaft at an angle of 15° to the arm. Once the needle is under the skin, release the artery forceps. Insert the blood bag needle into the vein for about 1–1.5 cm by a bold single prick to ensure smooth blood flow and secure on the arm with adhesive tape.
10. Instruct the donor to gently squeeze the ball/roller with the hand to improve blood flow.
11. If venipuncture fails, do not retry on the same arm. For the second trial, obtain the donor's permission. Use a new bag and discard the previous bag.
12. As soon as the blood enters the bag tubing, press the "start key" of the blood collection monitor. This will automatically measure the bag weight and the weight of CPDA solution so that the "display" will show only the volume of blood drawn. It also gently agitates the blood bag to properly mix the blood with the CPDA solution and prevent clotting.
13. When the collected blood volume reaches "programmed volume minus 5 mL," the rocker motor will stop its agitation, and when the collected blood volume reaches "programmed volume minus

3 mL," the clamp will automatically activate, and no blood will enter into the blood bag. The volume collected and the duration of bleeding are displayed on the first line of the monitor scale LCD (Liquid Crystal Display).

14. Remove the bag from the blood collection monitor scale tray and release the clamp at the end of collection.

15. Clamp the blood line of the blood bag in two different places and cut it in the middle. Collect blood in the pilot tubes from the tubing so that blood flows directly into the tubes from the donor arm.

16. Deflate the BP cuff and remove the needle gently from the donor's vein pressing the phlebotomy site. Place a sterile swab over the venipuncture site and apply pressure to the swab. Ask the donor to raise and fold the arm to prevent the swab from falling.

17. Seal the blood bag tube with a tube sealer. Grasp both ends of the tube and pass the tube through the slot provided in the electrode cover between the shutter electrodes. At the same time, push down the pipe detection lever. A movable electrode presses the tube against a fixed electrode. The "Seal" light-emitting diode (LED) lights up. The "Ready" LED goes out. The tube melts to form a sealed pattern. *Do not stretch the hose while sealing. This can cause leaks.*

18. After a certain period of time, the electrodes are removed, the 'Seal' LED goes out, and the "Ready" LED goes out. After a time delay, the electrode will release, the "Seal" LED goes OFF, and the "Ready" LED turns ON. Take out the sealed tube. In this way, make a number of segments in the tubing and use them for compatibility testing.

19. The blood samples of the donor are collected by inserting the vacutainer into the adaptor system of the Luer adaptor with holder (LAH). It ensures a closed system of blood sample collection. In addition to minimizing spillage and waste of collected blood, this makes handling and sampling of collected blood safer.

20. The needle from the bag along with the cut portion of the tubing is discarded in the red capped containers.

21. Freshly drawn blood units are stored at 4 ± 2°C in a blood center refrigerator intended for storage of untested blood units.

CLASSIFICATION OF ADVERSE DONOR REACTIONS

Adverse donor reactions can be classified into the following categories:

- Complications—mainly local symptoms
- Complications—mainly generalized symptoms
- Allergic reactions
- Serious complications
- Other reactions

Complications—Mainly Local Symptoms

These are related to the practice of needle insertion during the act of phlebotomy and the consequent response from the soft tissues, fascia, tendons, and neurovascular bundle harboring the vein, artery, and nerve. ADR mitigation for local complications includes the following interventions targeting mainly toward the training of blood transfusion services (BTS) staff:

- *Good phlebotomy technique*: The best practice includes induction training to new staff and regular refresher training and competence assessment.
  - Training of venous access available in antecubital fossa, with knowledge of the neurovascular bundle and the prominent nerves in the region
  - Technique of differentiating between nerve and a vein (collapsible nature)
  - The assessment of caliber of the vein with respect to the caliber of needle
  - The need to follow the "bevel up—aeroplane landing technique" on the side of the vein and then laterally insert the needle in a clean one-step procedure.
  - Anchor the needle safely with the adhesive tape without undue pressure of the needle and without any undue possibility of movement of needle from its position once the donor is asked to pump the handball.
  - The deflation of pressure by cuff/tourniquet to allow the free flow of blood
- The need to communicate the donor about the process of blood donation in order to make him/her comfortable when the staff is conducting the requisite intervention.

Complications—Mainly Generalized Symptoms

These complications include a more or less equal focus toward the donor and the BTS staff during the process of the donation. There are two approaches for this. The first is to improve donors psychologically and physiologically in their attitudes and the donation process. The other approach is to reduce vasovagal reactions and injuries in blood donors through predonation education, good setup and environment, staff supervision and skills, interventions, and postreaction treatment and instructions, although essential activities remain the same.

- *Improving the donor psychologically*:
  - First-time donor anxiety should be alleviated by establishing a communication channel with the donor, and a comfortable and friendly environment shall help in donor acclimatization with the process of donation.

- Predonation information, donor counseling, and medical screening should be provided to address the common concerns such as needle pain and weakness. Donor engagement using audiovisual gadgets and the applied muscle tension techniques can also reduce anxiety.

- *Improving the donor physiologically*:
  - Vasovagal reactions (VVR) are related to the proportion of blood withdrawn. The Association for the Advancement of Blood and Biotherapies (AABB) and Council of Europe have recommended 15% and 13–15% of the estimated volume, respectively. Even consideration of smaller blood bags may mitigate VVRs.
  - Fluid loading of the donor with water, isotonic fluids, and/or salt is recommended for mitigating VVRs. Gastric distention causes an increase in sympathetic discharge, leading to peripheral vasoconstriction and consequent diversion of central blood flow to maintain BP/isotonic fluid and salt increase the blood volume per say, and the effect is longer in comparison to the effect of plain water in mitigating.
  - Encouraging good hydration, usual meals, and salted snack intake a day before blood donation mitigates VVRs.
  - Muscle tension techniques are also known to alleviate VVR. Muscle tension in the lower body draws more blood from the large-capacity veins (peripheral heart) to the central heart, increasing stroke volume and therefore cardiac output.
  - Allowing a graduated rise from the donor couch also mitigates VVRs. The process of sitting with overhanging legs for a minute before being upright allows the blood volume to redistribute, preventing sudden pooling of blood in the peripheral heart.

- *Improving the donor's attitude*:
  - The predonation information material and the counseling of the donor prior to, during, and postdonation and provision of a neat and clean environment that is equipped with modern blood donation equipment improves the confidence of the donor on the BTS and allays anxiety in the first-time donors.
  - The friendly/joyful interaction of the BTS staff with the donor helps in coping with anxiety.
  - The information to the donor with emphasis on the value of the donation in terms of service to thalassemia, requiring regular blood transfusions.

- *Improving the process of blood donation*:
  - Trained professionals at workplace to deal with the blood donor comprehensively in the art of communication and practical processes such as finger-prick and phlebotomy.
  - Ambient temperature of the blood center

- Ability of staff to identify and delineate donors predisposed toward the development of VVRs such as:
  - ○ Lack of adequate sleep, water, or food intake
  - ○ First-time donor/female gender/young donor with low estimated blood volume
  - ○ Tachycardia or hypotension prior to donation
- Ability of the staff to identify and defer a donation due to "poor veins"
- Unidirectional flow and exit of donors with proper guidance at all workstations such as registration, predonation information, counseling, refreshment, donor management during donation, appropriate time of the donor couch, and oversight during the postdonation.
- The various work stations should be shielded from one another for the prevention of mass fainting episodes provoked by the sight of VVR or blood spill.
- Good postdonation information is more important for first-time successful donors to plan and optimize the next donation.
- Provision of salty snack, sweetened liquid, and water prior to donation
- Encourage the donor to stay for 15 minutes post refreshments under supervision for any adverse donor reaction.
- Thank the donor 3 times at least at reception, before phlebotomy, and postrefreshments.

COUNSELING DURING BLOOD DONATION

The above mitigating interventions in ADRs would translate the moral and ethical obligation of BTS in practice, apart from ensuring safety of the noble blood donors as far as possible with the present evidence available. The counseling during blood donation shall ensure the following:

- A history of previous allergies, phobias, and previous syncope episodes during injections or blood donations should be queried.
- The venipuncture procedure and the need to properly disinfect the skin and find a suitable vein
- The volume of blood to be collected and the time required for the procedure.
- Make sure that donor is comfortable.
- Assure the donor to relax
- Reduce his/her anxiety
- Assure the donor that the blood donation is very safe process.
- Postdonation personal care, including venipuncture site care and ways to prevent and treat acute and delayed donor reactions.

CHAPTER 11

Postdonation Care and Counseling

SCOPE AND APPLICATION

This standard operating procedure (SOP) includes postdonation care and counseling which are an integral part of quality donor services and care. Postdonation counseling is intended for all blood donors, but the content varies according to each donor's conditions and circumstances in order to achieve the following objectives:

- To describe the test results, the requirement of confirmation of results, the health implications of donors and discard of donated blood, and donor suitability of donors for future blood donations
- To otivate donors to provide all relevant information, including the possible sources of infection.
- To clarify donor questions or concerns
- To alleviate donor anxiety
- To provide information on precautions to avoid infecting others
- To provide information and donor referrals for further evaluation, treatment, and care, as appropriate.
- To collect demographic and risk exposure data from transfusion transmitted infection (TTI)-positive donors as part of a Haemovigilance program
- To emphasize the importance of a healthy lifestyle for nonresponsive donors and encourage regular blood donations
- To prepare a panel of rare blood types

RESPONSIBILITY

A counselor/medical officer is responsible for the postdonation care and counseling of the donor.

REQUIREMENTS

- Sterile cotton swabs
- Adhesive tape
- Thrombophob ointment
- Leaflet on postdonation instructions
- Counseling room providing safe and conducive environment

PROCEDURE

1. To avoid side effects, such as dizziness, instruct the donor not to get up from the chair for 5 minutes, even if they are perfectly fine.
2. Observe the donor for additional 10 minutes in the refreshment area while having refreshments.
3. Check the venipuncture site before the donor leaves the donor room. Do not tape until it leaks. If persistent bleeding occurs at the venipuncture site, apply pressure with a dry, sterile cotton swab. For a hematoma, gently apply antithrombotic ointment to the affected area after 5 minutes. The donor should be informed of the expected change in skin color. If pain persists, ask to apply ice.

POSTDONATION COUNSELING

Do's and don'ts shall be displayed in a postdonation/refreshment area to ensure donor safety.

- *Do's and Don'ts*
    - Drink plenty of water during the day.
    - Do not lift heavy objects or engage in strenuous activity with the donor's arms.
    - Do not smoke for the next 30 minutes.
    - Do not climb stairs for the next 30 minutes.
    - Do not drink alcohol for the next 6 hours.
    - Do not drive on the donation day.
    - No special dietary supplements are required. However, iron-rich foods such as green leafy vegetables, jaggery, dates, and meat (for nonvegetarians) are recommended.
    - Consult the nearest doctor or contact the blood center in case of swelling/bluish discoloration/pain at the venipuncture site.
    - Raise your arm and apply pressure in case of bleeding from the collection site.
    - Lie down with your legs raised above the head level if there is a feeling of faintness or dizziness. If the condition does not improve, consult the nearest doctor or contact the blood center.

- Resume all normal activities when no symptoms occur.
- Remove the bandage the next day.
- Counsel the rare blood group donors to make them aware about their blood group so that they are able to inform blood centers about their blood groups when relevant.
- Donors with nonreactive TTI results are counseled for proper self-care and maintaining a healthy lifestyle. Their generous blood donation must be acknowledged, and they are encouraged to donate blood in the future.
- Donors with positive TTI results will be counseled once test results are available. The counselor should:
  - Communicate results to the donor simply and clearly.
  - Give the donor time to review the information.
  - Make sure the donor understands the results.
  - Allow the donors to ask questions.
  - Help the donor deal with feelings arising from test result.
  - Address any immediate concerns and assist providers in finding close family and friends who can provide immediate support.
  - Describe follow-up services available in the health facilities and in the community, with a particular focus on treatment, care, and support.
  - Provide information to prevent further spread of infection.
  - Inform about other relevant preventive health measures such as a healthy lifestyle and proper diet.
  - Discuss disclosure of results, including when, how, and to whom.
  - Encourage and provide referrals for testing and counseling of partners and children.
  - Arrange specific dates and times for follow-up visits or referrals to treatment, care, counseling, support, and other services as needed.
- *Recall and deferral mechanism for seroreactive blood donors: The best place for postdonation counseling is a blood center where the counselors can create an atmosphere of safety and warmth and confidentiality.*
  - Donors who have consented to be contacted by the blood center in case of abnormal test result will be recalled to the blood center telephonically or by post. [**Annexure 11.1** in case of positive for human immunodeficiency virus (HIV) and **Annexure 11.2** in case of positive for TTI other than HIV].
  - Postdonation counseling is done, and consent for referral (**Annexure 11.3**) is also taken prior to contacting appropriate medical services to confirm diagnosis, follow-up, and treatment if necessary. The donor is given referral slip (**Annexure 11.4**).

- Donors who are negative for routine serological tests but are nucleic acid testing (NAT) reactive are also recalled and advised for clinical consultation.
- Donors seeking results should be informed of their TTI status and repeatedly advised to continue donating while negative, even if they are not seroreactive.

Annexures 11.1 to 11.4 are as per guidelines circulated by the National AIDS Control Organization (NACO) for recalling of TTI-positive donors.

ANNEXURE 11.1

Format for Letter for Intimation of TTI Status (HIV)

To   Date: _____

_____   Ref. No. _____

_____

_____

Dear blood donor

As you have offered the option of knowing your transfusion transmitted infection (TTI) status during your visit to this blood center for blood donation, you are requested to visit the blood center personally as some of the immediate results are not conclusive, and need to be confirmed for which you will be referred to Voluntary Counseling and Testing Center (VCTC).

Blood Center Officer

_____

_____

_____

ANNEXURE 11.2

Format for Letter for Intimation of TTI Status
(Other than HIV)

To   Date: _____

_____   Ref. No. _____

_____

Dear blood donor

As you have offered the option of knowing your transfusion transmitted infection (TTI) status during your visit to this blood center for blood donation, you are requested to visit the blood center personally as some of the immediate results are not conclusive, and need to be confirmed.

A fresh sample will be taken and tested. Afterwards you will be referred to the Physician.

Blood Center Officer

_____

_____

_____

ANNEXURE 11.3

Consent for Referral

I understand that
- During blood donation process I have been counseled regarding the importance of safe blood donation and have consented to testing of my blood and be informed of any abnormal test.
- These screening tests conducted at blood center are not diagnostic and may yield false-positive results.
- Any willful misrepresentation of facts could endanger my health or that of patients receiving my blood and may lead to litigation.
- I have been contacted, counseled and referred by the blood center for confirmation and management to appropriate facility.

_____   _____

Signature of referring blood center staff   **Signature of donor**

Place: _____

Date: _____

ANNEXURE 11.4

Referral Slip for Blood Donors
(To be filled by blood center staff)

Name and address of the blood center: _____

Date of referral: _____ Blood center ID: _____

Name of the donor: _____

Age: _____ Gender: _____ Phone number: _____ Contact details: _____

Name and designation of the referring person: _____

Reason for referral (to be ticked)	Date of testing	Assay used
Counseling and testing for HIV		
Testing for HBsAg		
Testing for HCV		
Testing of VDRL/RPR		
Testing of Malaria		

Address of the referral center: _____

Blood center seal with contact details: _____

(To be filled by ICTC/Laboratory and retained in record)

Name of the donor: _____ Date of performing test: _____

PID No./OPD No.: _____

Investigation done: _____

Result: _____

Seal of ICTC/Laboratory with contact details

Note: It is advised that Incharge ICTC/Laboratory should sign this before retaining in the record.

(To be filled by ICTC/Laboratory and returned to donor)

Name of the donor/Department: _____

Donor ID No.: _____ PID No./OPD Regd. No.: _____

Date of sample drawn: _____

Please come for retesting after 2 weeks on: _____

1. Result to be collected on: _____

2. Repeat test at ICTC on: _____

Seal of ICTC/Laboratory with contact details

Note: It is advised that Incharge ICTC/Laboratory should sign this before returning to the donor.

CHAPTER 12

Management of Adverse Donor Reactions

SCOPE AND APPLICATION

This standard operating procedure (SOP) describes how to deal with any of the adverse donor reactions that the donor may experience during the post-donation period.

RESPONSIBILITY

The medical officer and staff nurse of blood center are responsible for managing donor side effects after donating blood.

MEDICINES/MATERIALS REQUIRED

The following medicines/materials are required in case an emergency arises during the postdonation period:

Oral medication:
- Analgesic tablets, e.g., Paracetamol tablet IP 500 mg
- Calcium and vitamin C tablets
- Electrolyte replacement fluid [oral rehydration solution (ORS)] 22 gms sachet

Ointments:
- Thrombophob ointment
- Betnovate ointment
- Analgesic balm

Injections:
- Epinephrine (adrenaline) 0.18% w/v (1 in 1,000) 1 mL ampule
- Atropine sulfate 1 mg in 1 mL
- Mephentine 30 mg/mL (10 mL vial)
- Pheniramine maleate injection 22.75 mg/mL (2 mL ampule)
- Diazepam injection 5 mg/mL (2 mL ampule)
- Hydrocortisone 100 mg vial (to be dissolved in 2 mL sterile water for injection)

- Dextrose injection 25% w/v (100 mL bottle)
- Inj. Furosemide 25 mg/mL (2 mL ampule)
- Inj. Metoclopramide 5 mg/mL (2 mL ampule)
- Inj. Pheniramine Maleate (IP 22.75 mg)
- Inj. Sodium bicarbonate IP (8.4% w/v) 100 mL vial
- Sodium chloride 0.9% and dextrose 5% injection (500 mL bottle)
- Inj. Stemetil 12.5 mg/mL (1 mL ampule)

Miscellaneous:
- Bandages/dressings
- Band-Aid
- Spirit of ammonia
- Tongue depressor
- Disposable hypodermic syringes (2/5 mL) and disposable needles 24 G
- Clinical thermometer
- Oxygen cylinder
- Infusion set
- Paper bag

MANAGEMENT OF ADVERSE REACTIONS

- *Giddiness/syncope (vasovagal syndrome)*:
  - Make the donor lie down on the bed in a relaxed position.
  - Ask the donor to raise feet and lower head end.
  - Loosen tight clothing (belts, ties, etc.).
  - Maintain an adequate airway.
  - Check pulse and blood pressure.
  - Apply cold compresses to the forehead and back.
  - Administer inhalation of spirit of ammonia if needed. The donor should respond by coughing that raises the blood pressure.
  - *When bradycardia and hypotension*:
    - If bradycardia persists for >20 minutes, inject 1 mL atropine intramuscularly.
    - If hypotension persists, administer intravenous (IV) saline or glucose–saline infusion.
  - Inform such donor not to drive a vehicle or return to work or any hazardous occupations for 12 hours.
- *Convulsions*: True convulsions are very uncommon. However, if at all occurs, it is important to:
  - Tilt the head of the donor to one side
  - Prevent tongue biting
  - A tongue depressor or gauze is inserted between the teeth to keep the airway open.
  - Put screens around to maintain privacy
  - Check the pulse frequently

- Loosen the tight clothing
- Call a specialist if the spasm lasts longer than 5 minutes.
- After recovery, the provider should be given sufficient reassurance.
- Advise the donor tactfully not to donate the blood again.

- *Vomiting*:
  - Vomiting usually relieves symptoms and resolves on its own.
  - If vomiting persists and is severe, administer Stemetil injection intramuscularly.

- *Tetany/muscular spasm/twitching*:
  - These are usually the result of lowering/depletion of carbon dioxide due to hyperventilation of the anxious donor.
  - Ask the donor to inhale and exhale into the paper bag for immediate relief. Do not give oxygen.

- *Hematoma*:
  - Immediately remove tourniquet/compression cuff. Apply pressure to the venepuncture site and pull the needle out of the vein. Raise the arm above the head and hold for a few minutes. After about 5 minutes, gently apply an antithrombotic ointment around the phlebotomy site. Instruct the donor to apply ice to the phlebotomy site, if there is pain and inform about the expected change in skin color.

- *Eczematous reaction on the skin around the venepuncture site*:
  - Apply an ointment containing steroid, e.g., Betnovate ointment.

- *Delayed syncope*: These can occur 30 minutes to an hour after donation (usually after the donor leaves the blood center). Management is the same as described above for syncope.
  - The donor who gives a history of such attacks more than twice is permanently deferred.

- *Accidental puncture of the artery*: A rare complication in which blood flows very quickly. It is important to:
  - Stop the donation immediately.
  - Apply firm pressure to the puncture site for at least 15–20 minutes and raise the limbs above the heart level.
  - Reassure the donor and record the findings.
  - Allow the donor to go only when the blood center officer is satisfied about his well-being.

RECORD

Record all the adverse events and their treatments in the donor reaction register and submit online monthly adverse donor reaction report to the National Institute of Biologicals, Noida, Ministry of Health and Family Welfare, Government of India for monitoring under Donor Haemovigilance Programme of India (HvPI) and a copy of the report is also submitted to State Blood Transfusion Council.

CHAPTER 13

Assessing Suitability of Donor for Plateletpheresis

SCOPE AND APPLICATION

This standard operating procedure (SOP) describes the criteria for accepting donors for plateletpheresis to ensure the safety of both the donor and the recipient. The goal of the plateletpheresis procedure is to transfuse single donor platelets (SDP) to patients with thrombocytopenia and minimize the risk of multiple donor exposure.

RESPONSIBILITY

The medical officer is responsible for determining the suitability of the donor for plateletpheresis after evaluation of the medical history (in the donor questionnaire and health checkup form) and physical examination, including the results of the predonation screening test.

MATERIALS REQUIRED

- Blood donor questionnaire and health checkup form (apheresis) (Annexure 2.2)
- Writing pens
- General information in the form of pamphlets about blood donation and apheresis. The pamphlet should be designed by the blood center locally.

PROCEDURE

Healthy people do have excess platelets and the human body is constantly replacing them; therefore, removing platelets by apheresis has no adverse effects on donors. A properly screened healthy donor is selected for plateletpheresis. In addition to standard blood donation criteria as specified in the SOP no. 6, the following additional criteria are also taken care of:

- Age: 18–60 years

- Before the first plateletpheresis, the platelet count is not required or if 4 weeks or more have elapsed after the last plateletpheresis/procedure.
- The donor platelet count should be >150,000/μL, if the donation interval is <4 weeks.
- The interval between two platelet donations should be at least 48 hours after platelet/plasmapheresis but not more than 2 times a week and limited to 24 times in a year.
- Donor after whole blood donation should not be accepted before 28 days from the last plateletpheresis provided reinfusion of red cell was complete in the last plateletpheresis and if incomplete, the donor is not accepted within 90 days.
- A minimum of 3 months interval must be there for the plateletpheresis procedure unless the extracorporeal volume is <100 mL, if the donor has donated a unit of whole blood or if it became impossible to return the donor's red cells during previous plateletpheresis.
- Donors who are on antiplatelet medications (aspirin/aspirin-containing medications, piroxicam) or have taken these medicines within 3 days before donation are not accepted and donors who have taken Plavix/Clopidogrel and Ticlid/Ticlopidine are deferred for 14 days because these medicines affect platelets' ability to function properly.
- The donor is screened prior to the plateletpheresis procedure for all the mandatory infectious disease markers, i.e., human immunodeficiency virus (HIV), hepatitis B surface antigen (HBsAg), hepatitis C virus (HCV), Venereal Disease Research Laboratory (VDRL), and malaria parasite (MP) preferably by enzyme-linked immunosorbent assay (ELISA) a day prior to the procedure as for whole blood donation. Infectious markers are considered valid for 30 days to facilitate repeat targeted platelet/plasma donations.
- For urgent plateletpheresis, signed consent from the attending physician and patient should be obtained for rapid screening.
- Other donor parameters such as hematocrit, height, and weight must be entered into the machine.
- The donor should not be fasting before the procedure; however, he/she should avoid eating oily/fatty food.
- Written informed consent is obtained from the donor.
- Select a prominent and easily accessible antecubital vein on one of the arms for the apheresis.

RECORD

Enter all the details in the **Blood Donor Questionnaire and Health Checkup Form** (*apheresis*) (Annexure 2.2), donor register.

14

Plateletpheresis using a Blood Cell Separator (Dual Needle)

SCOPE AND APPLICATION

This standard operating procedure (SOP) describes a dual-needle PLT-5d program for plateletpheresis using a blood cell separator (COM. TEC version 4.02xx only). This SOP can be modified accordingly by the blood centers using other cell separators suitably to the manufacturer's specifications. In this program, platelets are separated in a continuous mode via two venous donor accesses. The C5L set is a closed system that allows platelets to be stored for up to 5 days. For this reason, the inlet needle is preinstalled in this set as well as sterile filters for the saline and acid-citrate-dextrose (ACD) lines. This SOP provides instructions for installation of apheresis set C5L, priming, separation, reinfusion, and removal of the apheresis set.

RESPONSIBILITY

The medical officer is responsible for determining the donor suitability for plateletpheresis. He/she must ensure that criteria are met after a physical examination including the evaluation of the medical history in the blood donor questionnaire and health checkup form and the results of the predonation screening tests.

MATERIALS REQUIRED

- COM.TEC blood cell separator version 4.02xx
- Double-needle closed system COM.TEC kit (C5L)
- Venipuncture supplies, i.e., alcohol swab, chlorhexidine solution, sterile cotton swab, etc.
- Ethylenediaminetetraacetic acid (EDTA) (lavender top) vacutainer for blood sampling
- Blood donor questionnaire and health checkup form (apheresis) (Annexure 2.2)

- Tube sealer
- Chewable calcium tablets
- Emergency medicine tray

PROCEDURE

Selection of the Platelet Program

1. Connect the COM.TEC blood cell separator to the power supply.
2. Press the I (power on) key in the front panel **(Fig. 1)**.

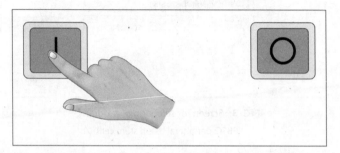

FIG. 1: Pressing power on.

3. Screen will display, showing software version. Press Continue **(Fig. 2)**.

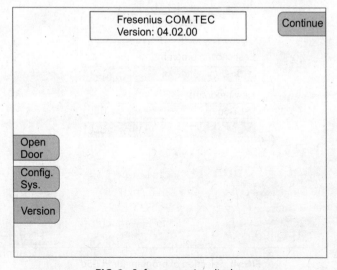

FIG. 2: Software version display.

4. Press Continue. The following screen will display **(Fig. 3)**.

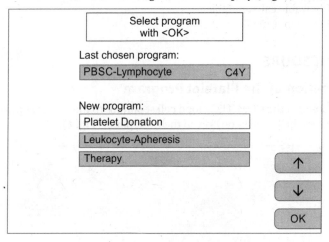

FIG. 3: Screen for selection of program.

(PBSC: peripheral blood stem cell)

5. Use the Up ↑ and Down ↓ keys to select the program group "Platelet Donation".

6. Press the OK key, and the following screen will display **(Fig. 4)**. Use the Up ↑ and Down ↓ keys to select the PLT-5d program. Press the OK key.

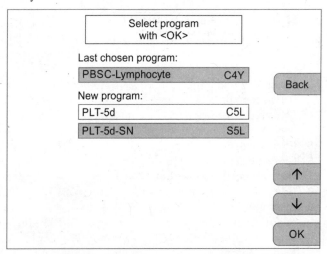

FIG. 4: Selection of program for PLT-5d.

(PBSC: peripheral blood stem cell)

Installation of the Apheresis Set (C5L)

7. After this, the screen for installation of kit will appear **(Fig. 5)**.

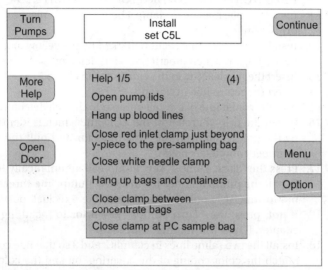

FIG. 5: Screen for installation of kit.
(PC: platelet concentrate)

7.1. The message "Install set C5L" will appear as above. Follow the on-screen help instructions for a total of five screens as follows.

7.2. Open all four pump lids. Press the Turn Pumps key. The threading pins automatically stop at the threading position (12 o'clock/ACD pump: 5 o'clock).

7.3. Hang up blood inlet/return lines onto hooks of intravenous (IV) rack on the right side of cell separator.

7.4. Close red inlet clamp just beyond Y piece to the presampling bag.

7.5. Close white needle clamp.

7.6. Close the platelet concentrate (PC) sample bag clamp.

7.7. Hang empty bag on the hook above return drip chamber.

7.8. Hang the plasma bag on the hook of clamp 4.

7.9. Install all four pump segments by inserting the top pump adapters into the color-coded pumps and holding them with your fingers, press Turn Pumps. The pumps will be loaded automatically. Close the pump lids on all the four pumps.

7.10. Install the RETURN DRIP CHAMBER at the AIR DETECTOR in such a way that DRIP CHAMBER is equally outside the DETECTOR on both TOP/BOTTOM side of DETECTOR.

7.11. Install the plasma line in clamp 4 between the Y-piece and the drip chamber.

7.12. Install the plasma line section marked by the yellow tabs into the hemoglobin/hematocrit (Hb/Hct) detector.

7.13. Insert the line leading to the empty bag in clamp 5.

7.14. Insert the return line in clamp 1.

7.15. Insert the inlet line of the cell pump into the cell detector.

7.16. Install the drip chamber of the ACD line which is identified by the green clamp in the ACD detector and pull the drip chamber completely down.

7.17. Press the "Turn Pumps" key. Pump will automatically load. Install the pump adapter for the ACD pump. The threading pin for the ACD pump should be in the 5 o'clock position. If not, press the "Turn Pumps" key prior to installing the adapter. Pump will automatically load.

7.18. Install the two saline lines in clamps 2 and 3 so that line colors match the color coding of the covering foil and the color of the roller clamps (red line clamp 2, blue line clamp 3).

7.19. Screw the filters of the red-coded pressure measuring lines onto the red-coded pressure measurement port for the inlet pressure.

7.20. Screw the blue-coded pressure measuring line for the return pressure onto the blue-coded pressure measurement port for the return pressure.

7.21. Hold the separation chamber with the top centrifuge adapter and allow the tubes to hang freely to the sides of the instrument without kinking.

7.22. Open the door of chamber holder. Push the circular adapter of the separation chamber into the groove of the central funnel. Close the door until it latches. The locking pin on the flat side of the chamber holder should not be visible.

7.23. Remove the empty package from the centrifuge door. Press the "Open Door" key. Slide open the centrifuge door. If "Open Door" key is not displayed, the door cannot be opened.

7.24. Turn the centrifuge rotor until one of the two line guides is on the right of the rotor. With the separation chamber installed, slide the chamber holder under the rotor with the line facing down.

7.25. Push the chamber holder onto the guide rail until it clicks into place. Rotate the locking flap down until it clicks into place. Pass the centrifuge tubing through the line guide. Push the upper centrifuge adapter with the narrow side first into the upper adapter holder.

Should the adapter be rotated slightly and then turn it in the direction in which the individual lines are twisted around each other? After the test spin, close the centrifuge door and perform another visual inspection. The door is properly locked if the "Open Door" key is displayed. Insert the Air Protect into the holder.

Caution

Make sure the centrifuge tubing is not pinched between the chamber holder and rotor.

Note:
- Manually rotate the rotor counterclockwise to ensure that it is installed properly.
- After a test revolution and another visual check, close the centrifuge door. The door will be locked when the "Open Door" key is displayed. Place the Air Protect into the holder.

Checks after Apheresis Set and Separation Chamber Installation (Fig. 6)

Visually verify the following:
- Make sure the red clamp on the inlet line below the branch to the presampling bag, the white needle clamp, the clamp between the concentrate bags, and the clamp on the concentrate sampling bag are closed. All other stop clamps in the set must be open.
- Make sure that the separation chamber is properly installed.
- Ensure correct installation of air detector and the ACD-A drip chamber in their holders.
- The ACD-A pump adapter and ACD-A tubing must be properly installed under the ACD-A pump drop counter.
- Make sure installation of the return line in clamp 1 and the saline lines in clamps 2 and 3.
- Make sure the plasma installation in clamp 4.
- Make sure installation of line leading to the empty bag in clamp 5.
- Make sure installation of the inlet line of the cell pump in the spillover detector.

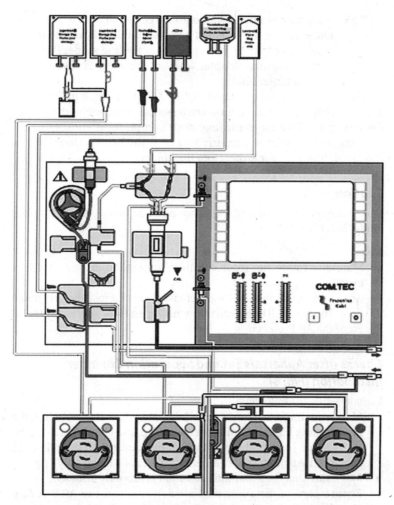

FIG. 6: Checks after apheresis set and separation chamber installation.
(For color version, see Plate 1)

Preparing for Priming

8. Press the "Continue" key; the following screen will display **(Fig. 7)**.
   A user manual is provided that explains how to connect the saline
   and ACD-A solutions prior to priming the set. Connect the ACD-A
   bag to the green connector and hang it onto the upper left hook
   on the front of the device. Break the cone of the ACD-A bag. Press
   the drip chamber to deaerate and adjust the level to approximately

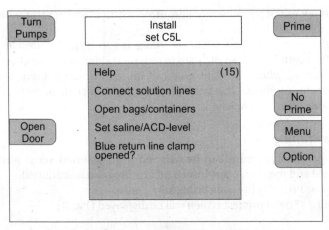

FIG. 7: Screen display after continuing on installation of set.

(ACD: acid-citrate-dextrose)

1 cm below the optical sensor. A saline bag is connected to the two transparent connectors. Hang the saline bag on the front left hook. Break the cones and adjust the fluid level in the two-drip chambers.

Priming

During priming, saline and ACD-A are pumped into the set to displace the air. The *Prime* program steps are divided into the following phases:

- *Detection of set and procedure*: The COM.TEC detects automatically the procedure selected and which set is suitable for that procedure. The additional ACD pump has a miniature contact which is actuated by the pump segment when the C5 set is installed. This contact does not work when using the C4 or PL1 set. If the contact positions are the same as those predicted by the software (activated for C5 method, not activated for C4 and PL1 methods), an ACD drip test is performed. If the actual position and the expected position are not the same, an error message is displayed (Failure: Wrong set).
- *Pressure test/test clamp 1*: With clamps 1 and 2 closed, the whole blood pump delivers until a negative pressure has developed at the inlet pressure monitor to see if the lines are installed in the clamps and if the clamps are closed tightly.
- *Priming phase V1*: The priming phase V1 usually ends as soon as the air detector is in a permanent alarm-free state and an increased volume of 100 mL is delivered into the empty bag. If the air detector

is not or not permanently alarm-free, a drip chamber error message will be displayed.

- *Priming phase V2/V3*: The centrifuge is accelerated or decelerated for a certain number of cycles to remove residual air in the chamber.
- *Priming phase V4*: The speed of the centrifuge is increased to operating speed. The interface detection is tested, as soon as this speed has been reached.

Skip Priming

The priming program can be skipped if an inserted set is already primed and the device was turned off or a program was aborted.

9.   Start Prime by pressing Prime key.

9.1.   The Alarm test screen will be displayed (**Fig. 8**).

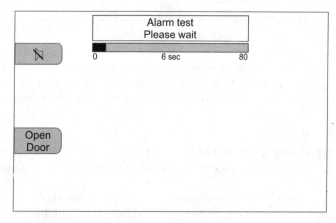

FIG. 8: Screen display during alarm test.

A bar graph indicates that the test is in progress. Start and end of the test are indicated by an audible alarm. The alarm test is performed automatically.

Note: Missed alarm messages are displayed as errors if the alarm system does not recognize them correctly. If there are multiple test errors, the first error is displayed. After correcting test errors, the alarm test should be repeated. The alarm test is repeated by pressing the Prime key again. After completion of the alarm test, priming is started automatically.

The following screen is displayed during priming (**Fig. 9**).

9.2.   Prime takes approximately 6 minutes to complete and on completion of priming, the following screen is displayed as shown in **Figure 10**.

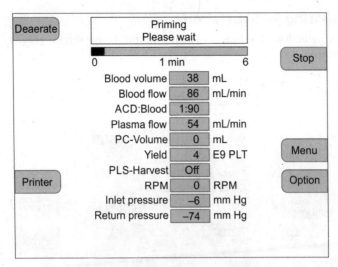

FIG. 9: Screen display during priming.

(ACD: acid-citrate-dextrose; PC: platelet concentrate; PLS: plasma; PLT: platelet)

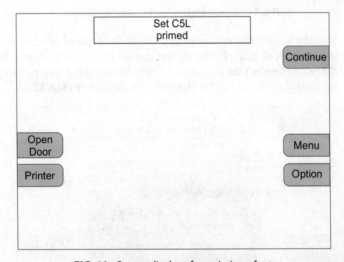

FIG. 10: Screen display after priming of set.

9.3. After the completion of automatic prime, a second priming can be performed by pressing the Prime key again. The option second priming is only available in the set primed screen.

9.4. When priming is completed, Prime Saline Diversion can be selected by using Up/Down keys to Donor or Waste Bag.

Preparing for Separation

After selection of saline diversion, the following screen **(Fig. 11)** is displayed.

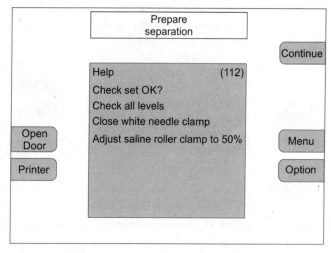

FIG. 11: Screen display for "Prepare separation."

10. Visually inspect the apheresis set. Check the level of the connected solutions in all drip chambers and correct if necessary. Ensure that the white needle clamp is closed. Close the two blue return clamps. Set the roller clamp to 50%. Press the Continue key **(Fig. 12)**.

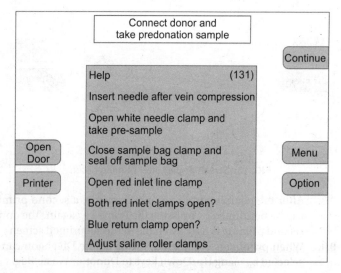

FIG. 12: Screen display for various checks.

Connecting the Donor and Collecting a Predonation Sample

11. Connect the donor after vein compression. Open the white needle clamp and collect at least 20 mL predonation blood sample. Close the clamp on the presampling bag and seal off the presampling bag. Open the red clamp on the inlet line and make sure that the two red clamps are open. Connect the return needle to the blue Luer lock connector. Deaerate and place the return needle. Open the blue return clamp. After pressing the "Continue" key, the display Donor values screen will appear **(Fig. 13)**.

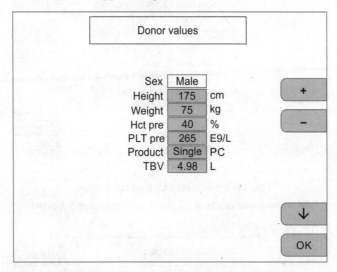

FIG. 13: Screen display for adding donor values.

(Hct: hematocrit; PC: platelet concentrate; PLT: platelet; TBV: total blood volume)

Menus

12. Donor values (height, weight, etc.) must be entered using the Up, Down, +, and – keys. After entering the data, press the "OK" key. The software will calculate the maximum blood flow possible based on the ACD rate and the donor value set in the Config. sys. The calculated values are displayed on the Procedure Menu screen **(Fig. 14)**.

Procedure Menu

13. Selected values can be changed by using the Up and Down keys to select the value to change. Use the + and – buttons to change the selected value. All values affected by this change will automatically

be adjusted. For example, changing the yield automatically recalculates the amount of blood processed.

14. Press OK; all the values are saved and the following screen will appear **(Fig. 15)**.

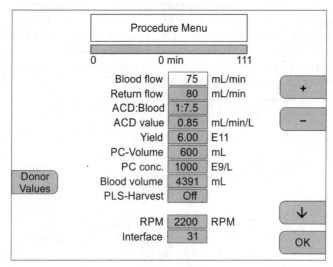

FIG. 14: Menu screen for calculated values.

(ACD: acid-citrate-dextrose; PC: platelet concentrate; PLS: plasma)

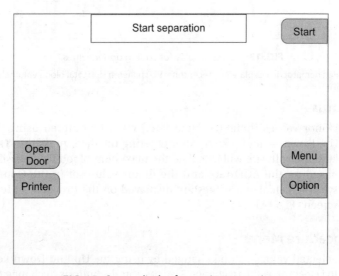

FIG. 15: Screen display for starting separation.

Separation

Before starting the program, all separation parameter changes should be made, but they can also be made at a later stage.

15. *Press Start*: Press the Start key. The device automatically performs a system pressure test to check the pressure measuring lines for tight connection and to verify correct position of all clamps at the return drip chamber.

Automatic Operation

The following display screen appears during the separation program (**Fig. 16**).

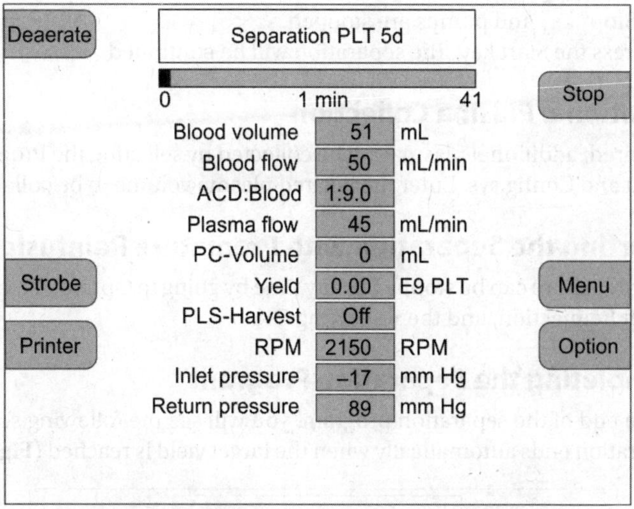

Deaerate		Separation PLT 5d	
	0	1 min	41	Stop
	Blood volume	51	mL
	Blood flow	50	mL/min
	ACD:Blood	1:9.0	
	Plasma flow	45	mL/min
	PC-Volume	0	mL
Strobe	Yield	0.00	E9 PLT	Menu
	PLS-Harvest	Off	
Printer	RPM	2150	RPM	Option
	Inlet pressure	−17	mm Hg
	Return pressure	89	mm Hg

FIG. 16: Screen display during platelet separation.

(ACD: acid-citrate-dextrose; PC: platelet concentrate; PLS: plasma; PLT: platelet)

The process runs completely automatically until the target volume is processed. The plasma pump is automatically controlled to maintain the resulting interface. In the C5 separation chamber, the blood is separated into red blood cells, buffy coat, and platelet-rich plasma.

The platelet-rich plasma is separated off behind a dam which holds back the red blood cells, and the PC is transported to the collection bag. At the end of the chamber channel, the platelet-poor plasma is returned to the donor by a plasma pump.

Throughout the entire separation procedure, the device is monitored by a complex alarm system. This ensures donor safety. In the event of an alarm or a malfunction, the device will automatically be switched to stop mode. The help menu provides troubleshooting and work-arounds to correct the problems.

Decomposition Phase

Before reaching the target volume of 20 mL on the PC, a beep sounds and the centrifugation speed is reduced by 100 rpm. The plasma and the cell flow are automatically controlled to decompose the interface until the end of the separation.

Pausing and Continuing the Separation Program

1. Press the Stop key. Separation stops. If the COM.TEC stops for >30 seconds, the centrifuge speed will drop to 1,000 rpm. Let the instrument stop for an additional 3 minutes and then reduce centrifugation speed to 600 rpm.
2. Clamp 1 is closed and clamps 2 and 3 are opened on pressing the "Stop" key and pumps are stopped.
3. Press the Start key. The separation will be continued.

Additional Plasma Collection

If desired, additional plasma can be collected by selecting the Programs menu and Config.sys. Enter the desired plasma volume to be collected.

Aborting the Separation with Premature Reinfusion

This procedure can be stopped at any time by going to Options, selecting Direct Reinjection, and then selecting OK.

Completing the Separation Program

At the end of the separation program, you will see the following screen. Separation ends automatically when the target yield is reached **(Fig. 17)**.

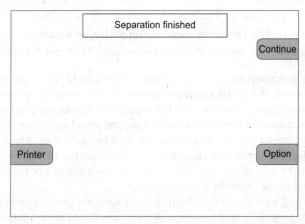

FIG. 17: Screen display after completion of platelet separation.

Reinfusion

At this stage, any remaining blood components in the line are returned to the donor. Disconnect the inlet line and add saline and ACD (120 mL of saline at a collection flow of 35 mL/min) to displace the blood from the line set and to return the blood to the donor via the return line. At the same time, the cell pump simultaneously transports the platelets still present in the separation chamber to the PC bag. Press Continue to display Reinfusion start menu **(Fig. 18)**.

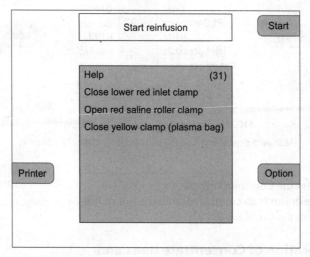

FIG. 18: Screen display guiding for the start of reinfusion.

Follow the instructions displayed on the screen:
1. The lower red inlet clamp is closed.
2. Open the red saline roller clamp completely.
3. The yellow clamp on the plasma collection bag is closed.
4. The donor is disconnected from the inlet line.
5. Press the Start key.
   Press the Start key. During reinfusion, the following screen **(Fig. 19)** will be displayed. If desired, you can end the reinfusion early by selecting Options and End Reinfusion and then selecting the OK key.

Terminating the Reinfusion
1. Display at the end of reinfusion.
2. Press the "Start" key to continue with another 30 mL reinfusion.
3. Press the "Stop" key to end the reinfusion.
4. The return line stopping clamp is closed.
5. The yellow clamp on plasma bag is closed.

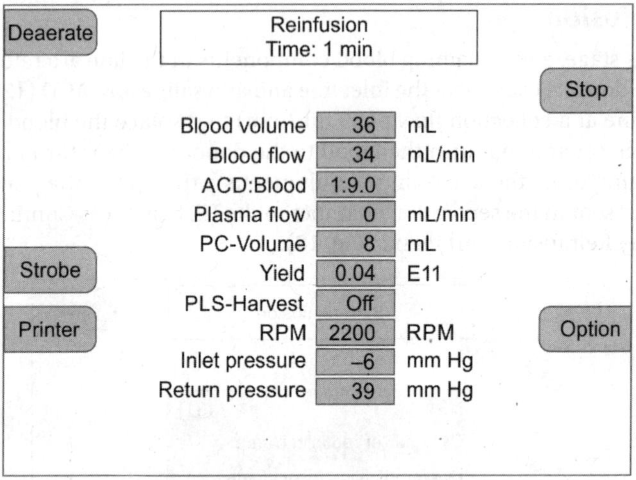

FIG. 19: Screen display during reinfusion.

(ACD: acid-citrate-dextrose; PC: platelet concentrate; PLS: plasma)

6. Press the Continue key.
7. The donor is disconnected from the return line.
8. Press the Continue key.

Deaeration of Concentrate Bags and Collection of Samples

The deaerating option is only available if the option of PC deaeration or PC deaerate (Volume) in the configuration is not deactivated.

Display (Fig. 20)

Use forceps to clamp both the red blood cell line leading to the drip chamber and the whole bloodline below the air separator:
1. The cell pump line segment is removed from the pump.
2. The concentrate bag by holding its connector up is removed.
3. Press the Start key.

Display (Fig. 21)

1. Deaerate the concentrate bag.
2. Once the concentrate bag is fully deaerated, press Stop.
3. If the concentrate bag has not been completely deaerated, press the Start key to remove additional 5 mL of air. Once deaeration is completed, press the Stop key.

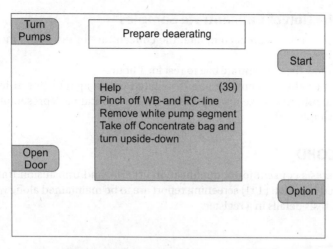

FIG. 20: Screen display for deaerating bags.

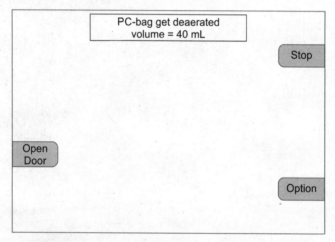

FIG. 21: Screen display on completion of deaeration of bags.

Removing Platelet Concentrate and Set

1. The set is removed after sealing off concentrate bag.
2. Press the Continue key.
3. Once the report is printed, the device is started for another separation by pressing the "Reset" key.
4. Press the OK key.
5. The device switches off.

Collection of Concentrate Samples

1. After reinfusion is complete, the concentrate in the bag is mixed thoroughly.
2. Allow the concentrate bag to rest for 1 hour.
3. Then the concentrate bag is agitated on an agitator for at least 30 minutes. Take a sample (make sure to obtain a representative sample).

RECORD

Apheresis consent form, qualification criteria, and transfusion transmitted infection (TTI) screening report are to be maintained along with apheresis details in a register.

Plateletpheresis using a Blood Cell Separator (Single Needle)

SCOPE AND APPLICATION

This standard operating procedure (SOP) describes a single needle (SN) PLT-5d-SN program for plateletpheresis using the COM.TEC Blood Cell Separator Version 4.02xx. This SOP can be modified suitably by the blood centers using other cell separators according to manufacturer's specifications. This program separates platelets in a continuous mode using the SN method. The S5L set is a closed system that can store platelets for up to 5 days. For this reason, sterile filters for the saline and acid-citrate-dextrose (ACD) lines as well as inlet needles are preconnected in this set.

This SOP provides instructions for installation of apheresis set S5L, priming, separation, reinfusion, and removal of the apheresis set.

RESPONSIBILITY

The medical officer is responsible for determining if the donor is suitable for plateletpheresis. He/she should confirm that the criteria are fulfilled after evaluation of Blood Donor questionnaire and health check up form (Annexure 2.2) including the results of predonation screening tests.

MATERIALS REQUIRED

- COM.TEC blood cell separator version 4.02xx
- SN closed system COM.TEC kit (S5L)
- Venepuncture supplies, i.e., alcohol swab, chlorhexidine solution, sterile cotton swab, etc.
- Ethylenediaminetetraacetic acid (EDTA) (lavender top) vacutainer for product samples

- Tube sealer
- Chewable calcium tablets
- Emergency medicine tray

PROCEDURE

Selection of the Platelet Program

1. Connect the COM.TEC blood cell separator to power supply.
2. Press the I (power on) key in the front panel **(Fig. 1)**.

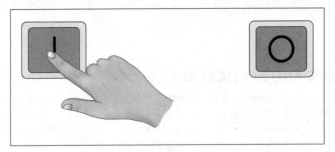

FIG. 1: Pressing power on.

3. Screen will display, showing software version **(Fig. 2)**.

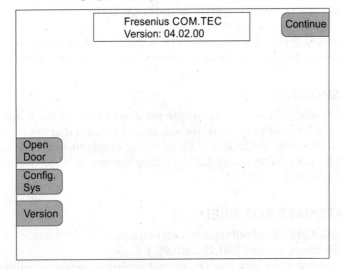

FIG. 2: Software version display.

4. Press Continue. The following screen **(Fig. 3)** will display.

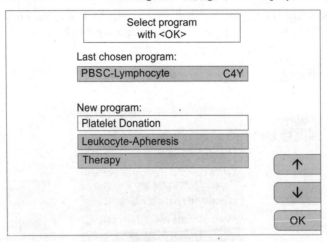

FIG. 3: Screen for selection of program.

(PBSC: peripheral blood stem cell)

5. Use the Up ↑ and Down ↓ keys to select a program group "Platelet Donation" **(Fig. 4)**. Press the OK key.

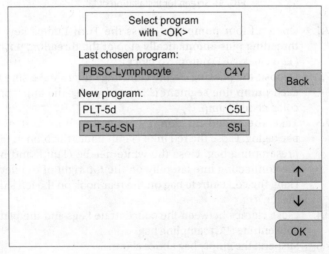

FIG. 4: Screen for selection of program.

(PBSC: peripheral blood stem cell)

6. Use the Up ↑ and Down ↓ keys to select the PLT-5d-SN program. Press the OK key.

Installation of Apheresis Set (S5L)

7. Message "Install set C5L" will display (**Fig. 5**). Follow the on-screen help instructions for a total of five screen pages as follows:

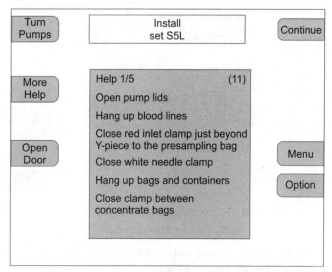

FIG. 5: Screen for installation of kit.

7.1. Open all four pump lids. Press the Turn Pumps key. The threading pins automatically stop at the threading position (12 o'clock/ACD pump: 5 o'clock).

7.2. Deposit the packing on the centrifuge door. Make sure that each pump line segment is located under the appropriate color-coded pump.

7.3. Take the rolled-up donor connecting lines out of the packaging. Close the red inlet clamp under the branch to the presampling bag, close the white needle clamp, and hang the connecting line laterally on the top right of the device. Hang the concentrate bag on the rear hook on the left side of the device.

7.4. Close clamps between the concentrate bags and the platelet concentrate (PC) sampling bag.

7.5. Suspend the empty bag above clamp 5.

7.6. Suspend the plasma bag above clamp 4.

7.7. Suspend the SN bag at the left side of the plasma bag.

7.8. Install all pump line segments so that the colors of pump adapter and the pump coding match. Make sure to push the pump adapter fully to the rear.

7.9. Press the Turn Pumps key. The pump lines will automatically be threaded into place.

7.10. Install the plasma line section leading to the bag behind the Y-piece in the upper part of clamp 4.

7.11. Install the section leading to the air detector drip chamber in the lower part of clamp 4.

7.12. Plasma line section, marked by the yellow tabs, is installed into the hemoglobin/hematocrit (Hb/Hct) detector.

7.13. Line leading to the empty bag is installed in clamp 5.

7.14. Return line is installed in clamp 1.

7.15. Inlet line of the cell pump is inserted into the spillover detector.

7.16. ACD drip chamber, which is identified by a green clamp, is inserted into the ACD detector and pull the drip chamber completely down.

7.17. Pump adapter for the ACD pump is installed. Before installing the adapter, one of the three set screws on the ACD pump must be in the 6 o'clock position if it is not already in the 6 o'clock position.

7.18. Press the Turn Pumps key. The pump lines are automatically threaded into place.

7.19. Install the saline line in clamp 2 (the S5L set is provided with one saline line only).

7.20. Install the SN collecting/return line in clamp 3 between the blue marks.

7.21. Install the line segment between the red-coded Y-piece and the encoded Y-piece on the left in clamp 6.

7.22. Install the other line segment over the red-coded Y-piece on the right side of clamp 6.

7.23. Screw in the filter onto the blue marked pressure gauge line for the return pressure.

7.24. Screw the red-marked inlet pressure gauge into the red-marked inlet pressure measurement connection.

7.25. Hold the separation chamber by the top centrifuge adapter so that the tubes hang down freely on the sides of the instrument without kinking. Open the hinged door of the chamber holder. Slide the circular adapter of the separation chamber into the groove of the central funnel. Close the hinged door till it clicks. You should not be able to see the locking pin on the flat side of the bolt holder. Remove the empty package from the centrifuge door. Press the "Open Door" key. Slide open the centrifuge door. If "Open Door" is not displayed, the door cannot be opened.

7.26. Turn the centrifuge rotor until one of the two line guides is on the right side of the rotor. With the separation chamber installed, push the chamber under the rotor with the lines facing down. Push the chamber holder onto the guide rail until it clicks. Rotate the locking flap down until it clicks into place. Pass the centrifuge tubing through the line guide. Slide the upper centrifuge adapter narrow side first into the upper adapter holder. If you need to rotate the adapter slightly, Do this so that each wire twists around itself.

7.27. Manually rotate the rotor counterclockwise one full turn manually to verify correct installation.

7.28. Close the centrifuge door after the test spin and another visual check. The door is properly locked when the "Open Door" key is displayed. Insert the Air Protect into the holder.

Checking Installation of Apheresis Set and Separation Chamber (Fig. 6)

Visually inspect the following:

- Ensure that red clamp on the inlet line below the branch to the presampling bag, the white needle clamp, the clamp between the concentrate bags, and the clamp on the sampling bag are closed. All other stop clamps in the set must be open.
- Ensure correct installation of air detector drip chamber and the ACD drip chamber in their holders.
- Ensure installation of return line in clamp 1.
- Ensure installation of saline line in clamp 2.
- Ensure installation of plasma line in clamp 4.
- Ensure installation of line leading to the empty bag in clamp 5.
- Ensure installation of inlet line for SN in clamp 6.
- Ensure installation of SN collecting/return line in clamp 3.

Preparation for Priming

8. Press the "Continue" key; following screen **(Fig. 7)** will display. Prior to priming the set, a user guide is available to assist with the connection of the saline and ACD-A solutions. Connect the ACD-A bag to the green connector and hang it from the upper left hook on the front of the device. Break the cone of the ACD-A bag. Deaerate the ACD-A drip chamber by pressing it and set the level to approximately 1 cm so that the fluid level is approximately 1 cm below the optical sensor. Connect the saline bag to the two transparent connectors. Hang the saline bag from the front left hook. Break the cones and set the fluid level in the two drip chambers.

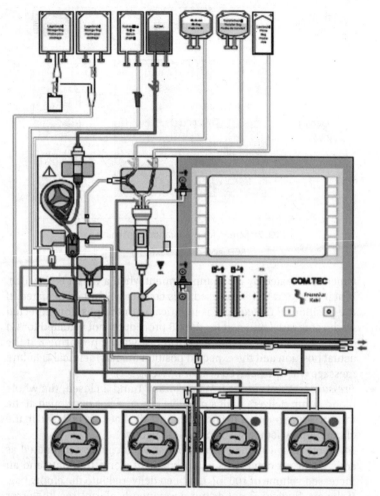

FIG. 6: Checks after apheresis set and separation chamber installation.
(For color version, see Plate 2)

Priming

During priming, saline and ACD-A are pumped into the set to displace the air. The Prime program steps are divided into the following phases:

- *Detection of set and procedure*: The COM.TEC automatically detects which procedure has been selected and which set matches the procedure. The additional ACD pump has a miniature contact

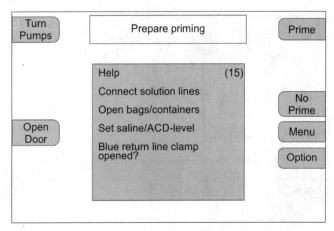

FIG. 7: Screen for preparation of priming.
(ACD: acid-citrate-dextrose)

which is actuated by the pump segment when a C5 set is installed. When a C4 or a PL1 set is used, this contact will not be actuated. If the position of the contact is identical with the position expected by the software (actuated for the C5 procedure, not actuated for C4 and PL1 procedures), the ACD drip test will be performed. If the actual position and the expected position are not identical, a failure message will be displayed (Failure: Wrong set).

- *Pressure test/test clamp 1*: With clamps 1 and 2 closed, the whole blood pump delivers until a negative pressure has developed at the inlet pressure monitor to check whether the lines are installed in the clamps and whether the clamps close tightly.
- *Priming phase V1*: The priming phase V1 is usually terminated as soon as the air detector is in a permanent alarm-free state and an increased volume of 100 mL has been delivered into the empty bag. If the air detector is not or not permanently alarm-free, the error message Drip chamber will be displayed.
- *Priming phase V2/V3*: The centrifuge is accelerated or decelerated for a certain number of cycles to remove residual air in the chamber.
- *Priming phase V4*: The speed of the centrifuge is increased to operating speed. As soon as this speed has been reached, the interface detection is tested.

Skip Priming

If an inserted set is already primed and the device was turned off or a program was aborted, the priming program can be skipped.

9. *Start Prime by pressing Prime key.*

   9.1. The Alarm test screen **(Fig. 8)** will be displayed.

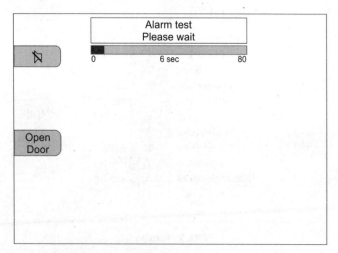

FIG. 8: Alarm test.

A bar graph indicates that the test is in progress. Start and end of the test are indicated by an audible alarm. The alarm test is performed automatically.

Note:

- If an alarm system fails to correctly detect an alarm, the alarm message which failed to occur will be displayed as an error. In case of several test errors, the first error which occurred is displayed. After correcting the test error, the alarm test must be repeated.
- The alarm test can be repeated by pressing the Prime key again.
- After the alarm test, priming is started automatically. The following screen is **(Fig. 9)** displayed while priming.

   9.2. Priming takes about 6 minutes for completion.

   9.3. A second priming can be performed by pressing the Prime key again after automatic prime has completed. The second prime option is only available on the Priming Settings screen **(Fig. 10)**.

   9.4. At the end of Prime, Prime Saline Diversion to Donor or Waste Bag can be selected using the Up/Down buttons.

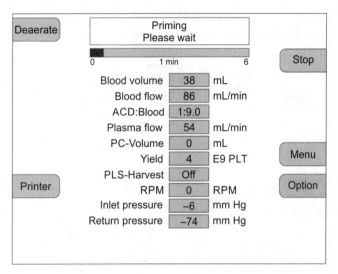

FIG. 9: Priming.

(ACD: acid-citrate-dextrose; PC: platelet concentrate; PLS: plasma; PLT: platelet)

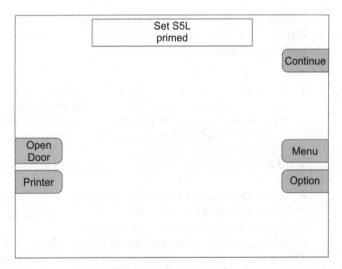

FIG. 10: Set S5L primed.

Preparing for Separation

After selection of saline diversion, the following screen **(Fig. 11)** is displayed.

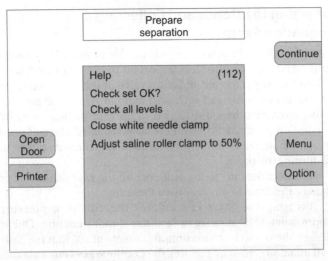

FIG. 11: Preparing separation.

10. Visually inspect the apheresis set. Check the level of the connected solution in all drip chambers and correct if necessary. Make sure that white needle clasp is closed and close if necessary. Close the two blue return clamps. Adjust the roller clamp to 50%. Press the "Continue" key **(Fig. 12)**.

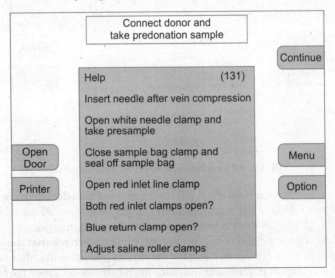

FIG. 12: Connecting donor.

Connecting the Donor and Collecting a Predonation Sample

11. *Applying the cuff*: Place the cuff on the donor's fully extended and relaxed upper arm. It is important to keep air out of the cuff. To do this, open the red deflation valve of the air-pressure pump and by pressing the cuff with your hand to remove all air. The red valve must then be closed again to prevent malfunctions in the separation program. When all the air is removed, the cuff pressure gauge should read 0 mm Hg. Subsequent adjustments can be made by turning the scale.

Connect the cuff to the cuff port on the rear connector panel being careful not to pinch or twist the cord.

Pressing the Start key inflates the cuff to a pressure of approximately 50 mm Hg to facilitate donor puncture. Due to its design, the pump has a maximum pressure of 100 mm Hg. Skip the cuff inflation screen by pressing the Continue key **(Fig. 13)**.

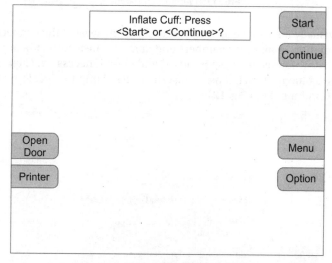

FIG. 13: Inflating blood pressure (BP) and Continue.

Insert the needle after vein compression. Open the white needle clamp and collect a predonation sample of at least 20 mL. Close the clamp on the presampling bag and seal off the presampling bag. Open the red clamp on the inlet line and check that the two red clamps are open. Connect the return needle to the blue Luer lock connector. Deaerate and place the return needle. Open the blue return clamp.

Press the Continue key and the screen for Donor Values appears **(Fig. 14)**.

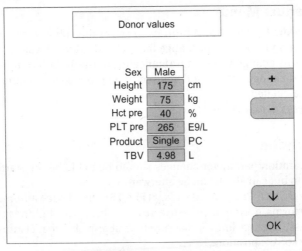

FIG. 14: Entering Donor values.

(Hct: hematocrit; PC: platelet concentrate; PLT: platelet; TBV: total blood volume)

Menus

12. Donor values (height, weight, etc.) must be entered using the Up, Down, +, and - keys. Once the donor values are entered, press the "OK" key. The software will calculate the maximum blood flow possible based on the ACD rate and the Donor Values set in the Config.sys. The calculated values are displayed in the Procedure Menu screen **(Fig. 15)**.

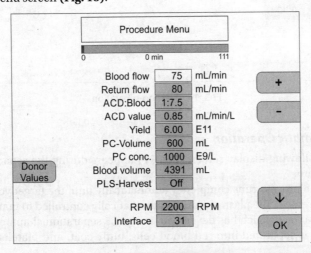

FIG. 15: Procedure screen.

(ACD: acid-citrate-dextrose; PC: platelet concentrate; PLS: plasma)

Procedure Menu

13. Use the Up and Down buttons to select the value to change. Use the + and – buttons to change the selected value. All values affected by this change will be automatically adjusted. For example, if the yield changes, the blood volume to be processed is automatically recalculated.
14. Press OK to save All Values.

Separation

All separation parameter changes should be made before starting the program but can also be made afterward:

15. *Press Start:* Press the Start key **(Fig. 16)**. The device automatically performs a system pressure test to check the tightness of the pressure gauge lines. Make sure that all drip chamber clamps are in the correct position.

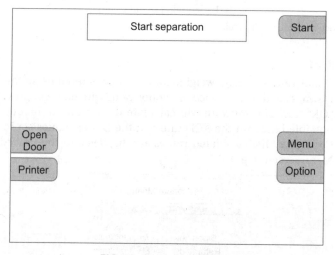

FIG. 16: Starting separation.

Automatic Operation

The following display screen **(Fig. 17)** appears during the separation program.

The process runs completely automatically until the target volume is processed. The plasma pump is automatically controlled to maintain the interface which has developed. In the C5 separation chamber, the blood is separated into red blood cells, buffy coat, and platelet-rich plasma.

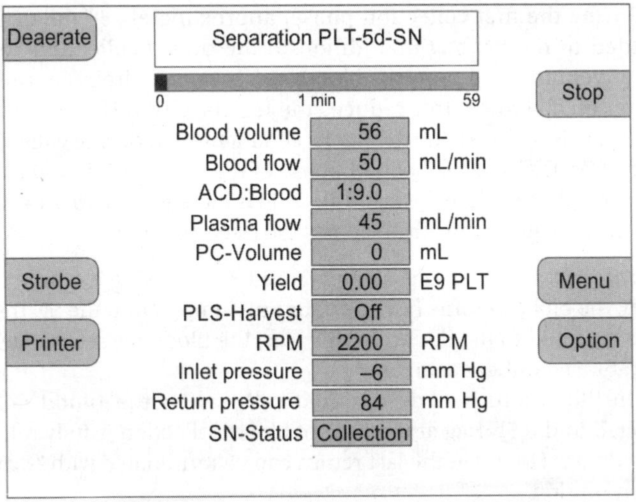

Deaerate	Separation PLT-5d-SN		
	0 1 min 59		Stop
	Blood volume	56	mL
	Blood flow	50	mL/min
	ACD:Blood	1:9.0	
	Plasma flow	45	mL/min
	PC-Volume	0	mL
Strobe	Yield	0.00	E9 PLT	Menu
	PLS-Harvest	Off	
Printer	RPM	2200	RPM	Option
	Inlet pressure	–6	mm Hg
	Return pressure	84	mm Hg
	SN-Status	Collection	

FIG. 17: Separation program.

(ACD: acid-citrate-dextrose; PC: platelet concentrate; PLS: plasma; PLT: platelet)

The platelet-rich plasma is separated off behind a dam which holds back the red blood cells, and the PC at the cell port is delivered into the collection bag. At the end of the chamber channel, the platelet-poor plasma is returned to the donor by the plasma pump.

During the entire separation procedure, the device is monitored by a complex alarm system. This ensures donor safety. In the event of an alarm or a malfunction, the device will automatically be switched into the stop mode. The help menu assists with troubleshooting and remedies to correct the problems.

Cycle Control

Collection cycle: The processed blood is sent to the SN bag during the collection phase.

At the beginning of the collection phase, inflate the cuff to a pressure of approximately 50 mm Hg. This will slightly compress the donor vein to avoid potential flow problems. Blood flow is reduced by 20% during cuff inflation.

The total extracorporeal volume will be 230 mL (set) + 150 mL (SN bag) + 250 mL (PC bag) = 630 mL (including ACD) at the end of the final collection phase of the standard separation procedure.

This extracorporeal volume, if not tolerated by the donor, can be changed by the attending physician at his discretion by decreasing the SN cycle volume Config.sys.

During the first collection phase, approximately 80 mL of buffer is added to the SN bag in addition to the preset collection volume (buffer volume) and prevents blood with a low Hct from entering the separation chamber. This reduces the interface (the Hct at the top of the SN bag is reduced due to platelet sedimentation during collection).

If COM.TEC's last collection phase of the COM.TEC is <50 mL, the collection phase before the last collection is increased up to a maximum of 50 mL and automatically becomes the last collection.

Return cycle: By reversing clamps 3 and 6 and using a whole blood pump, the blood volume (= cycle volume) pumped into the SN transfer bag is returned to the donor. In this way, the blood passes through the separation chamber again.

The final return ends automatically when the blood volume collected in the SN bag at the time of blood collection is fully returned to the donor. However, the last return can be terminated with "Exit Last Return" option.

Return blood flow: Return blood flow can be adjusted in the Procedure menu. Separation time can be shortened by increasing the return blood flow. Then increase the ACD infusion rate at this phase. The choice of appropriate return blood flow is left to the discretion of the treating physician. The blood return blood flow is combined with the collection flow. The maximum difference that can be set is 10 mL/min. By default, the return blood flow is 5 mL/min higher than the collection flow. Depending on other settings, the program will only allow a certain maximum flow rate. When the maximum permissible alarm limit is reached, the blood flow is reduced by 2 mL/min to prevent that the keys for changing the parameters are suppressed.

Change Options

Use the Up ↑ and the Down ↓ keys to select the parameter to change. Use the + and the – keys to change the selected parameter. Press OK key to confirm the change.

Options

- *Print parameters*: Parameter list is printed.
- *Direct reinfusion*: This key controls saline diversion at the start of the separation.
- *Cuff SN*: Controls automatic cuffing.
- *Chime SN*: This key controls the audible signal whenever the collection cycle is changed to return and vice versa.
- *Exit program*: Exit the program early if you are using the default program. For example, with a donation time of approximately

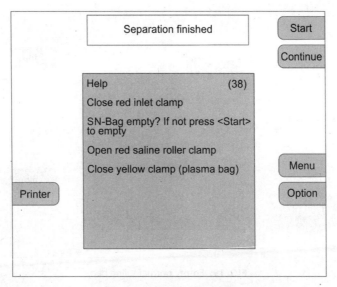

FIG. 18: Separation finished.

80 minutes, the donor's ACD load is approximately 375 mL. This corresponds to an average ACD rate of 4.7 mL/min which is the maximum since no fluid is infused to the donor during the collection phase.

Completing Separation Program

When the target yield has been achieved, the separation is terminated automatically **(Fig. 18)**.

Empty SN Bag

If the SN bag is not empty, press the "Start" key to continue SN return with an additional 20 mL each time. By pressing the Stop key, emptying of the SN bag can be stopped at any time. If the SN bag is not empty, SN return can be continued with an additional 20 mL each time the "Start" key is pressed. Emptying of the SN bag can be stopped at any time by pressing the "Stop" key **(Fig. 19)**.

Reinfusion

Separation Finished appears on the display when the target volume has been processed.

After pressing Next, the Post Reinfusion start menu **(Fig. 20)** is displayed as follows.

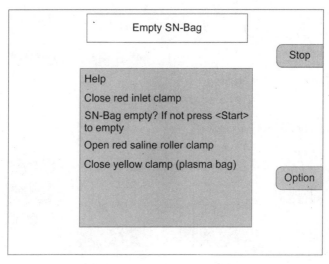

FIG. 19: Empty normal saline bag.

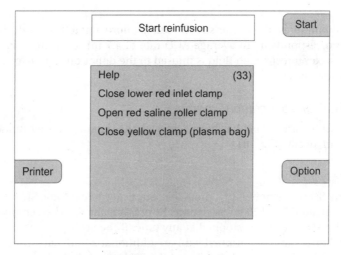

FIG. 20: Starting reinfusion.

Follow the on-screen instructions as follows:
- Close the lower red inlet clamp.
- Open the roller clamp on the saline line.
- Press the Start key.
- If desired, the reinfusion can be terminated early by selecting Option and End Reinfusion, followed by the OK key.

End of Reinfusion

- Close the return line closing clamp.
- Close the yellow stop clamp on plasma bag.
- Press the "Continue" key.
- Disconnect the donor.
- Press the "Continue" key.

Deaerate Concentrate Bags and Collection of Samples

The "Prepare Deaerate" option is only available if the option of PC deaeration or PC deaerate (Volume) in the configuration is not deactivated.

Display (Fig. 21)

Clamp both the red blood cell line leading to the drip chamber and the whole bloodline below the air separator with forceps. Remove the cell pump line segment from the pump. Lift the connector up and remove the concentrate bag. Press the "Start" key. The concentrate bag is being deaerated **(Fig. 22)**. When the concentrate bag is completely deaerated, press the "Stop" key. If the concentrate bag is not yet completely deaerated, press the "Start" key to remove another 5 mL of air. Press the "Stop" key when the deaeration is completed.

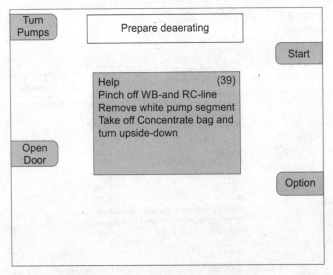

FIG. 21: Screen display for deaerating bags

Removing Platelet Concentrate and Set

- Remove the concentrate bag after sealing and set.
- Press the "Continue" key.
- Once the report is printed, the device is started for another separation by pressing the "Reset" key **(Fig. 23)**.

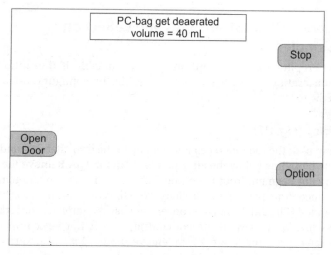

FIG. 22: Screen display on completion of deaeration of bags

Turn Pumps	Print out OK? Switch off	
	Separation result: COM.TEC Procedure PLT-5d-SN	Reset
	Separation time	– 0 min
	Blood volume processed	– 17 mL
	ACD (separation)	– 3 mL
	Blood volume-ACD (80 mL)	– 14 mL
Open Door	ACD to donor	– 2 mL
	PLT pre	– 265 E9/L
	PLT post (calculated)	– 264 E9/L
	PLT yield (prediction)	– 0.01 E11
	PC volume	– 0 mL
	ACD in PC	– 0 mL
	Plasma volume collected	– 0 mL
	ACD in plasma collected	– 0 mL
	Remaining ACD in set	– 3 mL

FIG. 23: Screening for switch off the cell separator.
(ACD: acid-citrate-dextrose; PC: platelet concentrate; PLT: platelet)

- Report will be printed as above on the Printer.
- Turn the device off by pressing "OK" key.
- Collection of concentrate samples.
- On completion of reinfusion, mix thoroughly the concentrate in the concentrate bag after completion of reinfusion.
- Allow the concentrate bag to rest for 1 hour.
- The bags are agitated on a suitable agitator for a minimum of 30 minutes.
- Obtain a representative sample after the lines are sufficiently rinsed with PC.

RECORD

Apheresis consent form, qualification criteria, and transfusion transmitted infection (TTI) screening report are to be maintained along with apheresis details in a register.

CHAPTER 16

Plateletpheresis using Blood Cell Separator (Trima Accel)

SCOPE AND APPLICATION

This standard operating procedure (SOP) describes the procedure specifically for plateletpheresis using the Trima Accel Cell Separator. Blood centers using other blood cell separators should modify SOP according to manufacturer's guidelines as such procedures are device-specific.

RESPONSIBILITY

The medical officer is responsible for determining donor suitability for plateletpheresis. He/she must confirm that the criteria are met after evaluating the blood donor questionnaire and health checkup form (apheresis), medical history, and physical examination, including the results of predonation screening tests.

MATERIALS REQUIRED

- Trima Accel Automated Blood Cell Separator/Collection System
- Trima Accel Automated Blood Collection System Tubing Set
- Anticoagulant Citrate Dextrose Solution, Solution A, Acid-citrate-dextrose (ACD-A), 500 mL
- Preprocedure sample collection supplies
- Venipuncture supplies, i.e., alcohol swab, chlorhexidine solution, sterile cotton swab
- Tube sealer
- Chewable calcium tablets
- Emergency medicine tray
- Blood donor questionnaire and health checkup form (apheresis) (Annexure 2.2)
- UID stickers
- Cell separator log book

PROCEDURE

Entering Donor Information

1. Turn the power "on."
2. The Trima Accel system completes a series of self-diagnostic tests and "The Donor information/Load system screen" displays **(Fig. 1)**.
3. Touch "donor info" on the main screen.
4. Touch the button corresponding to the donor's gender.
5. Touch "donor height" and enter the height using the number keypad. Touch "enter."
6. Touch "donor weight" and enter the weight using the number keypad. Touch "enter."
7. Verify the accuracy of the total blood volume calculation. Touch "confirm info."
8. Entering the donor's blood type is optional.
   If: Entering the donor's blood type,
   Then: Touch "blood type," enter the type on the letter keypad, and touch "enter."
   If: Not entering the donor's blood type, continue to step 8.
9. Touch "hematocrit." Enter the donor's hematocrit as a whole number using the number keypad. Touch "enter."
10. Touch "platelet precount" and enter the donor's platelet precount using the number keypad. Touch "enter."
11. Verify that the information is correct and then touch "confirm info."

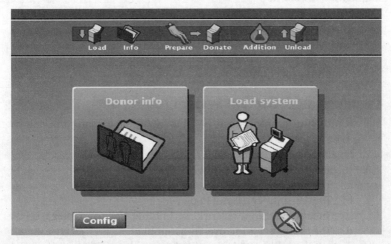

FIG. 1: Donor information/Load system screen.

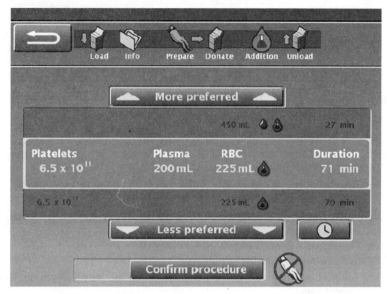

FIG. 2: Procedure selection screen.

(RBC: red blood cell)

Selecting Procedure

After confirming the donor information, the procedure selection screen displays **(Fig. 2)**.

This screen displays either a single optimal procedure or a list of desirable procedures, with the highest-priority procedure at the top highlighted in yellow.

1. If: Choosing the optimal procedure highlighted in yellow,
   Then: Touch "confirm procedure."
   If: Overriding the optimal procedure,
   Then: Select an alternative procedure in the list, and touch "confirm procedure."

Loading the Collection System Tubing Set

1. Choose the appropriate disposable tubing set for the components to be collected.
2. Open the tubing set package.
3. Inspect the tubing set. Do not use if:
   a. The needle cap is off,
   b. The AC spike cap is not in place,
   c. The tubing shows severe kinks or other signs of damage, or
   d. The tubing set is incorrectly assembled.
   Note: If the tubing set inspection fails, replace with a new set and repeat steps 2–3.

4. Touch "load system."
5. The Select REF screen displays.
6. Touch the REF button. Select the correct REF number from the list of numbers configured by your system administrator and then touch "enter." The Trima Accel system prompts you to verify that the REF number you selected matches the tubing set label.
7. Touch the "continue" button, and the status line displays a message specifying the REF number entered.
8. Open the tubing set package.
9. Remove the vent bag and the product bags and hang them on the intravenous (IV) pole. Position the bag tubing behind the display screen.
10. Remove the donor line from the package and remove the white paper tapes from the tubing.
11. Place the donor line in the indent on the left side of the machine.
12. Remove the cassette and position the bottom of the cassette on the bottom rail of the cassette holder, positioning the pump headers over the pumps.
13. Press the upper corners of the cassette to snap it into the cassette clamp.
14. Remove the channel from the package.
15. Open the centrifuge door by squeezing the handle to release the door lock and gently lower the door, and the centrifuge is displayed as per **Figure 3**.
16. Turn the metal arm of the centrifuge to the left, so that the loading port is open to the front.

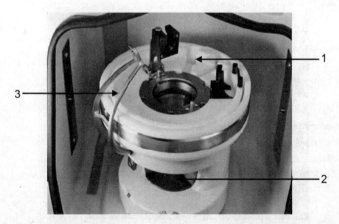

FIG. 3: Centrifuge of Trima blood cell separator showing filler (1), loading port (2), and centrifuge arm (3).

17. Raise the filler latch **(Fig. 4)** by pushing the pin toward the center of the centrifuge; while simultaneously pulling up on the filler latch.

18. Fold the channel in half and tuck the leukocyte reduction system (LRS) chamber (if applicable) to the folded channel aligning the chamber's length with the channel **(Fig. 5)**.

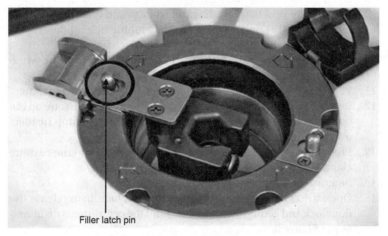

Filler latch pin

FIG. 4: Filler latch pin.

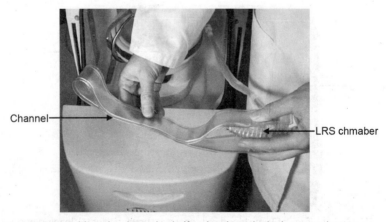

Channel

LRS chmaber

FIG. 5: Folding the channel in half and tucking the leukocyte reduction system (LRS) chamber.

19. Without stretching any of the tubes,
    a. Carefully feed the channel into the loading port and
    b. Gently pull the channel up through the opening at the top of the filler **(Fig. 6)**.
20. Lower the filler latch and press it to lock it into place.
21. Starting with the collection chamber on the left side, press the channel into the filler, loading the inlet port last **(Fig. 7)**.

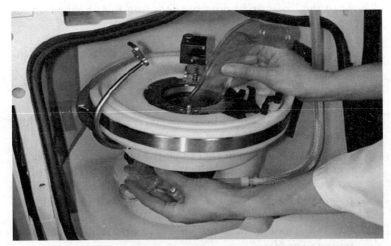

FIG. 6: Feeding the channel into the loading port and pushing it up through the opening.

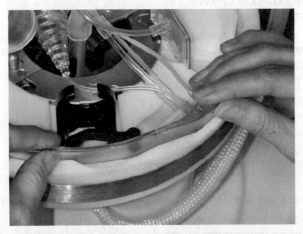

FIG. 7: Pressing the channel into the filler groove.

22. Load the LRS chamber into the bracket.
23. Ensure that the channel is properly seated and flush with the top edge of the filler and the LRS chamber is properly loaded into the bracket.
24. Position the centrifuge collar above the holder and push the collar into the holder.

    Note: You will hear a click when the collar locks into place in its holder.

25. Load the lower and upper bearings into their holders on the centrifuge arm.
    a. Load the upper collar.
        i. Insert the tubes into the holder with the collar below the holder.
        ii. Pull the tubing upward until the collar is fully seated in the holder.

    Note: The upper collar will be locked into place when the centrifuge door closes.

26. Rotate the centrifuge to check that the tubing and bearings are secure and not twisted. Verify that the locking pin is in its fully extended, locked position. Verify channel and LRS chamber are properly loaded.
27. Close the centrifuge chamber door.
28. Ensure that the lines to the product bags are not caught underneath the pump headers.
29. Touch "continue."

    Note: The cassette and pump headers will be lowered into place. The Trima Accel system automatically removes the air from the product bags.

30. Close the slide clamp on one platelet bag (if applicable).
31. At the prompt, close the white pinch clamps on the donor line and the sample bag line.
32. Touch "continue."

    Note: The Trima Accel system performs a tubing set test.

33. When the tubing set test is complete, insert the AC tubing into the AC sensor.
34. Touch "continue."
35. Verify that fluid is flowing into the AC drip chamber.

Connecting the Donor and Collecting the Components

1. Touch "begin donor prep."
2. Follow the prompts on the display and complete the prompted actions.

3. Perform the venipuncture.
4. Open the white pinch clamps
   a. On the donor line and
   b. On the tubing leading to the blood sample bag
5. Allow the blood sample bag to fill to the desired volume.
6. Close the white pinch clamp on the sample bag tubing.
7. Touch "start draw."
8. Permanently and hermetically seal the blood sample bag as close to the "Y" manifold as possible.
9. Draw samples as soon as possible from the sample bag using evacuated blood collection tubes.
10. After all samples are taken, discard the sample bag in an appropriate biohazard disposal container.
11. If adjustments are required during the procedure, refer to the *Trima Accel Automated Blood Collection System Operator's Manual* for instructions.
12. If an alert is observed during the procedure,
    a. Refer to the display for information on resolving the alert condition
    b. Refer to the *Trima Accel Automated Blood Collection System*
    c. *Operator's Manual* for additional instructions.

Performing the Postcollection Steps

1. When rinse back is complete, touch "continue."
2. Follow the system prompt, seal the collect lines just above the cassette, and remove the product(s) and AC bags.

   Note: Do not seal the vent bag.

3. Assure that the product bags are labeled with the donor identification number (e.g., unique blood unit number).
4. Close the white pinch clamp on the donor line.
5. Disconnect the donor and touch "continue."
6. Confirm that the donor is disconnected and touch "confirm disconnect."

Removing the Collection System Tubing Set and Blood Products

1. At the "remove" prompt, open the centrifuge door and remove the channel from the filler.
2. Remove the AC line from the AC sensor.
3. Remove any remaining bags.
4. Remove the cassette from the cassette holder by pressing the latch located in the upper right corner of the cassette.

Important: Remove the top edge of the cassette and then the bottom.

5. Discard the disposable tubing set in an appropriate biohazard container.
6. Touch "continue."
7. Touch "continue" to display the end-of-run summary screens.
8. Record procedure results.
9. Label the bags based on the display message and your center's SOPs.
10. Touch "next procedure."

RECORD

Apheresis consent form, qualification criteria, and transfusion transmitted infection (TTI) screening report are to be maintained along with apheresis detail in a register.

Plasmapheresis using an Automated Blood Cell Separator

SCOPE AND APPLICATION

This standard operating procedure (SOP) describes method for plasmapheresis using a blood cell separator (Trima Accel automated). It uses continuous-flow technology to separate various components from whole blood.

This SOP contains instructions for installation of apheresis kit, priming, separation, and removal of the apheresis kit. SOP can be modified for other types of blood cell separators being used by the blood center as per manufacturer's guidelines.

RESPONSIBILITY

The medical officer is responsible for determining suitability of donor for plasmapheresis. He/she should confirm that the selection criteria are fulfilled after evaluation of blood donor questionnaire and health checkup form, and medical examination, including the results of predonation screening tests.

MATERIALS REQUIRED

- Blood cell separator (Trima Accel automated or any other make)
- Kit for collection of plasma (specific to the blood cell separator)
- Acid-citrate-dextrose (ACD)-A solution, 500 mL
- Tube sealer
- Chewable calcium tablets
- Emergency medicine tray
- Venipuncture supplies, i.e., alcohol swab, chlorhexidine solution, sterile cotton swab
- Blood donor questionnaire and health checkup form (apheresis) (Annexure 2.2)
- UID stickers
- Trima Accel Automated Blood Collection System Operator's Manual, Version 6.1 or above

PROCEDURE

Loading the Trima Accel Collection System Tubing Set

1. Turn system "on."
2. Choose the appropriate disposable tubing set for collecting plasma.
3. Open the tubing set package.
4. Inspect the tubing set. Do not use if:
   a. The needle cap is off,
   b. The AC spike cap is not in place,
   c. The tubing shows severe kinks or other signs of damage, or
   d. The tubing set is incorrectly assembled.

   Note: If the tubing set inspection fails, replace with a new set and repeat steps 2–3.
5. Touch "load system."
6. Remove the vent, plasma, and platelet bags and hang the bags on the intravenous (IV) pole.

   Note: Number of bags in the set is dependent on the type of tubing set selected.
7. Remove the donor line from the package and the white paper tapes from the tubing.
8. Place the donor line in the indent on the left side of the machine.
9. Remove the cassette and position the bottom of the cassette on the bottom rail of the cassette holder.
10. Press the upper corners of the cassette to snap it into the cassette clamp.
11. Remove the channel from the package.
12. Open the centrifuge door.
13. Turn the centrifuge arm of the centrifuge to the left so that the loading port is facing to the front of the machine.
14. Raise the filler latch.
15. Fold the channel in half and tuck the LRS® chamber (if applicable) to the folded channel, aligning the chamber's length with the channel.
16. Without stretching any of the tubes,
    a. Carefully feed the channel into the loading port and
    b. Gently pull the channel up through the opening at the top of the filler.
17. Lower the filler latch and press it to lock it into place.
18. Starting with the collection chamber on the left side and press the channel into the filler, loading the inlet port last.
19. Load the leukocyte reduction system (LRS) chamber into the bracket.
20. Ensure that the channel is properly seated and flushed with the top edge of the filler and the LRS chamber is properly loaded into the bracket.

21. Position the centrifuge collar above the holder and push the collar into the holder.

    Note: You will hear a click when the collar locks into place in its holder.

22. Load the lower and upper bearings into their holders on the centrifuge arm.

23. Load the upper collar.
    a. Insert the tubes into the holder with the collar below the holder.
    b. Pull the tubing upward until the collar is fully seated in the holder.

    Note: The upper collar will be locked into place when the centrifuge door closes.

24. Rotate the centrifuge to check that the tubing and bearings are secure and not twisted. Verify that the locking pin is in its fully extended, locked position. Verify channel and LRS chamber are properly loaded.

25. Close the centrifuge door.

26. Ensure that the lines to the product bags are not caught underneath the pump headers.

27. Touch "continue."

    Note: The cassette and pump headers will be lowered into place. The blood cell separator (Trima Accel system) automatically removes the air from the product bags.

28. As per the system prompt, close the white pinch clamps on
    a. The donor line and
    b. The sample bag line.

29. Touch "continue."

    Note: The blood cell separator (Trima Accel system) system performs a tubing set test.

30. When the tubing set test is complete, system prompts to connect ACD solution.

31. Spike ACD solution, load the AC tubing into the AC sensor, and squeeze the drip chamber to ensure that it is half filled.

32. Touch "continue."

33. Verify that fluid is flowing into the AC drip chamber.

34. With successful kit priming, system disables "load system" button.

Entering Donor Information

1. Touch "donor info" button on the main screen.
2. Touch the button corresponding to the donor's gender.
3. Touch "donor height" and enter the height using the number keypad. Touch "enter."
4. Touch "donor weight" and enter the weight using the number keypad. Touch "enter."

5. Verify the accuracy of the total blood volume calculation. Touch "confirm info."
6. Entering the donor's blood type is optional.
   If: Entering the donor's blood type,
   Then: Touch "blood type," enter the type on the letter keypad, and touch "enter."
   If: Not entering the donor's blood type, continue to step 7.
7. Touch "hematocrit." Enter the donor's hematocrit as a whole number using the number keypad. Touch "enter."
8. Touch "platelet precount" and enter the donor's platelet precount using the number keypad. Touch "enter."
9. Verify that the information is correct and then touch "confirm info."

Selecting Procedure

The Trima Accel Collection System now displays the eligible procedures to be run based on the tubing set loaded.

1. If choosing the optimal plasma-only procedure highlighted in yellow,
   Then: Touch "confirm procedure."
   If: Overriding the optimal procedure,
   Then: Select an alternative procedure in the list, and touch "confirm procedure."
2. Select one of the procedures displayed.
3. Touch "confirm procedure."

Connecting the Donor and Collecting the Components

1. Touch "begin donor prep."
2. Follow the prompts on the display and complete the prompted actions.
3. Perform the venipuncture.
4. Open the white pinch clamps
   a. On the donor line and
   b. On the tubing leading to the blood sample bag.
5. Allow the blood sample bag to fill to the desired volume.
6. Close the white pinch clamp on the sample bag tubing.
7. Touch "start draw."
8. Permanently and hermetically seal the blood sample bag as close to the "Y" manifold as possible.
9. Draw samples as soon as possible from the sample bag using evacuated blood collection tubes.
10. After all samples are taken, discard the sample bag in an appropriate biohazard disposal container.

11. If adjustments are required during the procedure, refer to the *Trima Accel Automated Blood Collection System Operator's Manual* for instructions.
12. If an alert is observed during the procedure,
    a. Refer to the display for information on resolving the alert condition.
    b. Refer to the *Trima Accel Automated Blood Collection System Operator's Manual* for additional instructions.

Performing the Postcollection Steps

1. After rinse back is complete, touch "continue."
2. Follow the system prompts to seal the collect lines just above the cassette and remove the product(s) and AC bags.

   Note: Do not seal the vent bag.

3. Make sure that the product bags are labeled with the donor identification number (e.g., unique blood unit number).
4. Close the white pinch clamp on the donor line.
5. Disconnect the donor and touch "continue."
6. Confirm that the donor is disconnected and touch "confirm disconnect."

Removing the Kit Used for Collection of Plasma and Blood Component

1. When prompted to remove, open the centrifuge door and remove the channel from the filler.
2. Remove the AC line from the AC sensor.
3. Remove any remaining bags.
4. Press the top latch located in the upper right corner of the cassette and remove the cassette from the cassette holder.

   Important: Remove the top edge of the cassette and then the bottom.

5. Discard the disposable tubing set in an appropriate biohazard container.
6. Touch "continue."
7. Touch "continue" to view the summary screen at the end of the run.
8. Record procedure results.
9. Label the bag according to the display message and the SOP.
10. Touch "next procedure."

RECORD

Apheresis consent form, qualification criteria, and transfusion transmitted infection (TTI) screening report are to be maintained along with apheresis details in a register.

CHAPTER 18

Care of Platelet/Plasma Apheresis Donor during and after the Procedure

SCOPE AND APPLICATION

Although apheresis is a relatively safe procedure, it is not without potential complications for the donor. The various problems related to the apheresis procedure are:

- Anticoagulant use
- Fluid replacement
- Fluid and electrolyte imbalances
- Vascular access
- Hemolysis
- Air embolism
- Infections

Therefore, blood center staff should be trained to the highest standards of competence in the use of apheresis equipment and donor care.

RESPONSIBILITY

Blood center medical officer and blood center staff are responsible for caring of donors and managing side effects during and after the procedure.

MATERIALS REQUIRED

- *Oral medication:*
    - Analgesic tablets, e.g., paracetamol tablet IP 500 mg
    - Calcium and vitamin C tablets
- *Injection:*
    - Epinephrine (adrenaline) 0.18% w/v (1 in 1,000) 1 mL ampule
    - Atropine sulfate 1 mg 1 mL intramuscular (IM)
    - Calcium gluconate 10% w/v 10 mL intravenous (IV)
    - Pheniramine maleate injection 22.75 mg/mL (2 mL ampule)

- Diazepam injection 5 mg/mL (2 mL ampule)
- Hydrocortisone 100 mg vial (to be dissolved in 2 mL sterile water for injection)
- Dextrose injection 25% w/v (100 mL bottle)
- Metoclopramide 5 mg/mL (2 mL ampule)
- Sodium chloride 0.9% and dextrose 5% injection (500 mL bottle)
- Stemetil injection 12.5 mg/mL (1 mL ampule)
- Sodium bicarbonate 8.4 % w/v IV
- Deriphyllin (2 mL ampule IM)
- Furosemide injection 25 mg/mL (2 mL ampule)
- *Antiseptics*:
  - Savlon solution
  - Povidone iodine 5% solution
- *Miscellaneous*:
  - Bandages/dressings
  - Band-Aids
  - Heparin and benzyl nicotinate ointment (Thrombophob)
  - Spirit of ammonia
  - Tongue depressor
  - Disposable syringes (2/5 mL) and needles 24 gauge
  - Thermometer
  - Oxygen cylinder
  - Infusion set
  - Paper bag

GENERAL CARE DURING PROCEDURE

- Conduct a thorough evaluation of donor including:
  - Diagnosis and medical history
  - Vital signs and laboratory screening report
  - Special observations after last apheresis if any
- Many of the complications of apheresis can be attributed to the procedure itself or to primary or secondary donor medical conditions.
- Identifying preexisting medical conditions and determining potential impact on the donor during the apheresis procedure can help minimize or prevent adverse events.
- Donors should never be left alone in a room without trained personnel.
- Good vascular access is essential for a successful apheresis procedure. At least a good cubital fossa vein is required to draw whole blood from a donor. Steel needle of 16–17 gauge is used for the inlet/draw side to maintain blood flow rate of at least 40–50 mL/min. Lower arm or hand veins may be used for the return side. Steel needle of 17–18 gauge is used for the return side to support rapid flow of whole blood during the apheresis procedure.

- Knowing how to treat signs, symptoms, and side effects will help prevent mild reactions from becoming serious.
- Donors should be monitored at all times until they leave the facility.

COMPLICATIONS

Donor complications associated with the use of cell separators for platelet/plasmapheresis can be due to:
- Anticoagulant
- Vasovagal
- Allergy
- Vascular access
- Machine malfunction

Anticoagulant

Hypocalcemia (Citrate Toxicity)

Anticoagulants are used during the apheresis procedure to prevent clotting in the extracorporeal circuit. Acid-citrate-dextrose solution formula A (ACD-A) is used at a ratio of 1:12–1:15 (anticoagulant:whole blood). A calcium-binding citrate anticoagulant is used to prevent blood from clotting in the tubes of an apheresis machine.

A healthy adult liver metabolizes 3 g of citric acid every 5 minutes. The stored blood is anticoagulated using citrate [3 g/unit of packed red blood cells (PRBC)], which chelates calcium. Thus, transfusions at rates >1 unit every 5 minutes, impaired liver function, and anticoagulant lines of apheresis devices that are improperly attached to the rotary pump or removed during the procedure may require citric acid administration. Poisoning and hypocalcemia can occur. Citrate toxicity is most commonly observed in donors, associated with citrate anticoagulant infusions, and documented in up to 15% of procedures. The symptoms of citrate toxicity are given in **Table 1**.

Table 1: Symptoms of citrate toxicity.		
Mild	*Moderate*	*Severe*
Paresthesias	Lightheadedness	Tetany
Perioral (lips)	Muscle cramps	Laryngeal spasm
Peripheral (fingertips, legs)	Weakness	Seizures
Chills	Nausea	Arrhythmia
Shivering	Vomiting	Prolonged QT interval
"Crawling feeling"	Chest pain	Bradycardia

Prevention

Donors should be informed of symptoms of citric acid and encouraged to promptly report the occurrence of symptoms. Oral calcium supplementation during treatment can prevent the development of hypocalcemia.

Treatment of Citrate Toxicity

Mild:
- *Slow* down the procedure (inlet rate) to reduce the citrate infusion rate.
- Give oral or IV calcium replacement.
- Cover with warm blanket.
- Reassure the donor and monitor it closely.

Moderate:
- *Stop* the inlet blood pump.
- Initiate or increase calcium infusion.
- Weigh the risks and benefits of reinfusion.

Severe:
- *Terminate* the procedure.
- Do not rinse back.
- Start or continue IV calcium supplementation. If there is clinical and electrocardiographic evidence of hypocalcemia, 5 mL of 10% calcium gluconate can be given slowly to treat serious citrate reactions.
- Notify the doctor and the support team.
- Begin life support measures.

Inadequate Citration

This is due to kinking of the apheresis kit tubing. Insufficient levels of citrate can cause clotting in the extracorporeal cell separator circuit and reinfusion of materials with procoagulant activity, which can lead to disseminated intravascular coagulation (DIC) or hemolysis in the cell separator, and can cause reinfusion of hemolyzed blood.

Prevention

- Use the correct anticoagulant ratio recommended by the manufacturer.
- Monitor the anticoagulant pump, the rate of delivery from the drip chamber, and the amount of anticoagulant usage throughout the procedure to ensure consistent and accurate anticoagulant delivery.
- Monitor the return filter separation chamber for signs of clotting. Also, monitor the negative-pressure return line. This could be an early sign of clotting in the circuit.
- Monitor the color of the separated plasma for signs of hemolysis.

Treatment

- Check tubing for kinks.
- Increase anticoagulant:inlet ratio.
- In case of hemolysis, stop the procedure.

Vasovagal

Sudden fainting occurs due to low blood pressure caused by the nervous system's response to sudden emotional stress, pain, or trauma. This is common in whole blood donations and is also seen in apheresis procedures, although less frequently.

Symptoms

- Apprehension
- Lightheadedness
- Nausea
- Decreased pulse rate
- Low blood pressure
- Sweating
- May progress to cardiac arrest

Treatment

- *Terminate the procedure.*
- Raise feet and lower head end.
- Loosen tight clothing (belt, tie, etc.)
- Maintain an adequate airway.
- Check pulse and blood pressure.
- Apply a cold compress to forehead and back.
- Administer inhalation of spirit of ammonia if needed. The donor should respond by coughing, which will elevate the blood pressure.
- *For bradycardia and hypotension*:
  - If bradycardia continues for >20 minutes, administer atropine injection 1 mL IM.
  - If hypotension is prolonged, administer normal saline or dextrose saline infusions intravenously.

Allergic Reactions

Donors can be hypersensitive to:
- Povidine iodine—used for cleaning skin
- Ethylene oxide—used for sterilization of disposable sets
- Plastic disposable sets of replacement fluids.
- Latex

Table 2: Symptoms of allergic reactions.		
Mild	**Moderate**	**Severe**
Itching	Intense itching	Shortness of breath
Urticarial (rash)	Widespread urticarial	Hypotension
Rhinitis	Hives or welts	Diarrhea
Cough	Rhinitis	Laryngeal edema
Tearing	Wheezing	Cardiopulmonary arrest
	Tongue or facial swelling	

Symptoms

The symptoms are given in **Table 2**.

Treatment

Mild:
- Determine cause.
- Consider hydrocortisone as per advice of the physician.

Moderate:
- *Stop* the procedure.
- Maintain access for IV medication, i.e., hydrocortisone and epinephrine, as directed by the physician.

Severe:
- *Stop* the procedure.
- Medication as directed by the physician.

Complications of Vascular Access

The safest venous access is through venipuncture, most commonly through the antecubital vein. It can be accompanied by hematoma, bruising, and sometimes nerve damage. High return pressure can also cause hematoma. Poor vascular access may require rerouting the venipuncture or discontinuing the procedure. If these complications occur, the donor/patient should be carefully informed and appropriate treatment provided. Access complications include:
- Infection
- *Occlusion*: Mechanical or thrombotic
- Mechanical displacement
- Bleeding
- Air embolus
- Pneumo- or hemothorax

Prevention

- Careful selection of the vascular site is very important. A steel needle of 16–17 gauge is used for the inlet/draw side to maintain blood flow rate at least 40–50 mL/min. Lower arm or hand veins may be used for the return side. A steel needle of 17–18 gauge is used for the return side.
- Check for the kinks in the tubing.

Complications Due to Machine Malfunction

Machine failure leading to hemolysis, thrombus formation, air embolism, or leaking occurs in <0.5% of the procedures, but the consequences can be severe. This is usually due to improper manufacturing of the disposable set or improper assembly of the set. Newer devices have enhanced safety features to protect the donor and reduce these complications.

Hemolysis

Pushing blood through a narrow opening by a pump can cause hemolysis, especially if the blood is concentrated with a high hematocrit. Inadequate anticoagulant therapy is also associated with hemolysis.

Prevention

- Cell separators must be maintained according to the manufacturer's instructions. A planned maintenance schedule must be followed.
- The service technician must be available by phone during normal business hours in the event of a mechanical failure of the machine.
- All software should be carefully checked to ensure that there are no kinks or twists in the tubing before starting a procedure.
- Constant monitoring of plasma color should be done for the presence or absence of hemolysis.
- Constantly monitor the transmembrane pressure while using a filter.
- Special attention should be given to frequent low flow rates as these can lead to hemolysis.
- When there is any suspicion of hemolysis, the procedure must be terminated as the return of damaged red cells to the patient/donor could precipitate DIC and mimic a hemolytic transfusion reaction.

Air Embolus

- Most cell separators have an air detector device built into the reinfusion line. However, there is a risk of air embolism if all the lines are not fully primed while using blood warmers and other software beyond the machines' air detectors.

- Never rely entirely on "fail/safe" alarm systems. Occasionally, they may fail and all the reinfusion lines should be monitored constantly to prevent air embolism from occurring.

Infection
Equipment Contamination
- Never leave the cell separators and related equipment primed for longer than necessary.
- Apheresis equipment should be cleaned regularly with an appropriate decontaminating agent. Standard operating procedures should be in place for dealing with blood spillage.

Bacterial Infection
If bacterial contamination occurs during the setup and priming process, there is a risk of causing severe bacteremia, which can be fatal in immunocompromised patients. Usage of crystalloids, colloids, or albumin as replacement fluids during plasmapheresis also lowers the patient's immunoglobulin levels. The patients with low immunoglobulin levels and on immunosuppressive therapy are more susceptible to infections. Prophylactic administration of IV immunoglobulin in high-risk patients should be considered only under special circumstances.

POSTDONATION CARE
- Whenever possible, ensure that all donors/patients get the rest they need and drink at least one glass of liquid before leaving the apheresis site. If no side effects have occurred, this information is included in the appropriate notes.
- Adverse reactions must be handled promptly, appropriately, and in good faith and documented. Submit online monthly adverse donor reaction report to the National Institute of Biologicals, Noida, Ministry of Health and Family Welfare, Government of India for monitoring under Donor Haemovigilance Programme of India (HvPI), and SBTC. Donors should recover as fully as possible before being allowed to leave the venue.
- The attending physician/nurse must remain in the ward until the donor leaves the facility.

Blood Components Separation

INTRODUCTION

Human whole blood consists of red blood cells (RBCs), white blood cells, and platelets suspended in plasma. Instead of using human whole blood, modern blood transfusions optimally use human whole blood through on-demand component therapy. This is due to the fact that the preparation of blood components has been facilitated by the availability of plastic blood collection bags with integrated tubes, high-speed refrigerated centrifuges, deep freezers, and cell separators. Component separation maximizes the utility of the human whole blood units, as each blood component is used for different indications. Blood components can be prepared by the following two methods:

1. Centrifugation of whole human blood
2. Collection of individual blood components by apheresis

COMPONENTS PREPARATION BY CENTRIFUGATION OF WHOLE HUMAN BLOOD

The blood components are prepared by centrifugation of whole human blood, and due to differences in specific gravity, RBCs settle down to the bottom [packed red blood cells (PRBCs)], the liquid plasma rises above, and platelets form a layer in between these two layers. The functional efficiency of each component depends on appropriate processing and proper storage. Component therapy is universally applied for the proper and meaningful use of blood units. Preparation of PRBC and fresh frozen plasma (FFP) requires one-step heavy-spin centrifugation, whereas the preparation of platelet concentrate (PC), PRBC, and FFP requires two-step centrifugation. The separation algorithm using two methods is shown in **Flowcharts 1 and 2**.

Two blood components, PRBCs and FFP or factor VIII (F-VIII)-deficient plasma, are separated from human whole blood collected

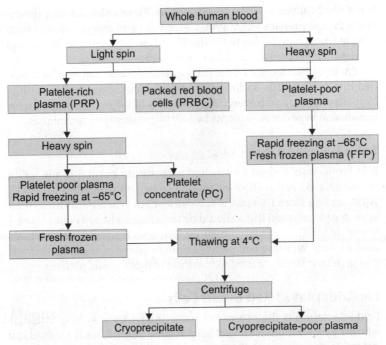

FLOWCHART 1: Component preparation by platelet-rich plasma (PRP) method.

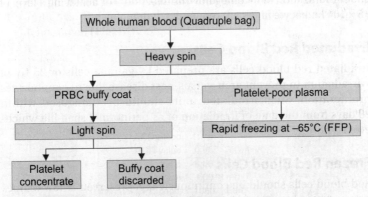

FLOWCHART 2: Component preparation by buffy coat method.

(FFP: fresh frozen plasma; PRBC: packed red blood cell)

in double bags. PRBCs, FFP, platelets or packed cells, F-VIII-deficient plasma, and cryoprecipitate are separated from human whole blood collected in triplicate bags. Plasma is frozen at –80°C and thawed at 4°C, leaving behind cryoglobulins as a precipitate called cryoprecipitate.

It mainly contains F-VIII and fibrinogen. Standard operating procedures for the preparation of PRBC, PCs, FFP, and cryoprecipitate from human whole blood collected in double, triple, or quadruple blood bags are described separately in Chapters 20 to 23.

Packed RBCs isolated from human whole blood can also be modified into semi-PRBCs, saline-washed RBCs, leukocyte-depleted RBCs, irradiated RBCs, and frozen RBCs. Aliquots of PRBCs are prepared for transfusion to pediatric patients by aseptic preservation techniques.

Saline-washed Red Cells

Red blood cells should be washed with sterile normal saline using an automated cell washer or manually by centrifugation at 2–8°C. Washing in a closed system is recommended. When performed in an open system, washed RBCs should be transfused within 24 hours, when stored at 4–6°C. A validated laminar flow bench should be used from time to time. Washing completely removes all the plasma, leukocytes, and platelets. These are used to transfuse to thalassemia patients.

Leukodepleted Red Blood Cells

Leukodepletion is the process of removing leukocytes from donated whole human blood. It should be prepared using known methods to reduce leukocytes to $<5 \times 10^8$ (required to prevent febrile reactions) in the final component and to $<5 \times 10^6$ for the prevention of alloimmunization or cytomegalovirus infection. For achieving a level of $>5 \times 10^6$, leukocyte filters are required.

Irradiated Red Blood Cells

Irradiated red blood cells are prepared by gamma cells or 25 Gy of x-irradiation to prevent graft-versus-host disease due to lymphocytes proliferation. Such irradiated units should be transfused within 28 days from the date of irradiation or as per normal shelf life whichever is shorter.

Frozen Red Blood Cells

Red blood cells should be continuously cryopreserved at low temperatures between –80 and –196°C in the presence of cryoprotectants. The RBCs must be washed prior to transfusion to remove cryoprotectants. Preparation, storage, thawing, and washing procedures should ensure recovery of at least 80% of the original RBCs or more depending on the procedure used. RBCs should generally be frozen within 6 days of blood donation and can be cryopreserved for up to 10 years. Glycerol is the most commonly used cryoprotectant and its concentration depends on the storage temperature.

Pooled Platelet Concentrate

A single unit of randomly donated platelets (prepared from whole human blood) is insufficient to achieve adequate hemostasis in adult patients. Therefore, up to six units of randomly donated, preferably ABO or Rh-matched platelets, are pooled into one bag of "Pooled Platelet Concentrate".

COLLECTION OF SINGLE BLOOD COMPONENT BY APHERESIS

Apheresis is the procedure of collecting the desired one or more blood components and returning the remaining blood components to the donor. The working principle of apheresis equipment is either centrifugation (different specific gravities) or filtration (different size). The most common equipment works on the principle of centrifugation and also offers leukodepleted products. In this method, a fixed quantity of blood is drawn into a bolus called an extracorporeal volume (ECV), the desired components (e.g., platelets) are separated into a collection bag, and the other components (e.g., RBCs, leukocytes, and plasma) are returned back to the donor. There are two types of centrifugation apheresis equipment—"intermittent type" and "continuous type."

Intermittent devices use a single venous line for both collection and return, whereas continuous devices use two simultaneous phlebotomy lines—one for collection and one for return. Plasmapheresis to obtain plasma, plateletpheresis to obtain PCs and granulocyte concentrates, leukapheresis to obtain lymphocytes and mononuclear cells, erythrocyte apheresis to obtain hematopoietic stem cells, therapeutic plasmapheresis, and cell apheresis are other procedures performed at blood centers.

Apheresis process is easier to perform, simpler, and with better quality components compared to the preparation of blood components by centrifugation, but it is expensive.

CHAPTER 20

Preparation of Packed Red Blood Cells and Fresh Frozen Plasma using Double Blood Bag

SCOPE AND APPLICATION

This standard operating procedure (SOP) describes the preparation of packed red blood cells (PRBCs) and fresh frozen plasma (FFP) using a double-bag system.

RESPONSIBILITY

It is the responsibility of the medical officer and blood center technician working in the blood component area to prepare PRBCs and FFP from whole human blood collected using the double-bag system.

MATERIALS REQUIRED

- Refrigerated centrifuge
- Plasma expresser
- Electronic weighing scale
- Double-pan weighing balance
- Double bags (450 mL)

PROCEDURE

1. Whole human blood is collected in primary bag (bag no. 1) of double-bag system **(Fig. 1)**.
2. Keep the blood units so collected vertically on a laminar flow table for 30–45 minutes. (process all units within 6 hours of blood collection)
3. Record the weight of bag no. 1 and enter it in the daily work register.
4. Keep the double-bag system in a bucket and balance it with dry rubber. Keep the equally balanced buckets with bags diagonally opposite in the refrigerated centrifuge ensuring that the position of the bags in the bucket is parallel to the spin direction.

5. Spin the double-bag system in refrigerated centrifuge after balancing the opposing buckets carefully at revolutions per minute (rpm) 5,000 × g (heavy spin) for 10 minutes at 4°C.
6. Carefully remove the blood bag system from the bucket after centrifugation. Blood bag no. 1 has red blood cells (RBCs) at the bottom and platelet-rich plasma (PRP) on the top **(Fig. 2)**.
7. Place blood bag no. 1 on the expresser stand and bag no. 2 on weighing balance under the laminar flow bench. Manually break the integral seal of the tube connecting it to satellite bag no. 2 and express the supernatant PRP into satellite bag no. 2 **(Fig. 3)** leaving 50–60 mL of PRP in the RBCs in primary bag no. 1, and this component is PRBCs.

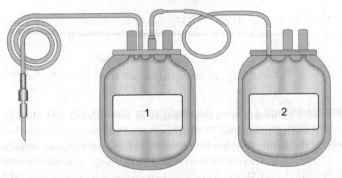

FIG. 1: Double bag for the preparation of packed red blood cell (PRBC) and fresh frozen plasma (FFP).

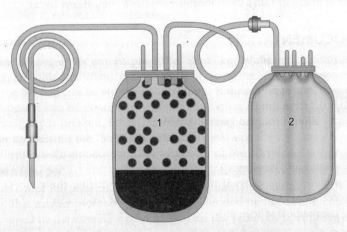

FIG. 2: Blood bag no. 1 contains red blood cell (RBC) at the bottom and platelet-rich plasma (PRP) on the top. **(For color version, see Plate 3)**

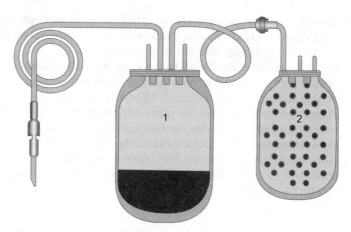

FIG. 3: Packed red blood cells (RBCs) in bag no. 1 and platelet-rich plasma in bag no. 2. (*For color version, see Plate 3*)

8. PRP contained in satellite bag no. 2 should be labeled as FFP if separated within 6 hours of collection and stored immediately below –30°C in deep freezer.
9. If PRP is separated after 6 hours of collection label, it is factor VIII-deficient plasma (F-VIIID).
10. Cut the tubing connecting bag no. 2 (or satellite bag) containing FFP/F-VIIID bags from bag no. 1 with the help of sealer.
11. Bag no. 1 containing PRBCs is then sealed and stored at 2–6°C in a blood center refrigerator. This has a shelf-life of 35 days.
12. Bag no. 2 (satellite bag) containing FFP/F-VIIID plasma is then kept at –30°C in a deep freezer. This has a shelf-life of 1 year.

DOCUMENTATION

- *Record the following details in the master record for blood/blood components*:
    - Date of preparation
    - Unit number
    - Blood group and serology results
- *Record in stock register*: Record the details of the PRBCs and FFP in the master record for blood/blood components after complete testing and labeling.
- *Incident reporting*: If there is a problem during the process of component preparation, create an incident report form and notify the medical officer.

CHAPTER 21

Preparation of Blood Components (Packed Red Blood Cells, Fresh Frozen Plasma, and Platelets) using Triple Blood Bag

SCOPE AND APPLICATION

This standard operating procedure (SOP) describes the preparation of packed red blood cells (PRBCs), platelet concentrates (PC), and fresh frozen plasma (FFP) using a triple-bag system.

RESPONSIBILITY

Preparation of PRBCs, platelets, and FFP using the triple-bag system is the responsibility of the medical officer and technical supervisor working in the component area.

MATERIALS REQUIRED

- Refrigerated centrifuge
- Plasma expresser
- Electronic weighing scale
- Double-pan weighing balance
- Triple-bag system (450 mL)

PROCEDURE

Preparation of PRBC, platelet concentrates, and FFP using the triple-bag system with or without additive solution:

1. The whole human blood is collected in a primary bag (bag no. 1) **(Fig. 1)**.
2. Process the collected whole human blood within 6 hours.
3. Let the units stand upright under laminar flow bench for 30–45 minutes.
4. Note the weight of the primary bag and enter it in daily work register.

5. Keep the blood bags of the triple-bag system in the buckets and balance them using dry rubber. Place evenly balanced buckets with blood bags diagonally opposite in the refrigerated centrifuge, ensuring that the position of the blood bags within the buckets is parallel to the spin direction.

6. After carefully balancing the opposing cups in a refrigerated centrifuge, spin the blood bags in refrigerated centrifuge at revolutions per minute (rpm) 2,000 × g (light spin at 1,750 rpm) for 10 minutes at 20–22°C (Adjust the speed and duration of centrifugation as per the manufacturer's instructions).

7. After centrifugation, carefully remove the blood bags (**Fig. 2**) from the bucket and place them on the expresser stand under the laminar flow bench. Manually break the integral seal of the tube connecting it to the satellite blood bag no. 2 and express the supernatant FFP into the satellite bag no. 2 (**Fig. 3**), leaving

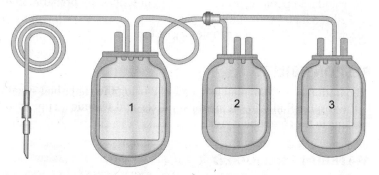

FIG. 1: Triple-bag system for preparation of packed red blood cells, platelet concentrates, and fresh frozen plasma.

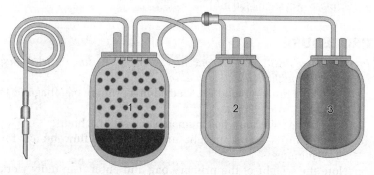

FIG. 2: Triple bag after centrifugation. (*For color version, see Plate 3*)

50–60 mL of plasma back along with the red blood cells in the primary bag no. 1, and this component is PRBC.

8. If the additive solution bag is used, remove all platelet-rich plasma (PRP) in satellite bag no. 2 before clamping and then unclamp bag no. 3 containing additive solution and allow additive solution to enter slowly into the primary bag containing PRBC.

9. Mix the contents of bag no. 1 thoroughly and seal the tubing between bag no. 1 and bag no. 2 using a dielectric sealer and detach bag no. 1 containing PRBC with additive solution in the blood center refrigerator (quarantine).

10. After carrying out mandatory testing of PRBC and negative results for transfusion transmitted infection (TTI), label bag no. 1, transfer it to a blood center refrigerator (for tested blood), and record in the master record for blood and components.

11. Spin the satellite bag no. 2 containing PRP and connecting bag no. 3 (from which additive solution was transferred to bag no. 1), at 22°C in refrigerated centrifuge at rpm 5,000 × g (hard spin at 3,750 rpm) for 5 minutes after balancing the buckets **(Fig. 4)**.

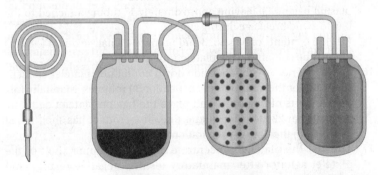

FIG. 3: Platelet-rich plasma (PRP) transferred to bag no. 2. (*For color version, see Plate 4*)

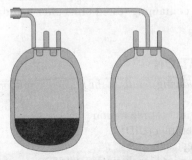

FIG. 4: Bag nos. 2 and 3 after centrifuge.

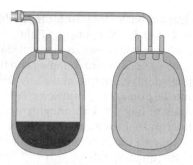

FIG. 5: Platelet-poor plasma in bag no. 3 and platelet concentrate in bag no. 2.

12. Place bag no. 2 containing PRP on the expresser stand under laminar air flow (LAF).
13. Express the supernatant platelet-poor plasma into the empty bag no. 3 leaving 50–60 mL plasma along with the platelet concentrates in bag no. 2 **(Fig. 5)**.
14. Seal the tubing using a dielectric sealer and cut the tubing of plasma bag no. 3, leaving approximately 1″ tubing attached to the bag to avoid breakage during storage.
15. Mix the contents of bag no. 3 and prepare a small segment (~8 cm) of the tube containing the platelets for quality control.
16. Leave bag no. 2 with label side down containing platelet concentrates under the laminar flow bench for 30 minutes. Manually mix the contents of bag no. 2 and place the bag on platelet agitator/incubator at 22–24°C for quarantine. The product has shelf life of 5 days from the date of preparation.
17. Transfer the platelet concentrate unit to the upper shelf of the platelet agitator after mandatory testing, negative results, and labeling.
18. Keep bag no. 3 containing platelet-poor plasma in the deep freezer (–30°C) under quarantine and transfer to the compartment of deep freezer containing tested units after mandatory testing and labeling.

DOCUMENTATION

- *Record the following details in the master record for blood and blood components*:
  - Date and time of preparation
  - Unique identifier (UID)
  - Type of bag used
  - Blood group and serological results

- *Record in stock register*: Record the details of the PRBCs, FFP and Platelet Concentrates in the master record for blood/blood components after complete testing and labeling.
- *Incident reporting*: If any problem is encountered during the process of component preparation, complete the incident reporting form and notify the blood center medical officer.

Blood Component Preparation by Buffy Coat Method using an Automated Component Extractor

INTRODUCTION

After centrifugation, the components are carefully separated using a manual plasma expressor or an automatic/semiautomatic extractor. Automated expression allows for standardization and consistency in the quality of blood components. Automation of blood components from whole blood is widespread. Automated processing reduces operator-dependent variability, controls the volume collected from the main blood bag to the satellite bag, and prevents red blood cell contamination of plasma and platelets. The result is high yield and consistently high-quality products. It helps streamline workflows and enforce manufacturing best practices.

These automatic component extractors are sold by many vendors, e.g., Span Healthcare Private Limited, Pyrotech Electronics Private Limited, Fresenius Kabi India Private Limited, and Terumo Penpol Limited, Macopharma. When choosing an automation partner, blood centers should also determine their customer support, training, and service needs. For better understanding, let us talk about Terumo Penpol Limited's automatic component extractor as the descriptions of all automatic component extractors from various vendors are not included in the preview of this book. The following two are automatic component extractors from Terumo Penpol Limited:

1. T-ACE II Plus
2. Archimede

T-ACE II PLUS

T-ACE II Plus **(Fig. 1)** is equipped with an internal microprocessor that processes information from the scales and the optical and mechanical sensors integrated in the device. Using the information gathered, T-ACE II Plus controls the pressure on the primary bag to direct the flow of

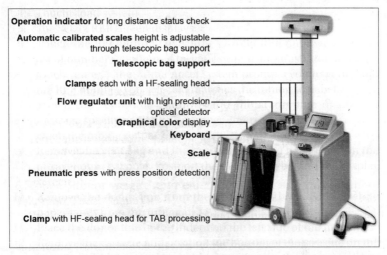

Operation indicator for long distance status check
Automatic calibrated scales height is adjustable through telescopic bag support
Telescopic bag support
Clamps each with a HF-sealing head
Flow regulator unit with high precision optical detector
Graphical color display
Keyboard
Scale
Pneumatic press with press position detection
Clamp with HF-sealing head for TAB processing

FIG. 1: T-ACE II Plus.

blood components extracted. It works according to defined protocols and is a highly flexible automatic blood component extractor for the standardized processing of blood components. This provides high-quality components.

Top and bottom bags are widely used for component preparation using the buffy coat method. The outlets at the top and bottom of the primary bag separate the collected blood into red cells, which go to the bottom bag with saline-adenine-glucose-mannitol (SAGM), and plasma, which goes to the top bag. The platelet is then prepared from the buffy coat, which is widely recommended for platelet preparation. Specially designed quadruple top and top bags of 350 mL and 450 mL capacity are also available for the buffy coat method to optimize blood donations.

ARCHIMEDE

Archimede automatic component extractor is a much more advanced and stand-alone tabletop instrument, unlike T-ACE II Plus, which has a separate air compressor. The extractor overview **(Fig. 2)** shows features of this automatic extractor including automatic cannula breaker, air removal from plasma bag, smart tube handling electric engine with 18 sensors, and advanced software bidirectional data transmission via local area network (LAN) and wireless local area network (WLAN), compatible with optional radiofrequency identification (RFID) and omnidirectional barcode reader, self-diagnostic program for remote service.

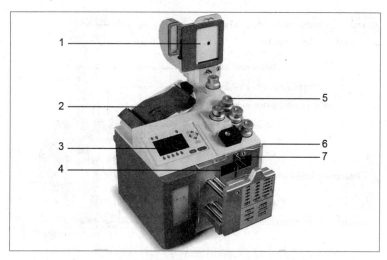

FIG. 2: Overview of Archimede automatic component extractor.

1. *Saline-adenine-glucose-mannitol press*: Automates the priming of in-line red cell filter with SAGM
2. *Automatic air removal from plasma bag*: Removes air from plasma bag quickly
3. *Graphical display*: Display of bag weights, plate force, and status of various operating phases
4. *High-precision separation*: Electric press with 18 optical sensors that detect the blood component interface for accurate separation
5. *Six clamps*: Colored tubing pathway next to each clamp for easy blood bag loading and automatic detection of correct tube placement
6. Highly accurate weight scale
7. Three cannula breakers

It has a user-friendly interface and is easy to load. A mechanical press in combination with an optical sensor applies pressure to the plasma bag to trigger clamping and sealing. There is a small plasma loss (2–5 mL) that is returned to the buffy coat. Blood component separation with the Archimede automatic component extractor is of high quality.

BLOOD COMPONENT PREPARATION USING T-ACE II PLUS

Scope and Application

This standard operating procedure (SOP) describes the preparation of packed red blood cells (PRBC), fresh frozen plasma (FFP), and cryoprecipitates using an automated component extractor (T-ACE

II Plus by Terumo Penpol). Blood components are prepared by the buffy coat method and leukofiltration after collecting 450 mL blood into quadruple blood bags (top and bottom bags with an integrated leukocyte filter) with additive SAGM solution.

Blood centers using other automatic component extractors (other than T-ACE II Plus of Terumo Penpol) should design their own SOP following the manufacturer's guidelines as such procedures are device-specific.

RESPONSIBILITY

A blood center technical supervisor working in the component area prepares PRBC, FFP, and platelets using an automated component extractor (T-ACE II Plus) under the supervision of the blood center medical officer.

MATERIALS REQUIRED

- Refrigerated centrifuge
- Centrifuge buckets
- Balancing dry rubber material
- Automatic component extractor
- Electronic weighing scale
- Penta in-line blood bags [top and bottom penta bags with an integrated leukocyte filter (450 mL) with additive SAGM solution]
- Quadruple blood bag with whole blood filter removing leukocytes and platelets

PROCEDURE

A. *Component separation using top and bottom penta blood bags with integrated leukocyte filter:* Top and bottom penta blood bags with integrated leukocyte filter are used for whole blood collection and separation of three different blood components (leukodepleted red blood cells, plasma, and platelets). The primary bag no. 1 contains citrate phosphate dextrose (CPD) solution and one satellite bag no. 3 is attached to a leukocyte filter which comes with SAGM solution for red cell preservation. Platelets are prepared from the buffy coat and are transferred to bag no. 5. The platelets are stored for 5 days.

- *Blood collection and preparation of components:*
  - 450 mL of blood is collected in the primary bag (bag no. 1) containing 63 mL of CPD and is kept at room temperature (22 ± 2°C) to process for blood components **(Fig. 3)**.
  - Collected blood must be processed within 6–8 hours after collection.

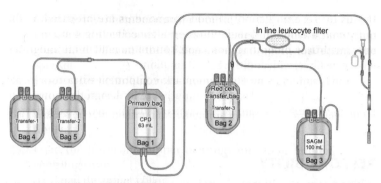

FIG. 3: Top and bottom blood bags with an integrated leukocyte filter.
(CPD: citrate phosphate dextrose; SAGM: saline-adenine-glucose-mannitol)

- Blood units collected in different blood bags are physically checked. Any discrepancies found must be entered into the register and notified to the technical supervisor and/or the blood center medical officer.
- Check the donor IDs of the primary and its satellite bags to make sure that they are the same.
- The decision to prepare the components of under/over-collected blood units is to be made after discussion with technical supervisor and/or blood center medical officer.
- Based on the selected blood bag for component preparation, enter the blood components to be prepared into the component register according to the donor ID number.
- Pack top and bottom penta bags in the centrifuge cup, weigh and balance it.
- Spin the bags at heavy spin (3,650 rpm for 10 minutes while using Cryofuge) at 22°C (*first spin*) **(Fig. 4)**.
- Carefully take out the cups containing blood bags as soon as the centrifuge stops and place on the working table.

1. *Preparing the automatic component extractor for separation of blood components:*
   a. Turn on the air compressor and wait until the pressure on air compressor reaches at least up to 6 bars. Watch the pressure on gauge provided at the rear side of the T-ACE II Plus also.
   b. Turn on the T-ACE II Plus.
   c. Wait until the "SELF CHECK" is completed.
   d. Once the self-test is complete, the door of the T-ACE II Plus gets open and START MENU is displayed.
   e. Select the desired program.
   f. Press "MENU"

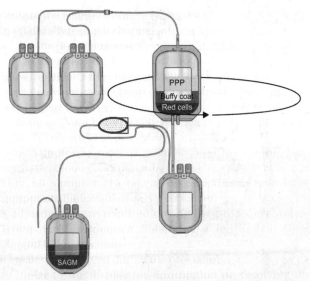

FIG. 4: Centrifuging whole blood with hard spin (first spin). **(*For color version, see Plate 4*)**

(PPP: platelet poor plasma; SAGM: saline-adenine-glucose-mannitol)

    g. Press "SCROLL" until the required program appears on the display.

    h. Press "STOP" to enter the selected program

2. *Separation of blood components* (**Fig. 5**):

    a. Place top and bottom bags after centrifugation on the scales of T-ACE II Plus as per graphical representation properly and hang the primary bag no. 1 on hanger making sure that the label of the bag faces to the door of the T-ACE II Plus.

    b. Route the tubing through seals and flow regulators. Ensure that the tubing moves freely inside clamps and flow regulators.

    c. Close the door of the T-ACE II Plus.

    d. *Open the click tips* of primary bag no. 1 and red cell transfer bag no. 2.

    e. Press "START" on the screen display to begin the separation. The equipment will now automatically separate the components. During the entire process, the operation indicator is illuminated.

    f. Concentrated red cells are transferred to the red cell transfer bag no. 2 in the bag system. Initially, 2–5 mL of plasma to the platelet bag no. 5 to avoid contamination of plasma with red cells and later on, the plasma is transferred to the plasma bag no. 4.

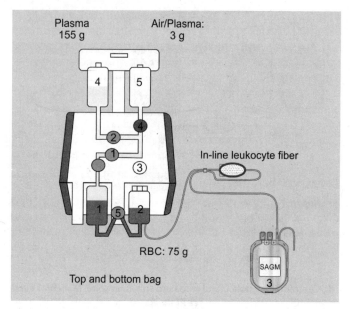

FIG. 5: Graphical placement of top and bottom penta blood bags. (*For color version, see Plate 5*)

(RBC: red blood cell; SAGM: saline-adenine-glucose-mannitol)

g. Buffy coat with some amount of plasma and platelets remains in the parent bag no. 1.

h. Follow the instructions displayed on the T-ACE at the end of separation and remove the plasma bag no. 4 and red cell bag no. 2 after these have been sealed by T-ACE II Plus.

i. Mix the buffy coat bag no. 1 and keep buffy bag in hanging position at least for minimum 1–2 hours after first separation.

j. Hang the buffy coat bag no. 1 on the hook of the centrifuge bucket. Centrifuge at low spin (1,050 rpm for 6 minutes, A/D 9/4) at 22°C (need to be optimized as per centrifuge make).

k. After centrifugation, place the bag on respective scales and follow the procedure for tube routing and program selection for platelets separation.

l. Equipment will automatically check the tube positioning and bags hanged on the scale. Press "START" for extraction of platelets from buffy. The platelets are collected in bag no. 5. The equipment will automatically seal the bag after separation.

m. A buffy coat containing some plasma remains in the primary bag no. 1. The T-ACE II Plus dilutes the buffy coat with plasma from satellite bag no. 4 and satellite bag no. 5. The machine will make a "click" sound when the process is completed and the operation indicator starts blinking. Follow the instructions displayed on the T-ACE II Plus at the end of separation.

n. When the process is complete, the display will show "remove the bag." Once the bag is removed, the T-ACE II Plus will return to its initial state and the "START" menu will be displayed again.

o. Gently mix the buffy coat in primary bag no. 1 and keep buffy bag along with satellite bag no. 5 in hanging position for at least 1 hour after the initial separation.

p. Hang the buffy bag along with the satellite bag on the hook of buffy stand provided in centrifuge cup, weigh and balance it.

q. Place the cups in the centrifuge and spin at 2000 × g (light spin at 1,050 rpm) for 6 minutes at 20–22°C (*second spin*).

r. After centrifugation, carefully take out the cups from centrifuge and place on the working table.

s. After selecting a program, place the bag on the respective scale of T-ACE II Plus. Follow the procedure for tube routing and program selection as per instructions mentioned above.

t. This equipment checks the tube positioning and bags hanged on the scale automatically. Press "START" to extract platelets from the buffy coat into the satellite bag no. 5. When the separation process is complete, the machine will automatically seal the bag.

u. Remove the bag after the sealing is complete.

v. Label expiry date on platelet concentrate, taking date of collection as zero day.

B. *Leukodepletion with top and bottom penta blood bags with an integral filter:* The procedure for separating of blood components remains the same as described above. However, the PRBCs are further processed as detailed below:

1. *Priming* (**Fig. 6**):

a. Hang the bag containing SAGM solution bag no. 3 on the stand.

b. First, open the clamp and then break off valve of SAGM bag.

c. Transfer the SAGM solution into the bag no. 2 containing separated red cells by passing the SAGM solution through the leukocyte filter.

d. Wait until the inlet side of filter collapses and then clamp the tube before changing the direction.

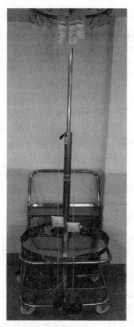

FIG. 6: Priming.

    e. Now, gently turn the bag no. 2 up and down to mix the red cells with the SAGM solution.

    f. During this time, ensure that the clamp is closed and hang the bag no. 2 upside down and open the clamp so that red blood cells start getting filtered into the SAGM bag no. 3.

2. *Filtration* **(Fig. 7)**:

    a. Filter the SAGM solution mixed with red cells through the integrated leukocyte filter and collect in a storage bag no. 3 **(Fig. 5)**.

    b. A dark red color on the surface of the filter inlet tube surface becomes clear as the endpoint of filtration is reached.

    c. Once the filtration endpoint is reached, clamp the tubing to seal it.

    d. Red blood cells mixed with SAGM solution after filtration in bag no. 3 are leukodepleted, labeled as leukodepleted PRBC and is stored at 2–6°C for 42 days.

3. *Record*:

    • Record the details of the leukodepleted PRBC in blood component register.

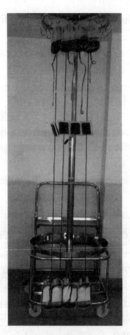

FIG. 7: Filtration.

C. *Component separation using quadruple blood bag with whole blood filter removing leukocytes and platelets* (**Fig. 8**):
1. Switch "ON" air compressor and wait for the pressure on air compressor to reach at least 6 bars. Watch the pressure on gauge provided at the rear side of the T-ACE II Plus also.
2. Switch "ON" the T-ACE II Plus.
3. Wait for the completion of "SELF CHECK."
4. Select the required program.
   a. Press "MENU".
   b. Press "SCROLL" till the required program is displayed.
   c. Press "STOP" to enter the selected program.
5. Whole blood (450 mL) is collected in the blood bag CPD 450 mL (bag no. 1).
6. Hang the blood bag no. 1 to suspend the filter in vertical position. Break the click tip of the tubing connecting bag no. 1 and the filter and place the post filter transfer bag no. 1 on a support to limit the filtration height to 90 cm.
7. The whole blood starts passing through the integrated filter and gets collected in transfer bag no. 1. The leukocytes and platelets

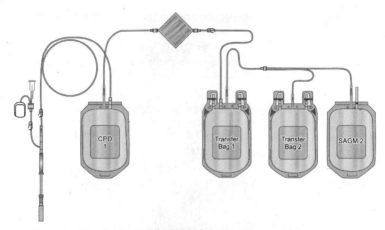

FIG. 8: Quadruple blood bag with whole blood filter removing leukocytes and platelets.

(CPD: citrate phosphate dextrose; SAGM: saline-adenine-glucose-mannitol)

are trapped inside the filter. A dark red color on the surface of the filter inlet tube surface becomes clear as the endpoint of filtration is reached.

8. Once the filtration endpoint is reached, clamp the tubing to seal the transfer bag no. 1.

9. Remove the bag from the stand and seal the filter outlet tube very close to filter and detach filter along with CPD bag no. 1.

10. Arrange the transfer bag no. 1 containing blood and transfer bag no. 2 and SAGM 2 bag into the centrifuge cup. Ensure that the blood bags are placed at the bottom of the centrifuge cup and no tubes are hanging out of the cup and the bag set is maintained straight into the cup. Weigh and balance it.

11. Perform hard spin (3,650 rpm for 10 minutes, A/D 9/4) at 22°C (to be optimized as per centrifuge make).

12. Place transfer bag no. 1, transfer bag no. 2 and SAGM 2 bag on the scales of T-ACE II Plus as per graphical representation properly, and route the tubes through sealers and flow regulator.

13. Ensure that tubes can freely move inside clamps and flow regulator.

14. Close the door.

15. Press "START" to begin the separation. Then, the equipment will automatically transfer the plasma to transfer bag no. 2. Detach the plasma bag.

16. Transfer the SAGM solution to the leukodepleted red cells and mix well.
17. Strip the post filter tube of the filled transfer bag no. 1 by means of a hand stripper to transfer the remaining leukodepleted blood in the tube to the transfer bag no. 1 and mix the content. Allow the tube to fill with blood again and make an appropriate number of segments necessary for testing.
18. Label the components as leukodepleted red cells and plasma and store at appropriate temperatures.

D. *Component separation using quadruple top and top bags of 350 mL (**Fig. 9**):* Quadruple top and top bags of 350 mL capacity are used for preparation of blood components by the buffy coat method to optimize blood donations for donors weighing 45–55 kg.
  1. Switch "ON" air compressor and wait for the pressure on air compressor to reach at least 6 bars. Watch the pressure on gauge provided at the rear side of the T-ACE II Plus also.
  2. Switch "ON" the T-ACE II Plus.
  3. Wait for the completion of "SELF CHECK".
  4. Select the required program
     a. Press "MENU".
     b. Press "SCROLL" till the required program is on display.
     c. Press "STOP" to enter the selected program.

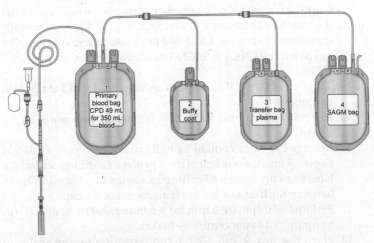

FIG. 9: Quadruple top and top bags of 350 mL.

(CPD: citrate phosphate dextrose; SAGM: saline-adenine-glucose-mannitol)

5. Whole blood (350 mL) is collected in the primary blood bag CPD 350 mL (bag no. 1).

6. Arrange bag no. 1 with blood set into the one half of the centrifuge cup so that the label faces the inner wall of the cup, while bag nos. 2, 3, and 4 with tubes in between the bags are placed in the other half cup of the centrifuge. Ensure that no tubes are hanging out of the cup and the bag set is maintained straight into the cup. Weigh and balance it.

7. Perform hard spin (3,250 rpm for 10 minutes, A/D 9/4) at 22°C (to be optimized as per centrifuge make).

8. Place bag no. 1 and other bags after centrifugation on the scales of T-ACE II Plus as per the graphical representation properly and route the tubes through sealers and flow regulator.

9. Ensure that tubes move freely inside clamps and flow regulator.

10. Close the door.

11. Open the click tips of bag nos. 1 and 4. Ensure that the click tips are opened completely by bending in either direction.

12. Press "START" to begin the separation. The equipment will now automatically transfer the components.

13. Initial 8–10 mL of plasma is transferred to bag no. 4 to avoid contamination of plasma with red cells. Thereafter, the plasma is transferred to bag no. 3. The T-ACE II Plus automatically clamps the tubing of bag no. 3 on the completion of plasma transfer. Thereafter, buffy coat is transferred to bag no. 2 and the tubing of bag no. 2 is clamped on completion of transfer of buffy coat. After the transfer of buffy coat, SAGM from bag no. 4 is automatically transferred to bag no. 1 and bag no. 1 containing concentrated red blood cell (RBC) in SAGM is sealed automatically by T-ACE II Plus.

14. The door of T-ACE II Plus opens up. Bag nos. 1 and 3 are labeled and stored.

15. Bag no. 2 containing buffy coat is hanged with ports up for 1 hour.

16. Arrange bag no. 2 containing buffy coat and the empty SAGM bag no. 4 into the one half of the cup of the centrifuge so that the label faces the inner wall of the cup. Ensure that the tubes are in between the bags and are not hanging out of the cup.

17. Perform light spin (950 rpm for 6 minutes, A/D 9/4) at 22°C (to be optimized as per centrifuge make).

18. Place bag nos. 2 and 4 after centrifugation on the scales of T-ACE II Plus as per the graphical representation properly and route the tubes through sealers and flow regulator.

19. Close the door.

20. Press "START" to begin the separation. The equipment will now automatically transfer the platelets to bag no. 4 and the door opens.
21. The empty bag no. 4 containing platelets gets sealed automatically on transfer of platelets.
22. The empty bag no. 4 containing platelets is labeled and stored in a platelet agitator cum incubator at 22–24°C for 5 days and bag no. 2 is discarded as per guidelines of biomedical waste rules.

DO'S AND DON'TS FOR T-ACE II PLUS

DO's

1. Switch on air compressor at least 1 minute before switching on the T-ACE II Plus.
2. Ensure a clean detector plate for efficient functioning.
3. Ensure no moisture outside the tubes.
4. Ensure proper insertion of tubes through clamps and flow regulator.
5. Place the primary bag with the label side visible (in front position).
6. Ensure that optical detectors (on the press plate) and sealing heads are clean and dry. Clean with tissue paper if blood/dirt is present on the detectors/sealing heads.
7. Use mild detergent for cleaning purpose.
8. The break-off valve on line donor tube should be opened completely during collection.
9. Packing should be done adequately such that the two hard sleeves at the base of primary bags should not come in between the primary and SAGM bags during centrifugation.
10. After priming, the clamp should be closed before mixing the red cell bag; otherwise, there is chance of air to enter the filter.

Don'ts

1. Do not switch on T-ACE II Plus before reaching specified air pressure range.
2. Do not close air outlet valve of compressor until any air tube removal is required.
3. Do not run air compressor if the oil level is insufficient.
4. Never use spirit to clean the detector plate. Use soap solution if necessary.
5. Do not disturb the bags on scales during process. System continuously checks these weights for its functioning.
6. Never apply more force to weighing scales while placing the bags since they are very sensitive.

7. Do not use the bags which are wet on the outside.
8. No label should be adhered to the backside of the primary bag; the sensor plate may not detect the layers.
9. Packing should be done adequately such that the two hard sleeves at the base of primary bags should not come in between the primary and SAGM bags during centrifugation.
10. After priming, the clamp should be closed before mixing the red cell bag; otherwise, there is chance of air to enter the filter.

DO'S AND DON'TS FOR OPERATION OF CRYOFUGE (6000i)

DO's

1. Check the input/output supply on the stabilizer before switching on the Cryofuge.
2. Wait for 2 minutes after switching on the Cryofuge to allow the time for self-testing.
3. Open the lid cover when the yellow light-emitting diode (LED) is lit up. This is only possible when the rotor is not rotating or has finished rotating and no error messages are shown.
4. Press the lid cover of the Cryofuge gently.
5. The hood should always be inserted in the holder provided for the purpose on the inner side of Cryofuge lid.
6. Clean the Cryofuge chamber daily after completion of the run.
7. Unlock the Cryofuge manually in case of power failure (as per the manufacturer's guidelines) after confirming that the Cryofuge is at standstill.
8. Lubricate the rotor buckets/hoods weekly.
9. Blood bags should be weighed out to a maximum tolerance of 5 g. The better counterbalance leads to better running performance of the Cryofuge and hence the improvement in the separation quality of components.
10. The bags must be placed firmly in the insert in order to avoid folding as this leads to formation of nests (accumulation of cells) evading sedimentation process, thereby leading to poor results.
11. The blood bags in case of double/triple or quadruple bags should be placed at the central area in the buckets next to the dividing wall.
12. Select the program as per requirement depending upon the use of double/triple or quadruple bags for separation of blood components.

Don'ts

1. Do not keep standing near the Cryofuge while it is in running condition.
2. The difference in the total weight of opposite-facing buckets should not exceed 10 g.
3. Do not open the lid manually when the rotor is moving.
4. No lubricant except as recommended by the manufacturer should be used.
5. Organic solvents, alkaline cleaners, or household cleaners containing scouring powder must not be used for cleaning.
6. Never place the hood outside the Cryofuge but should always be inserted in the holder provided in the inner side of the Cryofuge.

Preparation of Cryoprecipitate

SCOPE AND APPLICATION

This standard operating procedure (SOP) describes the preparation of cryoprecipitate from fresh frozen plasma (FFP).

RESPONSIBILITY

Preparation of cryoprecipitate from FFP using the triple-bag system under the supervision of the medical officer of blood center, is the responsibility of the technical supervisor working in the blood component section.

MATERIALS REQUIRED

- FFP ≥200 mL along with satellite bags
- Metal clips and hand sealer
- Refrigerated centrifuge
- Plasma expresser
- Electronic weighing scale
- Double-pan weighing balance

PROCEDURE

1. *Preparation of FFP*: The starting material is ≥200 mL platelet-poor FFP. Plasma must be free from red blood cells. Plasma separation should be started as soon as possible. Use FFP frozen at –65°C or below within 1 hour of preparation and should reach this core temperature within 7–8 hours of exposure to the target temperature. FFP stored in this way can be used for the preparation of cryoprecipitate within a year. Bags used for cryoprecipitate preparation require longer tube segments.

2. *Preparation of cryoprecipitate*:
   a. After freezing the FFP at −65°C or below for 3 days, thaw the frozen FFP overnight at 1–6°C in a blood center refrigerator.
   b. Put the bags in centrifuge buckets and balance the buckets on a weighing scale.
   c. Keep the bags parallel in the buckets.
   d. Spin the buckets at 5,000 × g (heavy spin at 3,650 rpm) for 10 minutes at 4°C.
   e. Using a plasma extractor, express supernatant plasma into another satellite bag leaving about 15–25 mL plasma and a whitish jelly-like precipitate called "cryoprecipitate" in the original bag. This cryoprecipitate is rich in factor VIII.
   f. Seal the tube and separate the bags containing cryoprecipitate and cryo-poor plasma (CPP).
   g. Store these two components, i.e., CPP and cryoprecipitate, at −70°C.

   Notes:
   • Cryoprecipitate can be prepared from FFP at any time up to 12 months after collection.
   • The expiration date of cryoprecipitate is 1 year from the date of blood collection, not from the date of its preparation.
   • Cryoprecipitate should be refrozen within 1 hour of thawing.

3. *Labeling*: *must contain the following information*:
   a. ABO and Rh grouping
   b. Original blood unit's number
   c. Components' name
   d. Date of collection of whole blood

DOCUMENTATION

Record the following details in the master record for blood and component:
• Preparation date
• Unique identifier (UID)
• Blood group, serological, and transfusion transmitted infection (TTI) results
• Date of collection and expiry

CHAPTER 24

Preparation of Saline-washed Red Blood Cells

SCOPE AND APPLICATION

This standard operating procedure (SOP) describes the procedure for preparing saline-washed red blood cells for use in the following patients:

- Febrile transfusion reactions that are not prevented by leukocyte reduction
- Immunoglobulin A (IgA) deficient with documented anti-IgA antibodies and when an IgA-deficient donor is not available
- History of a previous anaphylactic transfusion reaction
- Severe urticarial reactions that cannot be prevented by pretransfusion antihistamines.
- Potassium deficiency before transfusion to a fetus or a neonate with renal failure or when a large amount of red blood cell (RBC) component is needed for neonate (i.e., RBC exchange, dialysis, ECMO, etc.) when fresh RBCs are not available.

RESPONSIBILITY

Preparation of washed red cells is the responsibility of the laboratory technician working in the component area under the supervision of a technical supervisor and medical officer.

MATERIALS REQUIRED

- Refrigerated centrifuge
- Sterile connecting device
- Laminar flow bench
- Plasma expresser
- Electronic weighing machine
- Dry rubber balancing material
- Blood center refrigerator
- Crossmatched packed red blood cells (PRBC) unit
- Normal saline bag

PROCEDURE

1. Take crossmatched unit of PRBC.
2. Connect the PRBC bag to the cold (4 ± 2°C) normal saline bag under laminar flow and transfer 250 mL of saline in the PRBC bag and mix thoroughly.
3. Separate the PRBC bag from the normal saline bag by sealing the tubing using a dielectric sealer.
4. Check and record the batch number and expiry date of normal saline before use.
5. Centrifuge the PRBC bag at heavy spin at rpm 3,650 for 5 minutes (to be optimized as per manufacturer's instructions).
6. Transfer the supernatant saline into the transfer bag/waste receptacle using a plasma expresser under laminar flow bench.
7. Disconnect the transfer bag, seal, and discard.
8. Repeat the washing procedure using saline twice more (total three times) exactly in the same manner as described above in steps 2–7. In the end, keep 60–70 mL of saline with red cells in the bag.
9. Seal the bag containing finally saline-washed red blood cells.
10. Weigh the bag containing saline-washed red blood cells and store in the blood center refrigerator at 2–6°C.
11. Label and record the details in the master component register.

Note:
- Use the washed PRBC unit within 24 hours.
- Unit is discarded according to standard protocols when not used after taking a sample for sterility testing.
- Red cell viability and function are limited by removal of anticoagulant-preservative solution.
- Red blood cell (RBC) units washed with saline contain 10–20% less RBC than the original unit.
- Saline-washed RBCs take several hours to prepare, and the blood center should be ordered at least 24 hours in advance of anticipated demand.
- Since the washing process destroys up to 20% of the RBCs, patients who receive washed red blood cells usually require more units to achieve the same hematocrit (HcT) than patients given PRBC.

DOCUMEMTATION

Record the following details in the master record for blood and component:
- Preparation date
- Unique identifier (UID)
- Blood group, serological, and transfusion transmitted infection (TTI) results
- Date of collection and expiry

Labeling of Blood and Blood Components

SCOPE AND APPLICATION

Collected blood is held in quarantine and is released for transfusion only after negative/nonreactive testing for all mandatory tests, followed by labeling as per the provisions under the Drugs and Cosmetics Act 1940 and Rules 1945.

Blood unit labeling is a three-step process. The first step is performed by the staff nurse who labels the primary collection bag appropriately at the time of phlebotomy. The second step is performed by a blood center technician who labels the blood/blood component units with the donor's ABO/Rh type and the expiry date of the blood or blood components once the testing of blood grouping, transfusion transmitted infection (TTI) testing, and component preparation are completed. Finally, the third step is also performed by the blood center technician upon receiving of requisition of blood or blood components for transfusion. It involves labeling of details such as the name of the intended transfusion recipient and the results of the crossmatch test on the crossmatch label.

All labeling steps should be performed with precise attention. Mix-up of blood units during labeling can potentially lead to a patient's death from an ABO-incompatible transfusion reaction. Labels are required to identify and retrieve blood units for use, disposal, and follow-up in event of an adverse reaction.

RESPONSIBILITY

Ensuring proper labeling of blood units at the appropriate stages is the responsibility of nurses and laboratory technicians working in the blood center under the supervision of medical officer.

MATERIALS REQUIRED

- Unit number stickers
- One yellow-top and one purple-top vacutainers
- Preprinted adhesive labels confirming to regulatory requirements with color coding as per blood groups. Yellow label for Group A; pink label for Group B; blue label for Group O, and white label for Group AB (for both positive and negative Rh grouping)

PROCEDURE

1. A unit number sticker is placed on top of the donor base label just prior to blood collection. It should be noted that this unit number has never been used by a blood center before.
2. Write the blood collection date and expiration date on the donor-based label.
3. Paste one unit number sticker on the donor form.
4. Finally, blood sample vacutainers are labeled with the unit number sticker.
5. At this point, the blood collection bag is ready for the blood collection process.
6. After the collection and processing of whole blood, the blood units are stored in a blood storage refrigerator (quarantine).
7. After these blood units have been tested for blood group and TTI, place the tested bags on the table in a chronological order and discard any bags that are reactive/positive for TTI or are deemed unsuitable for use, in compliance with the Biomedical Waste Guideline.
8. The blood units found suitable for transfusion are affixed with green color self adhesive label mentioning nonreactive for HBsAg, Anti-HCV, Anti-HIV I/II and VDRL and negative for malaria parasite.
9. Clearly state on each label the unit number, collection date, expiry date, and quantity based on donor registration records.
10. Collection dates and expiration dates are very important. The expiration dates for blood collected in citrate-phosphate-dextrose-adenine (CPDA-1) bags are 35 and 42 days from the date of collection for triple and quadruple bags of additive solution, respectively.
11. After labeling the bag, second technician must cross-check the unit number and group of the bag with the donor's registry details.
12. After complete testing, screening, and labeling, the blood unit is stored in a blood center refrigerator dedicated to the tested blood units.

13. Label fresh frozen plasma (FFP), frozen-deficient plasma, and platelet concentrate in the same manner. Cryoprecipitate labels do not indicate blood type.
14. FFP and cryoprecipitate have one-year shelf life.
15. The shelf life of platelet concentrate is 5 days from the date of preparation.

DOCUMENTATION

Enter all labeled blood units with bag numbers in the blood stock register and ensure that there are no transcription errors.

Preservation of Blood and Blood Components

SCOPE AND APPLICATION

Blood and blood components are stored under mandatory storage conditions as specified under the Drugs and Cosmetics Rules 1945 to ensure their optimal viability and function.

RESPONSIBILITY

The responsibility of the blood center technicians working in the component area is to ensure that blood/blood component units are kept in quarantine pending mandatory testing and that units deemed suitable for transfusion are stored under appropriate conditions in respective storage areas (after processing and labeling).

MATERIALS REQUIRED

- Blood center refrigerator maintaining temperature 4 ± 2°C
- Deep freezers –40°C and –80°C
- Platelet incubator cum agitator

PROCEDURE

1. All untested blood/component units are stored under proper storage conditions in the quarantine refrigerator/plasma deep freezer/platelet agitator.
2. Once testing is complete, blood/blood component units fully tested and found suitable for clinical use are labeled as described in Chapter 25 and then transferred from the quarantine storage area to the tested storage area.
3. Any unit deemed unsuitable for use should be labeled biohazard and collected for separate disposal.

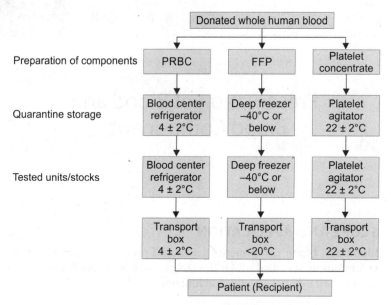

FLOWCHART 1: Blood cold chain from collection to transfusion.
(FFP: fresh frozen plasma; PRBC: packed red blood cells)

4. Store whole blood and red blood cell concentrates in trays in blood center refrigerators at 4 ± 2°C. Each tray is reserved for a specific blood group and has a label on the outside indicating the blood type. Arrange the blood bags in the tray chronologically, group-wise, and by expiry dates. Stack the trays in the refrigerator. This makes it very easy for the blood center technician on duty to remove the blood bags for issue.

5. Collected whole blood can be stored for up to 35 days in citrate-phosphate-dextrose-adenine (CPDA-1), up to 35 days in packed red blood cells (PRBC), and up to 42 days in PRBC suspended in additive solution.

6. Fresh frozen plasma, cryoprecipitate, and F-VIII deficient plasma bags should be stored in overlap bags in trays in a –40°C freezer, with a shelf life of 1 year for all these components.

7. The blood cold chain from collection to storage is shown in **Flowchart 1**.

8. Use fresh frozen plasma/cryoprecipitate as soon as possible after thawing to preserve labile factors.

9. Do not refreeze freshly thawed frozen plasma/cryoprecipitate.

10. Store platelets in a platelet incubator at 20–22°C with gentle shaking for up to 5 days.

11. Maintain sterility of blood/blood component units by maintaining cleanliness and sanitary storage conditions in storage areas.
12. Ensure adherence to prescribed storage conditions during storage at the transfusion center. Monitor temperatures in all storage areas with a continuous chart recorder. Change and save graphs/charts weekly. Check your alarm system monthly.
13. Conduct daily physical inventory checks against records.

DOCUMENTATION

Record all blood/blood component units issued for transfusion in issue register and master records for blood and its components. The blood/blood components found unsuitable (to be discarded) in the register meant for disposable units.

CHAPTER **27**

Preparation of Red Cell Suspension

SCOPE AND APPLICATION

This standard operating procedure (SOP) describes the method of preparation of red cell suspension of appropriate concentration for performing the following routine tests in a blood center:

- 5% red cell suspension of pooled cells for reverse grouping
- 5% red cell suspension of sample for direct antiglobulin test
- 5% red cell suspension of donor red cells for major crossmatch with the patient's sample

RESPONSIBILITY

It is the responsibility of a laboratory technician to prepare the red cell suspension for red cell serology. Suspensions of A, B, and O red cells are prepared daily by the blood center technician.

MATERIALS REQUIRED

- *Equipment*: Table top centrifuge machine
- *Reagent*: Low-ionic-strength saline (LISS) solution
- *Specimen*:
  - Anticoagulated blood specimen of donor
  - Anticoagulated blood specimen of patient
  - Anticoagulated blood specimens of known groups
- *Glassware*:
  - Test tubes
- *Miscellaneous*:
  - Micropipettes
  - Test tube stand

PROCEDURE

Principle

The ratio of serum to red blood cells (RBCs) can dramatically affect the sensitivity of agglutination tests. Consistently preparing a 1–5% RBC suspension is critical for agglutination studies.

Pooled Cell Suspension

1. Label the tubes with A, B, and O groups.
2. Add one drop of red cells from each of the three Group A sample tubes or segments into the A labeled tube.
3. Put one drop of red cells from each of the three Group B sample tubes or segments into the B labeled tube.
4. Put one drop of red cells from each of the three Group O sample tubes or segments into the O labeled tube.
5. Resuspend cells by filling all tubes 3/4 full with 0.9% saline.
6. Centrifuge the tubes at 2,000 rpm for 2 minutes. Decant the supernatant fluid.
7. Repeat steps 5 and 6 twice to properly wash the cells. The third washing should be in LISS solution.
8. Now, using a semi-automatic micropipette, take 10 µL of the packed RBCs and mix with 1,000 µL of LISS to make 1% suspension. To prepare 5% suspension of RBCs, take 25 µL of the packed RBCs and mix with 500 µL of LISS.
9. Test the pooled cells suspension thus prepared using antisera (anti-A, B, AB, and D).
    Donor/patients' cell suspension:
    a. Centrifuge the donor's blood sample at 2,000 rpm for 10 minutes.
    b. Take 10 µL of packed red blood cells (PRBCs) and mix in 1,000 µL of LISS to make 1% suspension.
    c. For making 5% suspension of PRBCs, take 25 µL of the PRBCs and mix in 500 µL of LISS.
10. Cells should be refrigerated at 4 ± 2°C when not in use.

Note:
- Hemolysis of PRBC due to improper washing can lead to erroneous results. Too heavy or too light a cell suspension can lead to false-positive or false-negative results. PRBCs are washed with isotonic saline to remove all traces of plasma or serum. They then need to be accurately diluted to prepare standard suspensions in saline/LISS solution.

- For automated immune-hematology analyzers, prepare a red cell suspension by washing with normal saline and mixing 40 μL of packed cells with 1,000 μL of normal saline to prepare 4% red cell suspension.

DOCUMENTATION

Record the donor unit IDs from which pooled cells are prepared in a register. Record the test results of testing the pooled cells with the antisera used in register. Mention the manufacturer's name and batch number of the antisera used for testing of pooled cells.

ABO Blood Grouping

SCOPE AND APPLICATION

This standard operating procedure (SOP) describes the method to determine an individual's ABO group correctly and ensure the reliability of the results. This procedure describes how to detect ABO antigens in the red blood cell and the reciprocal antibodies in the serum (Landsteiner's Law). It provides guidance for detecting weak variants, acquired antigens, Bombay (Oh) blood group, and irregular red cell antibodies using blood group reagents (antisera and standard red blood cells).

RESPONSIBILITY

The determination of ABO groups of donors and patients is the responsibility of the blood center laboratory technician under the supervision of the medical officer. Both red blood cell tests (forward grouping) and serum tests (reverse grouping) must be performed, except umbilical cord blood and peripheral blood typing for infants <4 months of age and red blood cell (RBC) unit confirmation, wherein only a forward grouping is performed. If these cells contain antigens for which cold-active alloantibodies other than anti-A or anti-B are present in the patient's plasma, a reaction with the reverse grouping cells is obtained. If possible, the reverse grouping must be repeated at a higher temperature or using reverse grouping cells that lack the implicated antigen. If the results of forward and reverse grouping do not match and reverse reactions differ, the "ABO discrepancy" should be further tested and resolved.

MATERIALS REQUIRED

- *Equipment*:
  - Refrigerator to store blood samples and reagents/diagnostic kits at 2–6°C
  - Tabletop centrifuge
  - Microscope
  - Incubator
- *Specimen*:
  - Clotted and anticoagulated blood samples of donor/patient
  - Test red cells suspension
- *Reagents*:
  - Anti-A, anti-B, and anti-AB sera
  - Groups A, B, and O pooled cells
  - 0.9% saline
  - Distilled water
- *Glassware*:
  - Serum tubes
  - Microtubes
  - Pasteur pipettes
  - Glass slides
- *Miscellaneous*:
  - Rubber teats
  - Disposal box
  - Sticks
  - Two plastic beakers
  - Test tube racks

PROCEDURE

Principle

The ABO system is the only system in which there is a reciprocal correlation between the antigens on the red blood cells and the naturally occurring antibodies in serum. Therefore, routine blood grouping of donors and patients should include both RBC and serum tests to serve as a cross-check each on the other. This method is based on the principle of agglutination of antigen-positive red blood cells in the presence of antibodies against the antigens. Three manual methods are available for blood grouping:

1. Glass slides or white tiles
2. Glass test tubes
3. Microwell plates or microplates

Glass slide or white tile method can be used for emergency ABO grouping or preliminary grouping, particularly in outdoor camps. However, it should always be supplemented with grouping of cells and serum by either tube or microplate techniques. It is not recommended for daily use due to unreliability in the following cases:

- Weakly reactive antigens on cells
- Grouping of serum with low titer anti-A or anti-B

It has always a drying effect that can cause aggregation of cells leading to false-positive results and weaker reactions that are difficult to interpret.

GLASS SLIDE OR WHITE TILE METHOD

1. Place one drop of anti-A reagent and one drop of anti-B reagent separately on a labeled slide or tile.
2. Add one drop of 20% red blood cell test suspension to each drop of the typing antiserum (suspension may be prepared by adding 20 parts of red blood cells to 80 parts of normal saline).
3. Mix cells and reagents with a clean stick. Spread each mixture evenly over an area of 10–15 mm diameter on the slide.
4. Tilt the slide and leave the test at room temperature (RT) (22–24°C) for 2 minutes. Then rock again to look for agglutination **(Fig. 1)**.
5. Record the results.

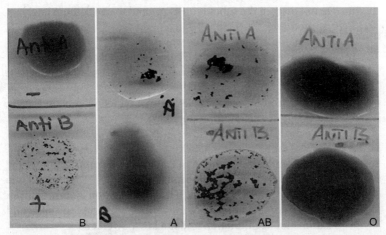

FIG. 1: Slide method for blood grouping. **(For color version, see Plate 5)**

Interpretation

Agglutination indicates positive results.

GLASS TEST TUBE METHOD

1. *Forward grouping*:
   a. Set the table and prepare the workbook.
   b. Verify the identity of blood samples on the labels, request forms, and workbooks.
   c. Prepare a 5% suspension of red blood cells in normal saline.
   d. Label three tubes as anti-A, anti-B, and anti-AB.
   e. Add one drop of antiserum to each labeled tube.
   f. Add one drop of red blood cell test suspension to each of the three tubes containing antiserum.
   g. Put up control to the fourth tube (add one drop of serum and test red cell suspension).
   h. Shake the tubes to mix well.
   i. Incubate for 10 minutes at RT.
   j. Centrifuge the tubes at 1,000 rpm for 1 minute, remove the tubes, and observe for hemolysis in the supernatant. Then, shake the tube to see if there is agglutination.
   k. If no agglutination is seen, transfer an aliquot of the contents of the tube to a microscope slide and examine for agglutination under a low-power lens.
   l. Record the grading of reaction on the worksheet.
   m. Do not discard the tubes (you may need to check them later).

2. *Reverse grouping*:
   a. Set the table and prepare the workbook.
   b. Label three tubes of A cells, B cells, and O cells.
   c. Add one drop of the unknown serum to be tested to each of these tubes.
   d. Add one drop of "pooled cells" from a panel of A1 cells, B cells, and O cells to the appropriate tubes.
   e. Shake the tubes to mix well.
   f. Incubate for 30 minutes at RT.
   g. Centrifuge the tubes for 1 minute at 1,000 rpm, remove the tubes, and observe for hemolysis in the tubes. Then, shake the tubes to see for agglutination. If no agglutination is seen, transfer an aliquot of the contents of the tube to a microscope slide and examine for agglutination under a low-power lens.
   h. Record the grading of reactions on the worksheet.
   i. Do not discard the tubes (you may need to check them later).

Defining the Strength of Reaction (Grading of Agglutination)

To record the difference in the strength of reaction, it is necessary to have a system of grading or scoring the reactions as depicted in **Table 1**.

INTERPRETATION

The interpretation of blood group is done as given in **Table 2**.

	Table 1: Degree of agglutination.
Grades	**Degree of agglutination**
4+	One solid agglutinate
3+	Several large agglutinates
2+	Medium-sized agglutinate with clear background
1+	Small agglutinates with turbid background
1+ w	Very small agglutinates with turbid background
W+ or +/–	Barely visible agglutination with turbid background
Zero/negative	No agglutination
mf	Mixtures of agglutinated and unagglutinated cells
H	Complete hemolysis (positive reaction)
Ph	Partial hemolysis, some red cells remain

Table 2: Interpretation of blood groups.							
Cell grouping (forward grouping)			**Forward interpretation**	**Serum grouping (reverse grouping)**			**Reverse interpretation**
Anti-A	**Anti-B**	**Anti-AB**		**A cells**	**B cells**	**O cells**	
+	–	+	A	–	+	–	A
–	+	+	B	+	–	–	B
–	–	–	O	+	+	–	O
+	+	+	AB	–	–	–	AB
–	–	–	O	+	+	+	Oh or any other irregular antibody

DISCREPANCIES BETWEEN CELL AND SERUM GROUPING RESULTS

Generally, the expected reactions for ABO red blood cell tests using anti-A and anti-B reagents are 3+ to 4+ agglutination reactions and ABO serum test results using reagent A1 cells and B cells are 2+ to 4+. ABO discrepancy is defined as discordance between results of red cell testing and results of expected serum testing or where expected reaction grading is more than grade 3 in the forward group and grade 2 in the reverse group or when there is discrepancy between historical results and current test results. In such cases, interpretation of blood group must not be concluded but the results should be recorded and further testing should be done to rule out "ABO discrepancies."

PRECAUTIONS

- Do not rely on your memory.
- If you get distracted during the test and do not remember where you put it, start the entire test over again.
- Always add serum to the tubes first, and check for its presence in the tube before adding the cell suspension to the same tube.
- If possible, have another person for double-check and record the results.

Rh Blood Grouping

SCOPE AND APPLICATION

Routine Rh grouping of red blood cells (RBC) involves a recipient's D-antigen testing and donor's D and Du-antigen testing. Testing for other important Rh antigens, such as C, c, E, and e, can be done with Rh genotyping if there is a specific reason to do so. The method of Rh grouping should be performed according to the manufacturer's instructions for the reagents used. However, this standard operating procedure (SOP) provides instructions for the use of anti-D blood group reagents.

RESPONSIBILITY

Blood center laboratory technicians are responsible for D-typing donors and patients using monoclonal and biclonal reagents under the supervision of medical officers. If there is a discrepancy between two batches of anti-D, another technician should repeat the test. If discrepancies persist, the medical officer should be notified. If the results of D typing of a blood donor are negative, perform the Du-typing procedure.

MATERIALS REQUIRED

- *Equipment*:
  - Refrigerator to store blood samples and grouping reagents at 2–6°C
  - Tabletop centrifuge
  - Microscope
  - Incubator

- *Specimen*:
  - Clotted or anticoagulated blood samples of donors
  - Clotted blood samples of patients
  - Red cells suspension
- *Reagents*: Different types of anti-Rh (D) sera
  - *Polyclonal human anti-D serum [immunoglobulin G (IgG)]*: Potentiating or enhancing substances such as albumin, enzymes, and antihuman globulin (AHG) reagents are used to bring about agglutination with human IgG anti-D.
    - o Anti-D serum (IgG) for saline or rapid tube test (high protein medium). This contains macromolecular additives and gives reliable results.
    - o There are two types of anti-D for saline tube testing:
      - i. Anti-D IgM
      - ii. Anti-D IgG-chemically modified
  - *Monoclonal anti-D reagents*:
    - o IgM anti-D monoclonal reagent
    - o IgM and IgG anti-D monoclonal reagent
    - o Blend of IgM monoclonal + IgG polyclonal reagent

    These antibodies are highly specific, react equally well at 20 and 37°C, and are reliable for slide and rapid test tube techniques. The monoclonal IgM anti-D reagent cannot be used for Du testing by indirect antiglobulin test (IAT), but IgM + IgG monoclonal reagent and blend of IgM monoclonal and IgG polyclonal can be used for Du testing. Use of potent anti-D reagents from two different manufacturers is recommended following the recommended technique.
  - *Controls for Rh (D) grouping*: Known O Rh (D) positive and O Rh (D) negative cells can be used as controls with monoclonal anti-D reagents.
  - Alternatively, AB serum or diluent control provided with the anti-D reagent or 22% bovine serum albumin can be used as a negative control with the test cells.
  - 0.9% saline
  - Distilled water
- *Glassware*:
  - Test tubes
  - Pasteur pipettes
  - Glass slides
- *Miscellaneous*:
  - Rubber teats
  - Plastic beakers
  - Wooden block to hold microtubes
  - Test tube rack
  - Rh view box

PROCEDURE

Three manual methods can be used for blood grouping:
1. Glass slide or white tile
2. Glass test tube
3. Microwell plate or microplate

SLIDE METHOD

This technique can be used for emergency Rh (D) typing when a centrifuge is not available. The slide test is not recommended for routine testing as it cannot detect weak reactions and may give negative results. A monoclonal IgM anti-D reagent is suitable for the slide method.

1. Take three slides and label as positive control, negative control, and test.
2. Place one drop of anti-D (monoclonal) reagent on each slide.
3. Add one drop of 20% test cell suspension to one drop of the typing antiserum. (A suspension can be prepared by adding 20 parts of RBC to 80 parts of normal saline).
4. Mix cells and reagent with a clean stick. Spread each mixture evenly on the slide over an area of 10–15 mm in diameter.
5. Place the slides on a view box surface (lighted) and tilt gently and continuously for 2 minutes.
6. Observe for agglutination **(Fig. 1)** and record the results. All negative results must be confirmed by microscopy.

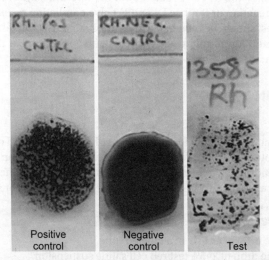

FIG. 1: Rh grouping showing agglutination in test and positive control.
(For color version, see Plate 6)

GLASS TEST TUBE METHOD

The method depends upon the type of the anti-D reagent used. Monoclonal anti-D will work in saline at room temperature, while others need to be incubated at 37°C. Therefore, instructions provided with the reagents by the manufacturers are to be followed.

Using Monoclonal Anti-D/Saline Agglutination Test

1. Add one drop of anti-D (Dl) to a clean tube labeled Dl and one drop of anti-D (D2) from another manufacturer in another clean tube labeled D2.
2. Add one drop of 22% bovine albumin/control reagent to the third tube labeled C.
3. Add one drop of 2–5% test cell suspension to each tube.
4. Mix well and centrifuge for 1 minute at 1,000 rpm (incubate if using IgG anti-D, incubate for 10 minutes at 37°C and centrifuge).
5. Resuspend the cell button and look for agglutination. All negative results are confirmed microscopically.

Interpretation

Positive test: Agglutination in anti-D both tubes and smooth suspension in control tube.

Negative test: Smooth suspension of RBC button in all the tubes (test and control).

Test is invalid: The test is invalid if both the test and control tubes give a positive reaction or if tubes Dl and D2 give conflicting results. In this case, the test should be repeated with saline IgM anti-D. Du testing must be performed for all microscopically negative reactions in the donor population.

ALBUMIN METHOD

Principle

Albumin increases the dielectric constant of the medium and decreases the zeta potential. This effect reduces the electrical repulsion between the RBC, leading to agglutination of cells. Normally, 22% bovine albumin is used because of rouleaux formation at higher concentrations.

Procedure

1. Put one drop of anti-D in a labeled tube.
2. Add one drop of 2–5% test red cell saline suspension.

3. Incubate for 45–60 minutes at 37°C.
4. Add one drop of 22% albumin along with wall of the tube. Albumin forms a layer on top of the red cells. Do not mix.
5. Incubate further for 15–20 minutes at 37°C.
6. Examine for agglutination after gentle shaking and confirm all negative results microscopically.

INTERPRETATION OF RESULTS (TABLE 1)

Antisera usually give a 2+ to 4+ reaction with the anti-D after immediate spin or a weak D test and negative reaction (O) in control cells. Tests not yielding 2+ to 4+ reaction require further investigation and testing.

The interpreted result may be *false positive* in the following cases:
- *Immunoglobulin coating of red cells*: In such cases, red cells are washed with normal saline and tested with saline-reactive anti-D.
- Poly-agglutinable red cells due to the presence of anti-T and anti-Tn antibodies in the serum. These cells are unlikely to affect the tests if commercial antisera are used.
- Contamination of anti-D with bacteria, foreign substance, or another antiserum
- If cells and antisera remain together for too long before the test is interpreted, the high protein medium may produce rouleaux resembling agglutination.

The results may be *false negative* in the following cases:
- Failure to add reagents
- Poor quality of reagents
- Incorrect cell-to-serum ratio
- Too heavy cell suspension in the tube may result in poor agglutination.
- Red cells having weak D antigen may not react well in the immediate spin-tube method.

Table 1: Interpretation of Rh grouping.			
Anti-D	**Rh control**	**Interpretation**	**Comment**
+*	0	Rh positive	
0	0	Rh negative	
+	+	Invalid test	The test is performed in saline-reactive anti-D
*If the strength reaction with the test cells is <2+, perform weak Du test on the red cells.			

CHAPTER 30

Testing for Weak Rh D Antigen

SCOPE AND APPLICATION

After the A and B antigens, serologic determination of D antigens status is the most important in blood transfusion practice and sometimes becomes problematic because of numerous factors like the use of different methods, use of reagents of various manufacturers, and the variability of the D antigen expression on some red blood cells (RBCs), leading to Rh typing discrepancies. The variants of the D antigen can be weak D (due to reduced number of D antigen sites on RBCs, but D antigen has all the epitopes) and partial D (qualitative variant, i.e., D antigen is characterized by the absence of one or more epitopes, but there is no difference in the number of sites on RBCs). It is important to identify a donor as partial D or weak D as the red cells of these donors could elicit an immune response if transfused to a negative recipient. But a recipient of partial D or weak D can be safely considered as Rh D negative and Rh-negative units can be used for transfusion. But at the same time, it is advisable to determine the correct Rh D status of patients because discrepancy in Rh D grouping will arise when these patients may become donors. At the blood center level, it can be difficult to distinguish between partial D and weak D, commonly referred to as weak D. This standard operating procedure (SOP) describes how all Rh D-negative individuals, whether slightly D or true Rh D-negative, are tested to determine their exact Rh D status.

RESPONSIBILITY

It is the responsibility of the blood center technician in the red cell serology laboratory to perform donor and patient Du typing by antiglobulin testing using a mixture of immunoglobulin M (IgM) + immunoglobulin G (IgG) monoclonal reagents.

MATERIALS REQUIRED

- *Equipment*:
  - Refrigerator for storing blood samples and grouping reagents at 2–6°C
  - Rh Du blood grouping
  - Tabletop centrifuge
  - Microscope
  - Incubator/dry bath
- *Specimen*:
  - A clotted or anticoagulated blood sample from a donor
  - A clotted blood sample from the patient
  - Test RBCs suspended in saline
- *Reagents*:
  - A mixture of monoclonal IgM + IgG reagents
  - Antihuman globulin (AHG—Coombs' reagent)
  - Known IgG-sensitized control cells
- *Glassware*:
  - Serum tubes
  - Microtube
  - Pasteur pipettes
  - Glass slides
- *Miscellaneous*:
  - Disposal box
  - Beakers
  - Wooden block to hold microtubes
  - Racks for holding serum tubes

PROCEDURE

1. Take two test tubes and label one tube "T" for test and the other tube "C" as a control.
2. Add two drops of anti-D (IgM + IgG monoclonal reagent) to the tube labeled "T."
3. Add two drops of normal saline as a control to another test tube marked "C."
4. Add one drop of a 5% suspension of washed RBCs to both tubes.
5. Mix both the test tubes and incubate at 37°C for 15–30 minutes.
6. Centrifuge at 1,000 rpm for 1 minute (or as specified by the manufacturer).
7. Carefully suspend the cell button and look for agglutination. If agglutination is present, the sample is Rh (D) positive and there is no need to proceed.
8. If negative, incubate at 37°C for an additional 30 minutes.

9. Centrifuge at 1,000 rpm for 1 minute. Check for agglutination.
10. Decant the supernatant, wash the cells with saline, and decant the supernatant three times.
11. Add two drops of AHG reagent (AHG—Coombs, reagent). Mix gently and centrifuge at 1,000 rpm for 1 minute.
12. Carefully resuspend the cell button and examine for agglutination. Record the grading of agglutination and interpret the results.

INTERPRETATION

For valid typing, the weak D control must be negative. Interpretation of Rh Du grouping is shown in **Table 1**.

Table 1: Interpretation of Rh Du grouping.		
Anti-D	*Control*	*Interpretation*
0	0	Rh negative
2+ to 4+	0	Rh positive
1+	0	Unable to determine—Additional test required
Positive	Positive	Unable to determine—Additional tests required

Note: All negative reactions should be confirmed by microscopy and by addition of known IgG-sensitized control cells, recentrifuged and reexamined for observing agglutination. The presence of agglutination confirms and validates the test results and indicates that the added AHG serum is reactive.

DISCREPANCIES AND PROBLEMS

- Improper and inadequate washing of RBC suspensions can lead to spurious agglutination due to the presence of serum macromolecules in suspension.
- Aggregation can occur when strong autoagglutinins are present in the serum of the recipient or donor. Proper washing and controls are designed to prevent or detect this problem.
- Antibody coating of the RBC [positive direct antiglobulin test (DAT)] can give rise to false-positive reactions, especially when tested for weak D. A DAT will detect this event.
- "Blocking phenomena" can lead to false-negative reactions. This is most common in hemolytic disease of the fetus and newborn (HDFN) due to anti-D. Antigenic sites on RBCs are thickly coated with maternal antibodies and may not react with antisera and hence the false-negative results.

- Technical errors can cause false-positive or false-negative reactions in the Rh test. RBCs reacting with one brand of anti-D reagent but not with another brand of anti-D reagent may have partial D antigen.

RESOLUTION

- If transfusion is required, transfuse Rh-negative RBC or whole blood before the conflict is resolved.
- When immediate spin results are invalid because of positive Rh control, the test is repeated with a new suspension of RBCs after washing twice with warm saline.
- When weak D test result is invalid because of positive DAT and a weak D determination is required, DAT is repeated after treating the patient's RBCs with chloroquine or glycine-ethylene-diaminetetraacetic acid (EDTA). Repeat the weak D test when DAT is negative.
- If weak D test agglutination <2+, patients are reported as Rh positive. Such patients are transfused with Rh-negative packed red blood cells (PRBCs) pending serological and clinical evaluation. In particular, a patient reacts with one manufacturer's anti-D reagent but not with another manufacturer's anti-D reagent; he/she may have a partial D antigen. Notify your immediate supervisor or blood center medical officer.
- Donors are labeled as Rh positive when agglutination is >2+ in weak D test.

CHAPTER 31

Antibody Screening

SCOPE AND APPLICATION

The purpose of antibody screening is to make sure that enough red blood cells will survive the transfusion for a sufficient period of time and that the blood is safe to transfuse. Blood grouping/crossmatching done alone may not be a suitable way to detect compatibility as this method hardly detects any incompatibility other than major mismatches. Undetected antibodies are responsible for adverse transfusion reactions that can manifest as immediate/delayed hemolytic transfusion reactions or could give rise to hemolytic disease of newborn. The antibody screen is done for people who:

- Require transfusion
- Are pregnant or postpartum women
- Are patients with suspected transfusion reactions
- are blood and plasma donors

Therefore, this standard operating procedure (SOP) describes how to detect clinically significant antibodies as early as possible so that blood centers have enough time to find matched blood.

RESPONSIBILITY

A blood center technician working in a serological laboratory is responsible to perform antibody screening of donors and patients. The medical officer of the blood center is informed in case of detection of unexpected blood group antibodies in any donor or patient.

MATERIALS REQUIRED

- *Equipment:*
    - Refrigerator for storing samples and reagents at 2–6°C
    - A deep freezer for storing enzyme papain cysteine in a frozen state

- Tabletop centrifuge
- Automated cell washer (for pretransfusion patients and prenatal testing)
- Microscope
- Incubator
- *Specimen*:
  - Clotted donor/patient blood samples
- *Reagents*:
  - Pooled group O cell/commercial antibody screening reagent red blood cells (two- or three-cell panel)
  - Papain cysteine
  - 22% bovine albumin
  - Antihuman globulin (AHG) reagent [anti-immunoglobulin G (IgG) + anti-C3d]
  - IgG-sensitized control cells
  - 0.9% saline
  - Distilled water
- *Glassware*:
  - Serum tubes
  - Coombs tubes (for pretransfusion patients and prenatal testing)
  - Microtubes
  - Pasteur pipettes
  - Glass slides
- *Miscellaneous*:
  - Disposal box
  - Beakers
  - Stand for microtubes
  - Racks for serum and Coombs tubes

PROCEDURE

Principle

In this test, pooled group O red blood cells or the antibody screening reagent red blood cells are combined with patient serum or plasma and incubated at 37°C. Addition of enzyme/albumin-enriched medium promotes the interaction of red blood cells with antibodies resulting in an antibody/antigen reaction. A positive test (hemolysis or agglutination) indicates the presence of alloantibodies or autoantibodies in the serum. A room temperature (20–25°C) saline test indicates the presence of cold antibodies (IgM) (anti-M, anti-N, anti-Le^a, anti-Le^b, anti-P, etc.) The enzyme technique enhances the reaction of Rh, Lewis, and Kidd antibodies, but certain antigens, i.e., M, N, S, Fy^a, and Fy^b, are weakened or inactivated. The indirect antiglobulin test (IAT) identifies the warm-reacting IgG and complement-binding allo- and autoantibodies.

The IAT which uses red blood cells suspended in low-ionic-strength saline (LISS) solution is considered optimal for detecting clinically relevant antibodies because of its speed, sensitivity, and specificity.

Donor blood is screened for antibodies with single cells and patients/recipient's blood is screened with the three-cell panel.

Method

1. Label test tubes with donor/patient and test identification.
2. Add two drops of test serum to each tube.
3. Add one drop of papain cysteine to all tubes labeled "enzyme" (if the enzyme method is being followed).
4. To each of the tubes labeled "saline" or "enzyme/albumin," add one drop of 2% pooled O red cell suspension (or 2% suspension of the antibody-screening reagent red cells).
5. Add one drop of 22% bovine albumin to tubes labeled "albumin" (if the albumin method is being followed).
6. Add one drop of 5% pooled O red cell suspension (or 5% suspension of antibody-screening reagent red cells) to tubes labeled "IAT," followed by two drops of 22% bovine albumin.
7. Mix the contents of the tubes gently and incubate for 1 hour for saline at room temperature (RT) and IAT at 37°C and incubate for 45 minutes for enzyme and albumin at 37°C.
8. Centrifuge saline, enzyme, and albumin tests tubes at 1,000 rpm for 1 minute.
9. Examine for hemolysis.
10. Gently resuspend the red cell button and examine for agglutination.
11. Examine all visually negative tests microscopically.
12. Grade and record test results immediately.
13. Proceed to perform antiglobulin phase of the IAT on tubes labeled "IAT."
14. Wash the cells three times with saline. Decant completely after last wash (washing can be done manually or using automated cell washer).
15. Add two drops of AHG reagent to the dry cell button.
16. Mix well and centrifuge at 1,000 rpm for 1 minute.
17. Read and record results.
18. Add one drop of IgG-sensitized cells to all test tubes with negative results. This shows a positive agglutination.

INTERPRETATION

- Hemolysis or agglutination in vitro may indicate the presence of unexpected antibodies. A positive antibody screen requires further testing to identify the antibodies.

- Absence of screening cells agglutination or hemolysis at any stage of the test is a negative test result and indicates the absence of a blood group antibodies in the serum or plasma sample.
- After adding IgG-sensitized cells to the negative test, the presence of agglutination indicates that the added AHG serum is reactive and the negative antiglobulin test is valid.
- If the IgG-sensitized cells added to confirm for anti-IgG activity show weak or absence of agglutination after centrifugation, the test is invalid and should be repeated.

Note: If the test reacts with all the reagent red blood cells, the possibility of spontaneous agglutination must be considered. Controls from cells washed three to four times and added to two drops of saline need not be reactive.

ANTIBODY IDENTIFICATION

Antibody identification follows a positive result of antibody screening. Antibody identification involves testing serum or plasma against a panel of reagent red blood cells. Panels such as the screening cells consist of group O reagent red cells populated for the most common antigens specificities. Commercially available cell panels are available in various antigen configurations of 10, 11, 15, 16, or 20 cells and can be viewed as advanced antibody screens. The use of auto control with the panel is recommended, especially if not routinely tested in screening cell panels.

After the test is completed, the results of each test phase are recorded on the antigram provided with the kit. The stage or reaction temperature at which agglutination occurs indicates that the antibody is IgG or IgM. IgM antibodies usually react at room temperature or immediately by centrifugation and IgM antibodies such as anti-Le^a, -Le^b, -M, -N, -I, and -P$_1$ are suspected. IgG antibodies react in the antiglobulin phase. Reactions in different phases indicate presence of multiple antibodies of both IgG and IgM types. After recording the results on the antigrams provided with the cell panel, the following steps identify the antibody.

- *Ruling out*: Antibodies can be ruled out using cells that are negative for all stages tested. If no antigen–antibody reaction occurs, indicating that the antibody does not react with the antigen present in the panel cells, the corresponding antigen can be ruled out to exclude the antibody. Heterozygous antigens should not be crossed out as antibodies may be too weak to react. This process is repeated for each negative cell.
- *Matching patterns*: The next step in panel interpretation is to examine positive reactions that match patterns. When a single antibody is present, the observed response pattern matches that of other cells.

- *Rule of three*: The rule of three requires that at least three antigen-positive red cells reactions and three antigen-negative red cells are observed.
- *Phenotyping the patient*: Individuals do not produce alloantibodies to antigens they carry. Another way to confirm antibody identification is to phenotype the patient's red blood cells to confirm that they are negative for the antigen corresponding to the identified antibody.

CROSSMATCH VERSUS ANTIBODY SCREENING

Crossmatching is often less reliable than antibody screening because some antibodies exhibit a dose effect. To illustrate the dose effect, let us look at an example of the Kidd blood group system, which has two major antigens Jk^a and Jk^b, as shown in **Table 1**.

In the above example, cell I retains the homozygous expression of Jk^a and expresses higher Jk^a antigen than the cell III, which retains the heterozygous expression of both Jk^a and Jk^b.

In crossmatching, the donor erythrocyte phenotype (antigenic configuration of red cells) is unknown, and it is possible that the patient has anti-Jk^a and donor red cells carry heterozygous expression of Jk^a. This gives compatible crossmatch even in the presence of corresponding antibodies.

For these reasons, an antiglobulin crossmatching with donor cells is not the most effective method for detecting serological incompatibility. Crossmatching detects the presence of antibodies in the patient's serum/plasma that correspond to antigens present on donor's red blood cells.

A negative or compatible crossmatch means that antibodies corresponding to the antigens of donor's red cells are absent in patient's serum/plasma. However, a compatible crossmatch does not mean that atypical antibodies are absent from the patient's serum/plasma.

Table 1: Kidd blood group system showing homozygous and heterozygous effect.			
Cell	*Jkª*	*Jkᵇ*	*Remarks*
Cell I	+	−	This cell is having homozygous expression of Jkª
Cell II	−	+	This cell is having homozygous expression of Jkᵇ
Cell III	+	+	This cell is having heterozygous expression of Jkª and Jkᵇ

DOCUMENTATION

- Record the results of the donor antibody screening in the donor grouping register
- Record the patient's antibody screening results in the patient grouping register
- All records are initialed by the blood center technician performing the test and by the technical supervisor verifying the results.

Pretransfusion Testing (Compatibility Testing)

SCOPE AND APPLICATION

The purpose of pretransfusion testing is to minimize the risk of transfusion reactions by selecting blood and blood components that have an acceptable transfusion survival rate and that the transfusion does not destroy the recipient's red blood cells (RBC).

The terms "compatibility testing" or "pretransfusion" and "crossmatching" are sometimes used interchangeably, but they are not. They should be clearly distinguished. Crossmatch is only part of the "compatibility test." It refers to the series of steps required before blood compatibility is confirmed and includes:

- Review of patient's past transfusion history and records [ABO and Rh blood groups]
- Recipient and donor ABO and Rh groups
- Antibody screening of recipient and donor sera
- Selection of blood for patient
- Crossmatching

Crossmatch is the final verification of ABO compatibility between donor and patient. This also ensures that no antibodies are present in the patient's serum and that antibodies in the patient's serum do not react with the donor cells during the transfusion. This procedure is used to assess tolerance in all patients requiring blood transfusions.

RESPONSIBILITY

A laboratory technician in the blood center is responsible for performing the crossmatch to find out the compatible blood for the patient.

MATERIALS REQUIRED

- *Equipment*:
  - Refrigerator for storing blood samples and reagents at 2–6°C
  - A deep freezer for storing enzyme papain/cysteine in a frozen state
  - Tabletop centrifuge
  - Microscope
- *Specimen*:
  - A clotted blood sample from a donor/patient
- *Reagents*:
  - Pooled group O cells/commercially available antibody-screening reagent RBCs (two or three cells)
  - Papain/cysteine
  - 22% bovine albumin
  - Antihuman globulin (AHG) reagent [anti-immunoglobulin G (IgG) + anti-C3d]
  - IgG-sensitized control cells
  - Normal saline (0.9%)
  - Distilled water
- *Glassware*:
  - Test tubes
  - Micropipettes
  - Glass slides
- *Miscellaneous*:
  - Beakers
  - Racks for serum and Coombs tubes

PROCEDURE

The crossmatch test procedure is divided into two parts:

1. A major crossmatch in which RBCs of the donor are mixed with the serum of recipient (patient)
2. A small crossmatch that mixes the donor's plasma with the recipient's (patient's) RBCs

Most blood centers avoid minor crossmatching because donor samples are prescreened for antibodies. The main crossmatch techniques are:

- Saline technique
- Albumin technique
- Enzyme technique
- Indirect antiglobulin technique

SALINE METHOD

Preparation of Donor Red Cell Suspension

Cut a segment of tubing from the donor unit to be crossmatched. Cut open the segment and add one drop of red cells into the test tube labeled only with the donor number and prepare 2–5% red cell suspension after washing with normal saline. Inspect the donor unit at this time. Any unit which appears contaminated (i.e., cloudy or discolored) should not be used.

Saline Crossmatching Method

1. Mark the two small test tubes as "major" and "minor."
2. Add a drop of the recipient's serum in the test tube marked "major."
3. Add one drop of the donor's serum to the test tube marked "minor."
4. Add one drop of the donor's RBC suspension to the test tube marked "major."
5. Add one drop of recipient's RBC (washed and suspended in saline to form suspension) in the test tube marked "minor."
6. Mix well and incubate at room temperature for 90 minutes (or at 37°C for 30 minutes).
7. For the immediate spin method, incubate for 5–10 minutes at room temperature, centrifuge for 1 minute at 1,000 rpm.
   Observe for agglutination. No agglutination means that donor and recipient blood is compatible.

Interpretation

- Presence of agglutination indicates an ABO mismatch. ABO blood grouping is repeated for the recipient and the donor.
- If there is absence of agglutination in the saline technique and no antibody screening is performed, proceed to the antiglobulin crossmatch.

BOVINE ALBUMIN METHOD

This test is similar to the "saline method" with the following differences:

1. Add one drop of bovine albumin (10–20%) to the test tube containing the recipient's serum to layer on the top of the serum.
2. Next, add the donor RBC suspension to this test tube. RBCs are allowed to sediment through the albumin before they come in contact with the serum.
3. Incubate and read as for "saline technique."

ENZYME METHOD

This test is similar to the bovine albumin test except that one drop of papain cysteine reagent instead of bovine albumin is added.

1. Incubate for 1 hour at 37°C
2. Look for agglutination. Agglutination should not occur if the donor and recipient blood are compatible.

Note: Autocontrol should be put up.

INDIRECT ANTIGLOBULIN METHOD

This test is performed similar to as described under "saline method" with the following additions:

1. After incubating the mixture of donor cells and recipient serum, wash the RBC with normal saline at least four times.
2. The cells are resuspended in a drop of normal saline.
3. Add a drop of Coombs serum (AHG serum).
4. Incubate at room temperature (RT) for 10 minutes and centrifuge at 1,000 rpm for 1 minute.
5. Look for agglutination both macroscopically and microscopically.
6. If there is no agglutination, add one drop of control IgG-coated cells.
7. Centrifuge at 1,000 rpm again for 1 minute.

Look for hemolysis or agglutination. The test is invalid and must be repeated if there is no agglutination.

INTERPRETATION

- The blood unit is serologically compatible with the patient if there is no agglutination/hemolysis at all phases of testing and can be reserved for the patient if other criteria are met.
- Hemolysis or agglutination at any stage of the test indicates an incompatibility between the donor's red cells and patient's serum. Further investigations are required and unit may not be released until the problem is resolved.
- The presence of agglutination on adding IgG-sensitized cells to a negative test indicates that the added AHG serum is reactive and the negative antiglobulin test is valid.

Causes of an Incompatible Crossmatch in Negative Antibody Screening

- Error in donor or patient ABO grouping.
- Presence of an antibody to a low-incidence antigen in the patient's serum or to another antigen not present in the screening cells (e.g., anti-Kp^a or anti-A$_1$, respectively).

- Direct antiglobulin test (DAT)-positive donor
- Presence of double dose of antigen (homozygous donor) in the donor cells, but the antibody screening cells contain antigen in a single dose. In case the patient's antibodies are not strong enough to react with single-dose screening cells, antibody screening test will be negative ("dosage effect") and crossmatch will be incompatible.

Note: Antibodies that give stronger reactivity with double-dose red cells than single-dose red cells are referred to as antibodies demonstrating dosage effect.

- Rouleaux
- Presence of cold allo- or autoantibody.

Incompatibility Resolution

Cold alloantibodies or autoantibodies are the most likely causes of positive crossmatches after negative antibody screening. However, errors in patient blood grouping or labeling error of blood unit should be ruled out immediately in cases of ABO incompatibilities.

If the patient's antibody test is negative and the immediate-spin (IS) crosscheck is positive, do the following:

- The unit and patient specimen are checked for any clerical error and confirm the blood grouping of the donor and the patient ABO. Both forward and reverse groupings are done to rule out the possibility of anti-A$_1$.
- Initiate a second prewarmed AHG crossmatch(s) after rouleaux formation is ruled out.
- If the donor's DAT is positive, repeat the crossmatch with new unit.

Perform antibody screening including identification of cold antibodies. If there are no discrepancies in the ABO blood grouping, DAT in the donor cells is negative, and there is no rouleaux.

Note:

- Blood units can be issued prior to completion of the workup without the need to sign an urgent blood request if an ABO incompatibility is ruled out, and both the antibody screening test and the IS crossmatch with prewarmed elements are negative;
- Resolve the antibody problem if the antibody screen is positive after the immediate spin crossmatch and complete all crossmatch(s) on the patient through the antiglobulin phase.

When indirect antiglobulin test (IAT) crossmatch(s) is positive in a patient with a blood group antibody using donor RBCs lacking the corresponding antigen:

- Antibody identification procedure is checked for any errors.
- Testing for additional antibodies to low-incidence antigen is performed.

After completion of the above test, select antigen-negative units and/or an appropriate crossmatch technique (e.g., use of autoadsorbed specimen or prewarmed technique) and repeat the crossmatch(s).

DOCUMENTATION

- Enter the results into the crossmatch register and compatibility report form.
- All records are initialed by the blood center technician who performed the tests and by the technical supervisor verifying the results.

Direct Coombs Test/Direct Antiglobulin Test

SCOPE AND APPLICATION

Antihuman globulin (AHG) serum recognizes immunoglobulin G (IgG) and/or C3d detects the presence of immune antibody (IgG) or the complement component (generally C3d) coated onto red cells. In the direct antiglobulin test, such sensitization of red blood cell (RBC) is tested when washed RBCs are incubated with AHG. Polyspecific AHG is most sensitive for detecting RBC sensitization as this is directed against both human IgG and complement. Monospecific antisera are used to detect only IgG or C3. When a direct antiglobulin test (DAT) is requested, an initial test using polyspecific AHG is performed. If this is positive, it is repeated using both monospecific reagents (anti-IgG and anti-C3) as a "reflex" test. The presence of human serum in the cell suspension will neutralize the AHG, leading to false-negative reactions. Therefore, RBCs must be washed repeatedly with saline to remove all serum before the addition of AHG. Verification of proper and complete washing is done by the addition of IgG-coated Coombs control cells ("check cells") to all negative AHG reactions.

RESPONSIBILITY

A laboratory technician in red cell serology laboratory is responsible for performing and documenting Coombs test result.

MATERIALS REQUIRED

- *Equipment:*
  - Tabletop centrifuge
  - Incubator
  - Microscope

- *Sample*:
  - Clotted blood sample of the patient
  - Ethylenediaminetetraacetic acid (EDTA)/citrate-phosphate-dextrose solution with adenine (CPDA) blood sample of the patient
- *Reagent*:
  - Low-ionic-strength saline (LISS) solution
  - Control cells (IgG-coated cells)
  - 2% suspension of reagent O cells
  - AHG reagent (Coombs serum)
- *Glassware*:
  - Glass test tubes
  - Glass slide

PROCEDURE

1. Set the table and label the test tubes. Prepare record books.
2. Add two drops of AHG reagent (Coombs serum) to a small tube after labeling it.
3. Check the identity of the specimen.
4. Make a 2% suspension of the red cells of the specimen in LISS after washing the cells three times.
5. Add one drop of the red cells to be tested to it. Mix by shaking.
6. Spin at 1,000 rpm for 1 minute.
7. Observe for agglutination with the naked eye. If no agglutination is seen, read the contents under a microscope (low power).
8. If the test is negative, add one drop of control cells (IgG-coated cells).
9. Mix and spin at 1,000 rpm for 1 minute and observe for agglutination.
10. Observe for agglutination with the naked eye. If no agglutination is seen, the result is invalid. Repeat the test.

    Repeat the test with monospecific reagents as when DAT is positive with polyspecific AHG, for all but cord blood workups.

Method using Monospecific Anti-IgG and Anti-C3

1. Label test tubes appropriately with patient ID and "IgG" and "C3."
2. Add one drop of the RBC suspension saline washed four times to each tube.
3. Add one or two drops of anti-IgG to the tube marked "IgG" and one or two drops of anti-C3 to the tube marked "C3" according to the manufacturer's instructions.

4. Mix and centrifuge at the appropriate speed and time according to manufacturer's instructions.
5. Observe the tubes for agglutination. If a reaction is equivocal or mixed field macroscopically, examine it under a microscope.
6. Record the results.
7. Add one drop of check cells as appropriate to any tube(s) with a negative reaction. Centrifuge and examine for agglutination

INTERPRETATION

- No agglutination means *negative direct Coombs test* (*DCT*)
- Presence of agglutination means *positive DCT*

DOCUMENTATION

Enter the results in investigation register.

CHAPTER 34

Indirect Coombs Test

SCOPE AND APPLICATION

Indirect Coombs test (ICT) is used to detect incomplete antibodies and complement binding antibodies in the serum of the patient. Red blood cells (RBCs) of O Rh positive group after washing are incubated with the serum of the patient. ICT is positive if agglutination occurs when centrifuged after addition of antihuman globulin (AHG) reagent. It is used to screen donor as well as recipient for atypical antibodies and screen pregnant women for immunoglobulin G (IgG) antibodies that cause hemolytic disease of the newborn after cross placenta into the fetal blood and to crossmatch the blood units for transfusion.

RESPONSIBILITY

It is the responsibility of the blood center technician in the red cell serology laboratory to perform ICT under supervision of the medical officer.

MATERIALS REQUIRED

- *Equipment*:
    - Tabletop centrifuge
    - Incubator
    - Microscope
- *Sample*:
    - Clotted blood sample of the patient
    - Ethylenediaminetetraacetic acid (EDTA)/citrate-dextrose solution with adenine (CPDA) blood sample of the patient
- *Reagent*:
    - Low-ionic-strength saline (LISS) solution
    - Control cells (IgG-coated cells)
    - 2% suspension of reagent O cells
    - AHG reagent (Coombs serum)

- 22% bovine albumin
- Papain/cysteine
- *Glassware*:
  - Glass test tubes
  - Glass slide
  - Pasteur pipettes
- *Miscellaneous*:
  - Test tube racks
  - Beakers

PROCEDURE

1. Add one drop of test serum in a pre-labeled test tube.
2. Add one drop of 2% suspension of reagent O RBC.
3. Incubate for 45–60 minutes at 37°C (for saline/albumin/enzyme) and the incubation time for LISS-suspended cells will be 10–15 minutes.
4. Observe for hemolysis or agglutination. Agglutination or hemolysis at this stage indicates presence of saline-reacting antibody.
5. Wash the cells four times in saline, if no hemolysis or agglutination.
6. Add one drop of AHG reagent to the washed cells and mix.
7. Centrifuge at 1,000 rpm for 1 minute.
8. Observe for agglutination. If no agglutination is seen, read the contents under a microscope (low power). Presence of agglutination means a positive ICT.
9. If the test is negative, add one drop of control cells (IgG-coated cells).
10. Mix and centrifuge for 1 minute at 1,000 rpm and observe for agglutination. If no agglutination is seen, the test is invalid and the test needs to be repeated.

Note: Auto-control is always put up with indirect antiglobulin test (IAT).

INTERPRETATION

- *No agglutination*: *IAT negative*
- *Agglutination present*: *IAT positive*

   Indirect antiglobulin test/indirect Coombs test is used to detect the presence of incomplete antibodies and complement-binding antibodies in the serum after coating these antibodies onto red cells in vitro in:

- Compatibility testing
- Screening for atypical antibodies in serum
- Detection of red cell antibodies not detected by other techniques (Le^a, K, Fy^a, Fy^b, Jk^a, Jk^b, etc.)

DOCUMENTATION

Enter the results in investigation register.

Saline Addition or Replacement Technique

SCOPE AND APPLICATION

A saline addition or replacement technique is used to distinguish rouleaux from true agglutination of red blood cells (RBCs). This method can be used in any test performed at 4°C, room temperature, or 37°C by direct agglutination, when rouleaux are suspected. Rouleaux are dispersed by the addition of saline or replacement with saline, whereas true agglutination will remain as such. A test that is negative after adding or replacing saline is considered negative.

RESPONSIBILITY

It is the responsibility of the blood center technician in the red cell serology laboratory to perform saline addition or replacement technique to distinguish between true agglutination and rouleaux formation.

MATERIALS REQUIRED

- Centrifuge
- Transfer pipettes
- 0.9% w/v saline
- Test tubes

PROCEDURE

Saline Addition Technique

1. After routine incubation and resuspension, proceed with the following steps in case the resuspended red cells suggest rouleaux formation.
2. Add one drop of saline to the test tube and mix gently.
3. Centrifuge for 15 seconds at 3,400 rpm.

4. Resuspend each test tube and read macroscopically.
5. Grade and record results
6. If the rouleaux persist, use the saline replacement technique.

Saline Replacement Technique

1. After routine incubation and resuspension, proceed with the following steps in case the resuspended red cells suggest rouleaux formation.
2. Centrifuge the test tube(s) for 15 seconds at 3,400 rpm.
3. Remove the plasma with a pipette.
4. Replace plasma with an equal volume of saline.
5. Mix the test tubes and centrifuge for 15 seconds at 3,400 rpm.
6. Resuspend each test tube and read macroscopically.
7. Grade and record results

INTERPRETATION

• Tests that are nonreactive after saline addition or replacement are considered negative.
• Tests that are reactive following saline addition or replacement are considered positive. Such test needs further investigation.

Note: Pseudoagglutination, called rouleaux, can be observed when RBCs are suspended in plasma or antiserum. This may be caused by the administration of plasma expanders or by protein abnormalities. Macroscopically, this agglutination is indistinguishable from true agglutination. Microscopically, it appears as distinctive "stack of coins" shape or as large, shiny rosettes. Rouleaux will disperse when suspended in saline. True agglutination is stable in the presence of saline.

Absorption and Elution
(for Weak Subgroups of A or B)

SCOPE AND APPLICATION

This is a method of checking for the presence of weaker antigens—A and B—on the surface of red blood cells (RBCs). The RBCs are incubated with the appropriate antisera to absorb antibodies, i.e., known antibody is incubated with unknown RBCs to see if the cells will take up the antibodies. The antigens on the red cells and the antibody present in the antiserum form antigen–antibody complex; in other words, the part of antibody is absorbed on the red cells. After absorption and subsequent washing away of unbound serum, bound antibody is eluted, usually by raising the temperature to about 56°C. The elute is then tested on the appropriate group of indicator cells. Agglutination indicates the presence of antigens with the same specificity as that of the indicator cells.

RESPONSIBILITY

It is the responsibility of the laboratory technician in the red cell serology laboratory to perform the absorption and elution test for detection of weak antigens of A or B group under direct supervision of a medical officer.

MATERIALS REQUIRED

- *Equipment*:
  - Refrigerator to store blood samples and reagents at 2–6°C
  - Tabletop centrifuge
  - Microscope
  - Incubator/dry bath
  - Water bath

- *Specimen*:
  - Clotted or anticoagulated blood samples
- *Reagents*:
  - Anti-A$_1$/anti-B
  - Pooled O group red cells
  - Pooled A$_1$ cells/pooled B cells
  - Normal saline
- *Glassware*:
  - Serum tubes
  - Microtubes
  - Pasteur pipettes
  - Glass slides
- *Miscellaneous*:
  - Rubber teats
  - Disposal box
  - Two plastic beakers
  - Wooden block to hold microtubes
  - Aluminum racks to hold serum tubes

PROCEDURE

Absorption and Elution

1. Wash 1 mL of cells to be tested at least three times with saline. Discard the supernatant after the last wash.
2. Add 1 mL of anti-A$_1$ to red cells if a weak variant of A is suspected or 1 mL of anti-B if a weak variant of B is suspected.
3. Mix the cells with antisera and incubate at room temperature for 1 hour.
4. Centrifuge the mixture and discard the supernatant antisera.
5. Wash the cells with 10 mL of normal saline five times, discarding the supernatant.
6. Save the supernatant of the fifth wash to test for free antibody.
7. Add an equal volume of saline to the washed and packed cells and mix.
8. Elute the adsorbed antibody by placing the tube at 56°C in water bath for 10 minutes and mix the red cell saline mixture at least once during this period.
9. Centrifuge and remove the cherry-colored elute and discard the cells.

Testing the Elute

1. If anti-A was used, test the elute against three different samples of A$_1$ cells and three group O cells at room temperature at 37°C.

2. If anti-B was used, test the elute against three different samples of B cells and three group O cells at room temperature at 37°C.
3. Test the fifth saline wash in the same manner to show that the washing has removed all antibody not bound to the cells.

INTERPRETATION

- If the elute agglutinates or reacts with specific A or B cells and does not react with O, then the tested cells have active A or B antigens on their surface that can bind with specific antibody.
- If the elute also reacts with O cells, it indicates nonspecific reactivity of elute and the result is invalid.
- Elution test results are not valid if the fifth saline wash reacts with A and B cells. This indicates that there was an active antibody in the medium that was not bound to the cells under test.

Automation in Immunohematology

CONVENTIONAL VERSUS AUTOMATION IN IMMUNOHEMATOLOGY

Conventional immunohematology testing techniques prior to transfusion are very cumbersome. The most commonly used conventional tube technology remains the gold standard but has many limitations, especially in busy blood centers. The inherent drawbacks of the manual tube method are as follows:

- Variation in red blood cell concentration in the red blood cell suspension that affects the antigen to reagent/antibody ratio.
- Elution of low-affinity antibodies during washing by centrifugation
- Inconsistent agglutination grading and subjective results interpretation
- Human errors

In response to current good manufacturing practices, automated systems have emerged that provide blood centers with accurate and reproducible testing techniques using:

- Microplate method
- Column agglutination technology (CAT)
- Solid phase red blood cell adherence assay (SPRCA)
- Molecular blood grouping

These new technologies are automatable, both fully or semiautomated, and user friendly. Semiautomated and fully automated equipment have been developed for immunohematology testing with variable throughput. One can select the desired system depending on the workload and the tests to be performed in the blood center. These systems can perform ABO and Rh phenotyping, unexpected antibody detection and identification, major and minor crossmatching, antibody titration in both saline phase and antihuman globulin (AHG) phase, direct antiglobulin test (DAT) and indirect antiglobulin test, weak D test, extended antigen phenotyping, etc. The automated platforms

BIO-RAD, Ortho-Clinical Diagnostics, and Grifols are based on CAT. The IMMUCOR platform is based on the SPRCA principle and DIAGAST is based on the innovative erythrocyte magnetized (EM) technology. Equipment selection depends on the following factors:

- Installation-related issues (additional requirements and issues during installation, such as time from completion of installation to normal use of actual equipment, air conditioning, electrical upgrades for water purification systems, etc.)
- Training of staff
- Backup of automation equipment
- Customer service support (handling times for customer service calls, competence of provider's customer service representatives, personnel training, etc.)
- Reagent supply chain
- Other end-user issues

Column agglutination technology is described here as an introduction to automation. CAT has the following advantages over traditional tube methods:

- Forward and reverse grouping is performed simultaneously.
- Delivers clear objective results
- Agglutination patterns are easy to read.
- Reaction patterns are stable and can be stored for several days with the image of the reaction.
- Cells not required to be washed for antigen typing or for DAT
- Procedural controls are integrated into the cards.
- Ensures standardization with consistent results
- Saves time
- Revolutionized blood center work and gained wide acceptance

The CAT system consists of a plastic card containing six to eight microtubes for easy labeling. The top of the microtube contains a large reaction chamber and the bottom contains a matrix of microbeads. It uses the principle of controlled centrifugation of red blood cells through a matrix of prearranged microbeads and appropriate reagents predispensed in specially designed microtubes. A measured volume of serum or plasma and/or red blood cells is dispensed into the reaction chamber of a microtube. The card is centrifuged after incubation. If agglutination is present, the red blood cells are trapped in the microbead matrix according to the degree of agglutination. Unagglutinated red blood cells will pellet at the bottom of the microtube.

INTERPRETATION OF RESULTS

The agglutination reactions are graded from 0 to 4+ as shown in **Figure 1**.

This technology is marketed by many manufacturers. One such automated system manufactured by Ortho Clinical Diagnostics (OCD)

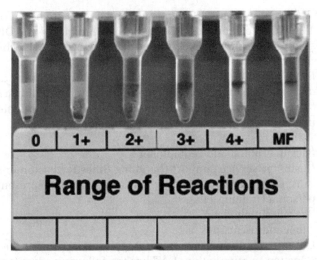

FIG. 1: Range of reaction grading. (*For color version, see Plate 6*)

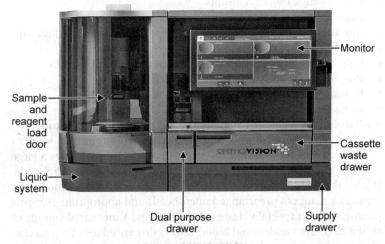

FIG. 2: ORTHO VISION.

is ORTHO VISION **(Fig. 2)**. The Ortho-Workstation (semiautomated) is also provided for performing various immunohematology tests with improved efficiency.

This system uses CAT, but the difference is that the microtubes have a glass microbead matrix instead of a gel bead matrix. The ORTHO VISION analyzer is an automated immunohematology analyzer that gives blood centers the flexibility to perform highly stressful transfusion scenarios in a simpler and reliable way. It provides accurate results. It runs blood types, antibody screens, immunoglobulin G (IgG) crossmatches, indirect Coombs test (ICT), direct Coombs test (DCT), antibody panels, antigen typing, and dilutions. All of these immunohematology testing methods have reduced the manual input and improved efficiency. Technicians do not have to worry about forgetting maintenance because the machine would not run without maintenance.

Assay processing functions, including liquid pipetting, reagent handling, incubation, centrifugation, reaction grading, result interpretation, and data management requirements, are automated using cards and digital image processing with the ORTHO VISION analyzer. The ORTHO VISION analyzer can be used as a stand-alone instrument or connected to the user's laboratory information system (LIS).

Automation has brought quality to immunohematology testing with following advantages:

- A barcode system prevents errors in sample and reagent identification and processing
- Helps to minimize the error opportunities as the manual steps are limited in the process
- Helps to improve precision and accuracy in samples, reagents, and red cells metering
- Prevents human error when interpreting results
- Prevents transcription errors when documenting the results

Explaining the operation of all automated analyzers is beyond the scope of this book. To understand the process of automation, the operation of the ORTHO VISION analyzer with standard operating procedures (SOPs) is described below.

OPERATION OF ANALYZER

Switch on the System

The system may be off, idle, or processing. If the system is off, you will need to start it and load system fluids and supplies.

1. Confirm that the system is connected to a power outlet.
2. Press the "ON" switch located on the lower right side of the system.

If the system is idle or processing, review the status screen and respond to any needs or errors.

Note: On startup, there is a short time period for log on with maintenance permissions (Field Service or Key Operator as directed by Service). Note that the system does not initialize after the Service Log in, leaving the system in a maintenance state.

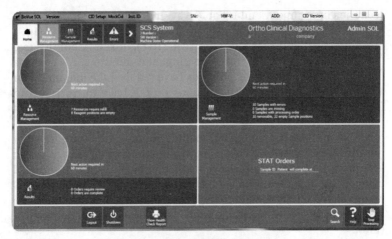

FIG. 3: Screen status for any error (red color) and review status (yellow color).
(*For color version, see Plate 7*)

A normal system startup leaves the system in an operational state. The system will perform device and consumable inventories. The system will post an error for the incubator (37°C) module until the required temperature is attained. It will also post an error that requests the saline/deionized (DI) water to be filled and the liquid waste to be emptied.

If starting up after an urgent shutdown, any orders in the work list/database with status running will be flagged as aborted. The system will discard any cards or cassettes found onboard and perform an inventory. *Warning*: The system assumes that fluid reservoirs are full on any startup (**Fig. 3**).

Screen Status

Log on to the system:
1. Touch anywhere on the home-dashboard status screen to log on.
2. Enter the username (as assigned) and password (as assigned).
3. Press Enter.

After LOG on screen view (**Fig. 4**).

Setting User-defined or Third-party Reagents/Reagent Red Cells to Use in ORTHO VISION

1. Click on stop processing on the bottom right of the screen.
2. In the new window, click on "Stop processing" icon.
3. Touch Set up.
4. Touch "Testing" under Tools.

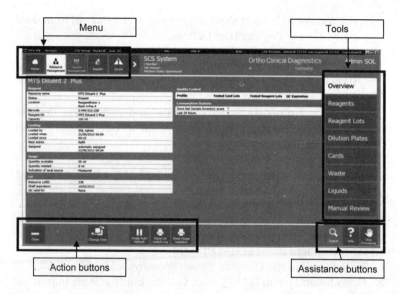

FIG. 4: Screen view after Log on.

5. Touch Reagent kits (*register user-defined reagent kit and link to an OCD reagent kit*).
6. Touch Show details (*select appropriate OCD reagent kit from the list on the left side of the screen*).
7. Add user-defined kit (*enter reagent kit name that you want to create*).
8. Touch Save.
9. Touch Back.
10. Select user-defined/created reagent from the list shown on the left side of the screen.
11. Touch Resume processing.

Registration of Reagent Lots

1. For registering the new reagent lots, Touch "Reagent Lots" under Tools button.
2. For OCD reagents with barcodes, select "Register OCD Lot."
3. In the new window, scan the barcode of the reagent and the second input of the barcode or manually enter the barcode number twice.
4. Touch "Verify." System will show the Lot No. and Exp date of the reagent.
5. Click "Register Lot." Now the reagent lot will be registered and displayed.

6. For registering user-defined reagent lots or reagent lots from third party, Touch "Register User Defined."
7. Select the "User-defined Reagent kit" from the list displayed.
8. Scan the barcode of the Reagent if available, or enter the Reagent ID twice for all the reagents and Touch Next.
9. Enter the Lot ID twice, Touch "Verify" > "Next."
10. Enter the expiry date, Touch "Validate" and then Touch "Register Lot." Now the user-defined reagent lot will be registered and displayed.

Load Saline, Deionized Water, Reagents, and Cassettes

Check Fluids/Waste

(*Note*: If you have stopped processing, the empty waste buttons are inactive; for adding inventory, Touch resume processing > Yes and wait for the Instrument status as operational.)

1. To Refill saline and DI water, Touch *Resources > Liquids > Refill.*
2. Open liquid system (LSYS) door, pull the bottle release button for saline/distilled water container and remove the container.
3. Refill the containers with 4,700 mL of saline and 900 mL of distilled water. Load the container using the bottle insertion tool and close the door.
4. To empty liquid waste, Touch *Resources > Waste > Empty.*
5. Discard the liquid waste down the drain and clean with tap water.
6. Reload the empty liquid waste bottle using the bottle insertion tool and close the door.
7. To empty used cassettes, Touch *Resources > Waste > Empty Dry.*
8. Open the access door to waste tray and remove the cassette waste container.
9. Discard the used cassettes, clean the waste tray, and reload the tray in the system.

Load Consumables

1. For loading cassettes, Touch *Resources > Cassettes > Load/Unload.*
2. Wait for the cassette loading area (CCLA) door to unlock. Open the CCLA, load the cassettes as required, and close the door.
3. The system takes the inventory.
4. For loading Reagents, Touch *Resources > Reagents.*
5. Select the position to load the "Reagent rack." Reagent red cells in the agitating position 1 or 2 or 3; for BLISS or red cell diluent, select nonagitating position 4.
6. For loading reagents, place the reagents in the specified tray after removing the caps.

7. For the red cell reagents, the vials can be capped with pierceable caps, which helps in enhancing the on-board stability of the red cell reagents, such as reverse grouping cells and antibody screening or identification cell panels.
8. Select "Load/Unload" icon.
9. Wait for the door to unlock.
10. Open the door, load the reagent rack in the specified position, and close the door.
11. System recognizes the bar-coded reagents and takes the inventory.

Loading non-bar-coded reagents:
1. After loading the non-bar-coded reagents as mentioned above, the system showed the vial position in red color, as it could not recognize the reagents.
2. Touch the vial position in red color.
3. Touch "Assign to Position" and open the door as specified by the system.
4. Select the specific reagent from the drop-down list.
5. Select the lot that is already registered from the drop-down list.
6. Select the reagent and close the door.
7. System takes the inventory and now the reagent position will be green in color.
8. For loading dilution trays, touch "Dilution trays" under Tools button.
9. Touch the position between 1 and 6 for loading Dilution trays and then Touch Load/Unload button.
10. Wait for the door to unlock. Open the door; load the dilution tray in the specified position.
11. To load diluent tray in other positions, select the desired position. The rotor moves to that position.
12. Load the dilution tray in the position and close the door.

Processing Samples

1. For Sample Processing, select "Samples" icon.
2. Samples can be processed using "Create order" or "Batch Order"
3. For processing using "Create Order," click on "Create Order."
4. Click on "Sample ID" and enter Sample ID details twice.
5. Select Sample type, if it has to be changed from "Cent blood" to "Packed cells," "3 Cells," "0.8 cells," or "Plasma."
6. Click on "Assigned Profiles" and select the profiles for the particular sample ID.
7. If it is an urgent/STAT sample, select "Priority" and select "STAT."
8. Click on "Save and Start."

9. If the Assigned Profile is crossmatch, click on "Add donor Sample." For single donor, click once.
10. Select "Donor ID 1" and enter donor details twice.
11. Select "Sample type" as Cent blood or Packed cells.
12. Click on "Add donor sample" if the second donor is to be added or click on "Save and Start."
13. For processing using "Batch order," click on "Batch Order."
14. Select Sample IDs from the list of samples loaded on the Instrument.
15. Click on "Assigned Profiles" and select the profiles for the particular sample ID.
16. Click on "Save and Start."
17. For loading samples, select "Samples."
18. Touch the position between 1 and 6 for loading sample trays and then Touch "Load/Unload" button.
19. Wait for the door to unlock. Open the door and load the sample tray in the specified position.
20. To load in another position, select the desired position; the rotor moves to that position. Load the sample tray and close the door.
21. System recognizes the bar-coded samples and starts processing as per the order.
22. For the nonbar-coded samples, the system shows the vial position in red color.
23. Touch the vial position in red color.
24. Touch "Assign to Position" and open the door as specified by the system.
25. Enter the patient/donor details twice and click on validate.
26. Close the door, and the instrument scans the sample, and the sample will be processed for the assigned tests.

Reviewing Results

1. For result reviewing, Touch "Results" icon.
2. To view a particular result, select the sample ID and click on "Show details."
3. To view colored image of the result, i.e., cassette/column, click on "Change to color."
4. To view the other side view of the cassette/column, click on "Change to back."
5. For report printing, select "Results" icon. Reports can be printed as "Order report" or as "Lab report."
6. To print report of a particular sample ID, select the sample ID and click on "Show Order Report" and in the new window, click on "Print."

7. To print a list of all the results currently displayed in "Results" icon, click on "Show Lab Report" and in the new window, click on "Print."
8. To archive a result, select sample ID and click on "Archive Order."

System Shut Down

1. For system shut down, Touch "Home > Shut Down."
2. In the new window, click on "Yes"; the instrument state would be "Shutdown Cleanup."
3. Wait for the system to unlock all the doors, and the monitor to become blank.
4. Wait until the indicator in the bottom of the Touch screen monitor blinks and then switch off the system.

CHAPTER 38

Forward and Reverse Blood Grouping

SCOPE AND APPLICATION

This standard operating procedure (SOP) describes an automated method for the detection of ABO/Rh antigens on the red blood cells and generally expected reciprocal antibodies in the serum related to the ABO blood group system (Landsteiner's law) to determine the ABO/Rh blood group status of the patient or donor correctly by an automated method.

RESPONSIBILITY

Blood center laboratory technicians in serology are responsible for performing patient/donor ABO typing. The technical supervisor is responsible for reviewing and approving groupings. A medical officer will oversee the procedure and will be responsible for testing to rule out blood group mismatches.

MATERIALS REQUIRED

- *Reagents*:
    - BioVue forward and reverse grouping cassettes
    - A1 cell (3–5% suspension in saline)
    - B cell (3–5% suspension in saline)
- *Materials*:
    - Sample rack
    - Reagent rack
    - Dilution tray
    - Evaporation caps
- *Equipment*:
    - Fully automated analyzer
    - Refrigerator to store samples (2–6°C)
    - Refrigerator to store reagent (2–8°C)
    - Laboratory centrifuge with timer

- *Type of sample*: Anticoagulated whole human blood collected in 4/6 mL ethylenediaminetetraacetic acid (EDTA) evacuated tubes or anticoagulated blood from blood bags with citrate phosphate dextrose (CPD)/acid citrate dextrose (ACD) anticoagulated may also be used.

Do not use specimens with the following conditions:
- Hemolyzed blood samples
- Obvious contamination (microbial or any other body fluids)

PROCEDURE

1. *To load sample*:
   a. After loading all the consumables (forward and reverse cassettes, A1 and B cells, dilution tray), load samples into a sample rack. Samples > Load/Unload.
   b. Place the rack on the loading station and close the door.
   c. The system checks inventories and selection of samples: Samples > Create Order (or Create Batch) > (Select Samples to be included and choose the test requirements).
   d. For barcoded samples, scan the new sample barcode(s) with the hand-held scanner or type manually twice for the double-blind sample ID entry. Select the profile—"BLOOD GROUPING."
2. *To initiate the process*:
   a. Touch the save and start button.
      (Testing is initiated on samples when all test conditions and system requirements are met.)

INTERPRETATION

Interpretation of test result is done automatically by ORTHO VISION ANALYZER software as soon as the assay is completed. The interpretation of test along with a picture of cassette can be seen in Result area by touching the "Results" icon. The computer screen will show reaction of all columns of cassette used in a particular assay with the interpretation of test with gradation of reactions [4+, 3+, 2+, 1+, 0.5, 0, mixed field (MF)].

To edit result, go to result icon and then open the particular result view. Edit the result by touching gradation of reaction area and add comments in comment area.

Note: All the discrepant results are to be handled very carefully.

DOCUMENTATION

Sample report printout:

Click on "Results" > Click on "Show Lab Report" > Click Preset > Click on Current/Daily/Weekly/Monthly > Print

Or

Click on "Results" > Click on an individual test result > Show details > Click image > Send to LIS > Click on "TRACES" folder > Open and Copy the Link and Then go to folder "Report Export" > Paste the link copied in search > Result image will open > Copy the image > Paste on Desktop > Rename

Then Open HIS > Click on LIS > Click on Blood Center > Click on Report Status > Select Patient name > Click on Test and enter the result > Upload the image from the desktop > Click on Save > Click on Finalization > Verify the particulars of the Patient > Click on Finalize

Then go to result printing > Preview the report and print

The sample of the report generated is given in **Annexure 38.1**.

Report printout:

All the test results should be rechecked by another technician and finally approved by the medical officer.

Note: If there is an ABO discrepancy/invalid result, this is resolved by performing blood grouping on the same sample using another standardized method (using the tube method).

Quality Control Procedure

- *Internal:* Anti-A and anti-B present in forward and reverse grouping cassettes are tested daily against reference cells (A1 and B). Anti-D is tested daily against negative control and positive control cells.
- *External:* BEQAS—(*Blood Bank External Quality Assessment Scheme*): Participation in external quality control program should be ensured once in 4 months.

ANNEXURE 38.1

Name:	MR No:	Sample Date:
Sex/Age:	IP. No.:	Receiving Date:
Ward/Bed No.:	Dept Ref:	OPD/IPD: IPD

Test Report Status: Final

Department of Blood Center

Investigation	Test Result
Blood Grouping with Reverse Grouping (Method: Column Agglutination Technology)	

ANTI-A	ANTI-B	ANTI-D	CTL	A1 CELL	B CELL	ANTI-H
–	–	4+	–	3+	4+	4+

(For color version, see Plate 7)

Observation

Blood grouping with reverse grouping "O" Rh positive.

Interpretation of Results

Positive reactions in the microtube are indicated by RBC agglutinates trapped anywhere in the microtube column. Positive reactions can be graded from 1+ to 4+.

A 4+ reaction is indicated by a solid band of RBCs on top in the microtube column.

A 3+ reaction displays agglutinated RBCs in the upper half of the microtube column.

A 2+ reaction is characterized by RBC agglutinates dispersed throughout the length of the microtube column.

A 1+ reaction is indicated by RBC agglutinates mainly in the lower half of the microtube column with some agglutinated RBCs pelleted at the bottom.

Negative reactions display a pellet of RBCs at the bottom of the microtube column and no agglutinates within the matrix of the microtube column. Mixed-field reactions can also be observed in the microtube column test. These reactions are more commonly encountered during RBC typing procedures, rather than during serum or plasma testing methods, but in either case they are easy to recognize. Antigen positive RBCs, in this case, are completely agglutinated by the specific antisera present and they lie at the top of the microtube column, whereas the remainder of the RBCs that are antigen negative do not agglutinate and pellet at the bottom.

-------------**End of Report**-------------

....
Technologist   **Technical Supervisor**   **Consultant Blood Center**

- This report is of the sample received along with Test Requisition Form (TRF) for the patient, the particulars of which are given in the TRF and the report. In case the result does not correlate with the opinion/findings given/inferred in the report, the patient/ referring doctor may check for any sampling error and contact the Blood center immediately for reconfirmation by repeating the investigation.
- The blood and other samples received are presumed to be of the patients, the details of which are given on the sample tubes and TRF.
- This report is not valid for medico-legal purposes.

METHOD USING SEMIAUTOMATED WORKSTATION

Sample and Material Required
- Blood sample in EDTA
- Micropipettes
- A1 and B cells (4%)
- Disposable pipette tips
- Workstation
- Blood grouping cassette

Procedure
1. The control in blood grouping cassette is very important as in this case when red blood cells (RBCs) are coated with antibodies or any interfering proteins, the control will be positive and the forward grouping will be invalid. The forward grouping is to be repeated after washing the cells.
2. Make 4% suspension of pooled A1 and B cells (1,000 µL normal saline + 50 µL packed red cells).
3. Take out blood grouping cassette (ABD control reverse grouping cassette).

4. Label the cassette with the patient's name or Medical Registration (MR) number.
5. Open the wells of the blood grouping cassette.
6. Add 40 µL of plasma/serum in columns 5 and 6.
7. Add 10 µL of 4% RBC suspension (patient) in columns 1, 2, 3, and 4.
8. Add 10 µL of A1 and B cells (4%) in columns 5 and 6, respectively.
9. Centrifuge the cassette for 5 minutes in workstation.
10. Read and grade the reaction of the result and scan the cassette.
11. Upload in HIS and generate the report as per sample given in **Annexure 38.1**.
12. Enter the results of the patient/recipient grouping in the requisition form.

Discrepancies between Cell and Serum Results

If there is a discrepancy between the forward and reverse grouping, when the reactions in the forward grouping do not match the reactions in the reverse grouping or where expected reaction grading is less than grade 3 in the forward group and grade 2 in the reverse group or where there is discrepancy between historical results and current test results, an interpretation must not be entered but the results must be recorded and the "ABO discrepancy" must be resolved by further testing.

39

Major Crossmatch

SCOPE AND APPLICATION

This standard operating procedure (SOP) describes the steps to follow for operating the automated analyzer for crossmatching using cassettes based on column agglutination technology. This helps in determining compatibility between donors and patients requiring transfusions.

RESPONSIBILITY

Blood center laboratory technicians working in the serology section are responsible for performing the crossmatch and documenting the results. If incompatibility is detected, he/she will inform the blood center medical officer.

MATERIALS REQUIRED

- *Reagents*:
    - Antihuman globulin (AHG) polyspecific cassettes
    - BLISS solution
    - Donor's red blood cells (RBCs)
    - Patient's serum
- *Materials*:
    - Sample rack
    - Reagent rack
    - Dilution tray
    - Evaporation caps
- *Equipment*:
    - Fully automated analyzer
    - Refrigerator to store samples (2-6°C)
    - Refrigerator to store reagent (2-8°C)

PROCEDURE

1. *To load sample*:
   a. After loading all the consumables (AHG polyspecific cassettes and BLISS), load samples (both donor RBCs and patient sera) into a sample rack separately. Samples > Load/Unload.
   b. Place the rack on the loading station and close the door.
   c. The system checks inventories and selection of samples: Samples > Create Order (or Create Batch) > (Select Samples to be included and choose the test requirements).
   d. For barcoded samples, scan the new sample barcode(s) with the hand-held scanner or type manually twice for the double-blind sample ID entry. Select the profile—"MAJOR XM."
   e. Select the donor sample icon to input the donor ID (either manually or by scanner).
   f. Put the required details for the donor sample and press ok to continue.
2. *To initiate the process*:
   a. Touch the "Save" and "Start" button.
   (Testing is initiated on samples when all test conditions and system requirements are met.)

INTERPRETATION

Interpretation of test result is done automatically by ANALYZER software as soon as the assay is completed. The interpretation of test along with a picture of cassette can be seen in Result area by touching "Results" icon. The computer screen will show reaction of all columns of cassette used in a particular assay with the interpretation of test with gradation of reactions [4+, 3+, 2+, 1+, 0.5, 0, mixed field (MF)].

To edit result, go to result icon and then open the particular result view. Edit the result by touching gradation of reaction area and add comments in comment area.

Note: All the discrepant results are to be handled very carefully and only to be edited when sure about the edited result.

DOCUMENTATION

Sample report printout:
Click on "Results" > Click on "Show Lab Report" > Click Preset > Click on Current/Daily/Weekly/Monthly > Print

Or

Click on "Results" > Click on an individual test result > Show details > Click image > Send to LIS > Click on "TRACES" folder > Open and Copy the Link and Then go to folder "Report Export" > Paste the link copied in search > Result image will open > Copy the image > Paste on Desktop > Rename

Then Open HIS > Click on LIS > Click on Blood Center > Click on Report Status > Select Patient name > Click on Test and enter the result > Upload the image from the desktop > Click on Save > Click on Finalization > Verify the particulars of the Patient > Click on Finalize

Then go to Result printing > Preview the report and print

The sample of the report generated is given in **Annexure 39.1**.

Report printout:
All the test results should be rechecked by another technician and finally approved by the doctor.

Note: If there is an ABO discrepancy/invalid result, this is resolved by performing blood grouping on the same sample using another standardized method (using the tube method).

QUALITY CONTROL PROCEDURE

- *Internal*: Can be done by doing crossmatching between two known samples to get a desired result, which will prove the quality of the AHG reagent in the cassettes.
- *External*: Participation in external quality control program is recommended once in 3 months.

ANNEXURE 39.1

MR No.:	Investigation No.:
Name:	OPD/IPD:
Sex/Age:	Crossmatch Date:
Consultant:	Diagnosis:
Blood Group: A Rh POSITIVE	

Department of Blood Center

Investigation	Test Result
Crossmatch Method: Polyspecific AHG Technique	

0792-21   0826-21   0898-21

(For color version, see Plate 8)

Report

The crossmatch put up in the AHG POLYSPECIFIC CASSETTE as shown above displays NEGATIVE reaction as evidenced by presence of a distinct pellet of RBCs at the bottom of the Micro Column indicates that the following DONOR UNIT/S is/are compatible with the blood sample of the patient and is/are suitable for Transfusion.

Important Note

- Crossmatched blood will be kept in reserve for the said patient only up to 72 hours.
- Fresh blood sample of patients requiring repeated blood transfusion must be sent every 72 hours for antibody screening/crossmatching to avoid blood transfusion reaction due to atypical antibodies developed on account of previous transfusion.

Unit No.	Blood group	Segment No.	Blood component	Expiry	Date and time of issue	Sign. of technician
792-21	A Rh positive	OJVS1987	PRBCS (leuko-depleted)			
826-21	A Rh positive	OKCJ1267	PRBCS (leuko-depleted)			
898-21	A Rh positive	OJPY2482	PRBCS (leuko-depleted)			

....

Signature of Technologist

Note: Blood unit once issued will not be taken back after 30 minutes from the time of issue.

METHOD USING SEMIAUTOMATED WORKSTATION

Materials Required

- Clotted blood sample of the patient
- Ethylenediaminetetraacetic acid (EDTA)/citrate phosphate dextrose adenine (CPDA) blood sample of the patient
- Tabletop centrifuge
- BLISS
- Micropipettes
- Disposable pipette tips
- Workstation
- Anti-immunoglobulin G (IgG), C3d polyspecific cassette

Procedure

1. Make 4% suspension of donor cells (washed once in saline) (1 mL normal saline + 50 µL pooled donor cells).
2. Take out anti-IgG, C3d polyspecific cassette.
3. Label the cassette with the patient's name or Medical Registration (MR) number.
4. Open the well of the cassette.
5. Add 50 µL of BLISS to each column.

6. Add 10 μL of the 4% donor's RBC suspension.
7. Add 40 μL of the patient's serum/plasma.
8. Incubate for 10 minutes at 37°C in a workstation incubator.
9. Centrifuge the cassette for 5 minutes using workstation centrifuge.
10. Read and grade the reaction of the result and scan the cassette.
11. Upload in HIS and generate the report as per **Annexure 39.1**.

A *positive reaction* is recorded when red cells are retained in or above the column after centrifugation. The reaction is graded and the unit is incompatible.

A *negative reaction* is recorded (as 0) when a distinct button of cells sediment to the bottom of the column after centrifugation and the blood unit is compatible.

ABO, Rh Blood Grouping and Direct Antiglobulin Testing of Newborn

SCOPE AND APPLICATION

This standard operating procedure (SOP) describes method for automated detection of the presence of ABO/Rh antigens on neonatal and antibodies on the surface of red blood cells (RBCs).

RESPONSIBILITY

Blood center laboratory technicians are responsible for performing neonatal ABO/Rh typing and direct antiglobulin testing (DAT). A technical supervisor is responsible for reviewing and approving the results. The medical officer is responsible for overseeing the procedure and finalizing the results.

MATERIALS REQUIRED

- *Reagents*:
  - Newborn [A, B, AB, D, control, antihuman globulin (AHG) anti-immunoglobulin G (IgG)] cassette
  - A1 cell (3–5% suspension in saline)
  - B cell (3–5% suspension in saline)
  - AB cell (3–5% suspension in saline)
  - BLISS solution
- *Materials*:
  - Sample rack
  - Reagent rack
  - Dilution tray
  - Evaporation caps
- *Equipment*:
  - Fully automated analyzer
  - Refrigerator to store samples (2–6°C)

- Refrigerator to store reagent (2–8°C)
- Laboratory centrifuge with timer
- *Type of sample*: Anticoagulated whole human blood collected in a 1 mL ethylenediaminetetraacetic acid (EDTA) evacuated tube.

Do not use specimens with the following conditions:
- Hemolyzed blood samples
- Obvious contamination (microbial or any other body fluids)

PROCEDURE

1. *To load sample*:
   a. After loading all the consumables New-born (A, B, AB, D, control, AHG anti-IgG) cassette, dilution tray], load samples into a sample rack. Samples > Load/Unload.
   b. Place the rack on the loading station and close the door.
   c. The system checks inventories and selection of samples: Samples > Create Order (or Create Batch) > (Select Samples to be included and choose the test requirements).
   d. For barcoded samples, scan the new sample(s) barcode(s) with the hand-held scanner or type manually twice for the double-blind sample ID entry. Select the profile—"New-born DAT."
2. *To initiate the process*:
   a. Touch the Save and Start button.
      (Testing is initiated on samples when all test conditions and system requirements are met.)

INTERPRETATION

Interpretation of test result is done automatically by ORTHO VISION ANALYZER software as soon as the assay is completed. The interpretation of test along with a picture of cassette can be seen in Result area by touching "Results" icon. The computer screen will show reaction of all columns of BioVue cassette used in a particular assay with the interpretation of test with gradation of reactions [4+, 3+, 2+, 1+, 0.5, 0, mixed field (MF)].

To edit result, go to result icon and then open the particular result view. Edit the result by touching gradation of reaction area and add comments in comment area.

Note: All the discrepant results are to be handled very carefully and edited when sure.

DOCUMENTATION

Sample report printout:
Click on "Results" > Click on "Show Lab Report" > Click Preset > Click on Current/Daily/Weekly/Monthly > Print

Or

Click on "Results" > Click on an individual test result > Show details > Click image > Send to LIS >Click on "TRACES" folder > Open and Copy the Link and Then go to folder "Report Export" > Paste the link copied in search > Result image will open > Copy the image > Paste on Desktop > Rename

Then Open HIS > Click on LIS > Click on Blood Center > Click on Report Status > Select Patient name > Click on Test and enter the result > Upload the image from the desktop > Click on Save > Click on Finalization > Verify the particulars of the Patient > Click on Finalize

Then go to Result printing > Preview the report and print

The sample of the report generated is given in **Annexure 40.1**.

Report printout:
All the test results should be rechecked by another technician and finally approved by the doctor.

Note: If there is an ABO discrepancy/invalid result, this is resolved by performing blood grouping on the same sample using another standardized method (using the tube method).

Quality Control Procedure

- *Internal*: BioVue® newborn (A, B, AB, D, control, AHG anti-IgG) cassettes are tested daily against reference cells (A1, AB, and B) and anti-D is tested daily against negative control and positive control cells.
- *External*: Participation in external quality control program should be ensured once in 4 months.

ANNEXURE 40.1

Name: B/O	MR No: 310870	Sample Date:
Sex/Age: Female/00 Y/ 0 M/	IP. No.:	Receiving Date:
11D Ward/Bed No.:	Lab No:	Report Date:
Referred By:	Dept Ref No: 108743	OPD/IPD: IPD

Department of Blood Center

Investigation	Test Result
New Born ABO/Rh/DAT (Method: Column Agglutination Technology)	

ANTI-A	ANTI-B	ANTI-AB	ANTI-D	CTL	DAT	ANTI-H
–	–	–	4+	–	–	4+

(For color version, see Plate 8)

Observation	
1. Blood Group:	"O" Positive
2. DAT:	Negative

Interpretation of Results

Positive reactions in the microtube are indicated by RBC agglutinates trapped anywhere in the microtube column. Positive reactions can be graded from 1+ to 4+.

A 4+ reaction is indicated by a solid band of RBCs on top of the microtube column.

A 3+ reaction displays agglutinated RBCs in the upper half of the microtube column.

A 2+ reaction is characterized by RBC agglutinates dispersed throughout the length of the microtube column.

A 1+ reaction is indicated by RBC agglutinates mainly in the lower half of the microtube column with some unagglutinated RBCs pelleted at the bottom.

Negative reactions display a pellet of RBCs at the bottom of the microtube column and no agglutinates within the matrix of the microtube column.

Group A and B antigens are not fully developed at birth, weaker reactions may occur with red cells of newborns than of adults and subgroups often cannot be identified. The serum of adults contains antibodies directed against the A and B antigens absent from their own red cells. Both antibodies appear after the first 4–6 months of life. As a result, reverse grouping is not usually undertaken on newborn blood samples. **Therefore, Repeat Blood Grouping is advised after 6 months of age for confirmation of ABO/Rh.**

Direct Coombs Test on newborn blood samples has become a standard procedure, since it is of importance to know if the newborn's red cells have been coated with maternal antibodies (IgG) in utero or the complement generally C3d in cases of hemolytic disease of newborn (HDN). It is also done in cases of autoimmune hemolytic anemia (AIHA), drug-induced red cell sensitization, and hemolytic transfusion reactions to detect antibody coating of red cells.

--------------**End of Report**-------------

....

Technologist   Technical Supervisor   Consultant Blood Center

- This report is of the sample received along with test requisition form (TRF) for the patient, the particulars of which are given in the TRF and the report. In case the result does not correlate with the opinion/findings given/inferred in the report, then the patient/referring doctor may check for any sampling error and contact the Blood Center immediately for reconfirmation by repeating the investigation.
- The blood and other samples received are presumed to be of the patients, the details of which are given on the sample tubes and TRF.

CHAPTER 41

Antibody Screening (with Pooled "O" Cells)

SCOPE AND APPLICATION

This standard operating procedure (SOP) describes antibody screening through AutoAnalyzer system using cassette-based column agglutination technology. Antibody screening rules out the presence of unwanted antibodies in patient/donor samples. Antibody screening may further help in investigation of unwanted antibody.

RESPONSIBILITY

Blood center laboratory technicians are responsible for performing antibody screening (using pooled "O" cells) along with technical supervisor for reviewing and approving the results. Medical officer oversees the procedure and the results.

MATERIALS REQUIRED

- *Reagents*:
  - Antihuman globulin (AHG) polyspecific cassettes
  - BioVue low-ionic-strength saline (BLISS) solution
  - Pooled screening cell (3%)
  - Donor's serum
- *Materials*:
  - Sample rack
  - Reagent rack
  - Evaporation caps
- *Equipment*:
  - Fully automated analyzer
  - Refrigerator to store samples (2–6°C)
  - Refrigerator to store reagent (2–8°C)

PROCEDURE

1. *To load sample*:
   a. After loading all the consumables (AHG polyspecific cassettes, Ortho BLISS, pooled screening cells), load samples into a sample rack—Samples > Load/Unload.
   b. Place the rack on the loading station and close the door.
   c. The system checks inventories and selection of samples: Samples > Create Order (or Create Batch) > (Select samples to be included and choose the test requirements).
   d. Scan the new barcoded sample(s) barcode(s) with the handheld scanner or type manually twice for the double-blind sample ID entry. Select the profile—"AB SCREEN 'O' CELLS."
2. *To initiate the process*:
   a. Touch the save and start button. (Testing is initiated on samples when all test conditions and system requirements are met.)

QUALITY CONTROL PROCEDURE

a. *Internal*: AHG antisera present in AHG polyspecific cassettes are tested daily against reference serum (presence of known antibody) with the SURGISCREEN to get the desired result.
b. *External*: BEQAS—Participation in external quality program once in 4 months is required.

INTERPRETATION

ANALYZER software interprets the test results automatically as soon as the assay is completed. Interpretation of test, along with picture of cassette, can be seen in result area by touching results icon. The computer screen will show reaction of all columns of cassette used in particular assay with the interpretation of test with gradation of reactions [4+, 3+, 2+, 1+, 0.5, 0, mixed field (MF)].

To edit result, go to result icon and then open the particular result view. Edit the result by touching gradation of reaction area and add comments in comment area.

Note: All the discrepant results are to be handled very carefully.

DOCUMENTATION

Sample Report Printout

Click on "Results" > Click on "Lab Report" > Click on Print

Or

Click on "Results" > Click on an individual test result > Click on report to take individual printout

Report printout: All the test results should be rechecked by other blood center technicians and finally approved by the medical officer on duty before printing out.

Note: If there is any discrepancy/invalid result, it is resolved by performing the same test of the same sample with some other standardized method (by the tube method).

METHOD USING A SEMIAUTOMATED WORKSTATION

Materials Required
- Clotted blood sample of the donor
- Ethylenediaminetetraacetic acid (EDTA)/citrate-phosphate-dextrose-adenine (CPDA) blood sample of the donor
- Tabletop centrifuge
- BLISS
- Micropipettes
- Disposable pipette tips
- ORTHO workstation
- Anti-immunoglobulin G (anti-IgG), C3d polyspecific cassette
- "O" pooled cells (in-house or commercial cells)

Procedure
1. Make 4% suspension of pooled "O" cells (washed once in saline) (1 mL normal saline + 50 μL pooled "O" packed cells). Otherwise, use commercially available pooled "O" cells.
2. Take out anti-IgG, C3d polyspecific cassette.
3. Label the cassette with donor ID.
4. Open the wells of the cassette.
5. Add 50 μL of BLISS to each column.
6. Add 10 μL of the 4% suspension of "O" pooled cells.
7. Add 40 μL of the donor serum/plasma.
8. Incubate for 10 minutes at 37°C in ORTHO Workstation incubator.
9. Centrifuge the cassette for 5 minutes using workstation centrifuge.
10. Read and grade the reaction of the result and scan the cassette.

A *positive reaction* is recorded when red cells are retained in or above the column after centrifugation. The reaction is graded and is interpreted as positive for atypical antibodies.

A *negative reaction* is recorded (as 0) when a distinct button of cells sediment at the bottom of the column after centrifuge and is interpreted as negative for atypical antibodies.

Record
Record the results in a donor register.

42

Antibody Screening (with Three-cell Panel)

SCOPE AND APPLICATION

This standard operating procedure (SOP) describes the steps to operate the AutoAnalyzer system to perform antibody screening using the cassette-based column agglutination technology. Antibody screening can exclude unwanted antibodies present in patient/donor samples. This screening may aid in further investigation of this unwanted antibody.

RESPONSIBILITY

Serology department technicians are responsible for performing antibody screening (using three-cell panel). The technical supervisor is responsible for reviewing and approving the results. The medical officer is responsible for overseeing the procedure and finalizing the results.

MATERIALS REQUIRED

- *Reagents*:
    - Antihuman globulin (AHG) polyspecific cassettes
    - BioVue low-ionic-strength saline (BLISS) solution
    - SURGISCREEN (3%) cell panel
    - Patient's serum
- *Materials*:
    - Sample rack
    - Reagent rack
    - Evaporation caps
- Equipment:
    - Fully automated analyzer
    - Refrigerator to store samples (2–6°C)
    - Reagent refrigerator to store reagent (2–8°C)

PROCEDURE

1. *To load sample*:
   a. After loading all the consumables (AHG polyspecific cassettes, Ortho BLISS, SURGISCREEN cells), load samples into a sample rack. Samples > Load/Unload
   b. Place the rack on the loading station and close the door.
   c. The system checks inventories and selection of samples: Samples > Create Order (or Create Batch) > (Select samples to be included and choose the test requirements).
   d. Scan the new barcoded sample(s) with the handheld scanner or type manually twice for the double-blind sample ID entry. Select the profile "AB SCREEN 3 CELLS."
2. *To initiate the process*:
   a. Touch the Save and Start button. (Testing is initiated on samples when all test conditions and system requirements are met.)

QUALITY CONTROL PROCEDURE

- *Internal*: AHG antisera present in AHG polyspecific cassettes are tested daily against reference serum (presence of known antibody) with the SURGISCREEN to get the desired result.
- *External*: BEQAS—Participation in external quality control program is required once in 4 months.

INTERPRETATION

Interpretation of test result is done automatically by ANALYZER software as soon as the assay is completed. The interpretation of test, along with picture of cassette, can be seen in Result area by touching *Results* icon. The computer screen will show reaction of all columns of cassette used in particular assay with the interpretation of test with gradation of reactions [4+, 3+, 2+, 1+, 0.5, 0, mixed field (MF)]

To edit result, go to result icon and then open the particular result view. Edit the result by touching gradation of reaction area and add comments in comment area.

Note: All the discrepant results are to be handled very carefully and edited only when sure.

DOCUMENTATION
Sample Report Printout

Click on "Results" > Click on "Lab Report" > Click on Print
Or
Click on "Results" > Click on an individual test result > Click on report to take individual printout

Report printout:

All the test results should be rechecked by another technician and finally approved by the doctor on duty before printing out.

Note: If there is any discrepancy/invalid result, that is resolved by performing the same test of the same sample with some other standardized method (by the tube method).

METHOD USING A SEMIAUTOMATED WORKSTATION

Materials Required

- Clotted blood sample of the patient
- Ethylenediaminetetraacetic acid (EDTA)/citrate-phosphate-dextrose-adenine (CPDA) blood sample of the patient
- Tabletop centrifuge
- BLISS
- Micropipettes
- Disposable pipette tips
- ORTHO workstation
- Anti-immunoglobulin G (anti-IgG), C3d polyspecific cassette
- Reagent Red Cells Panel (Surgiscreen)

PROCEDURE

1. Take out anti-IgG, C3d polyspecific cassette.
2. Label the cassette with patient's name or medical record (MR) number.
3. Open three wells of the cassette and label I, II, and III.
4. Add 50 µL of BLISS to each column.
5. Add 10 µL of each 4% commercial three-cell panel to the respective columns.
6. Add 40 µL of the patient's serum/plasma.
7. Incubate for 10 minutes at 37°C in a workstation incubator.
8. Centrifuge the cassette for 5 minutes using workstation centrifuge.
9. Read and grade the reaction of the result and scan the cassette.
10. Upload in hospital information system (HIS) and generate the report.

A *positive reaction* in each column is recorded when red cells are retained in or above the column after centrifugation. The reaction is graded for each column and interpreted for the presence of atypical antibodies as per antigram chart provided with the commercial cells.

A *negative reaction* is recorded (as 0) for each column when a distinct button of cells sediment to the bottom of the column after centrifuge. When the reaction is negative in all the columns, atypical antibodies are not present.

43

Direct/Indirect Coombs Test

SCOPE AND APPLICATION

This standard operating procedure (SOP) describes direct and indirect Coombs test (DCT and ICT) through autoanalyzer system using cassettes based on column agglutination technology. The DCT detects the coating of red cells in vivo with antibody [immunoglobulin G (IgG)] or C3d, whereas ICT detects the presence of incomplete autoantibodies/complement-binding antibodies in the serum of the patient.

RESPONSIBILITY

Blood center laboratory technician is responsible for DCT/ICT using cassettes based on column agglutination technology, while technical supervisor checks and approves the result, and medical officer supervises the procedure and finalizes the results.

MATERIALS REQUIRED

- *Reagents*:
  - Antihuman globulin (AHG) polyspecific cassettes
    o For ICT:
      - Pooled screening cell (3%)
      - Patient serum/plasma
    o For DCT:
      - Patient red cell (3–5% suspension in saline)
      - BLISS solution
- *Materials*:
  - Sample rack
  - Reagent rack
  - Evaporation caps

- *Equipment*:
  - Fully automated analyzer
  - Refrigerator to store samples (2–6°C)
  - Refrigerator to store reagent (2–8°C)

PROCEDURE

1. *To load sample*:
   a. After loading all the consumables (AHG polyspecific cassettes, Ortho BLISS, Ortho pooled SURGISCREEN cells), load samples into a sample rack. Samples > Load/Unload.
   b. Place the rack on the loading station and close the door.
   c. The system checks inventories and selection of samples: Samples > Create Order (or Create Batch) > (Select samples to be included and choose the test requirements).
   d. For barcoded samples, scan the new sample(s) barcode(s) with the hand-held scanner or type manually twice for the double-blind sample ID entry. Select the profile—"DCT/ICT or DCT and ICT."
2. *To initiate the process*:
   a. Touch the "Save" and "Start" buttons. (Testing is initiated on samples when all test conditions and system requirements are met.)

QUALITY CONTROL PROCEDURE

- *Internal*: AHG antisera present in AHG polyspecific cassettes are tested daily against reference serum (presence of known antibody) with the SURGISCREEN to get the desired result.
- *External*: Participation in external control is required once in 4 months.

INTERPRETATION

ORTHO VISION ANALYZER software interprets the results automatically as soon as the assay is completed. The interpretation of test, along with a picture of cassette, can be seen in Result area by touching "Results" icon. The computer screen will show reaction of all columns of BioVue cassette used in particular assay with the interpretation of test with gradation of reactions [4+, 3+, 2+, 1+, 0.5, 0, mixed field (MF)].

To edit result, go to result icon and then open the particular result view. Edit the result by touching gradation of reaction area and add comments in comment area.

Note: All the discrepant results are to be handled very carefully.

DOCUMENTATION

Sample report printout:

Click on "Results" > Click on "Show Lab Report" > Click Preset > Click on Current/Daily/Weekly/Monthly > Print

Or

Click on "Results" > Click on an individual test result > Show details > Click image > Send to LIS > Click on "TRACES" folder > Open and Copy the Link and Then go to folder "Report Export" > Paste the link copied in search > Result image will open > Copy the image > Paste on Desktop > Rename

Then Open HIS > Click on LIS > Click on Blood Center > Click on Report Status > Select Patient name > Click on Test and enter the result > Upload the image from the desktop > Click on Save > Click on Finalization > Verify the particulars of the Patient > Click on Finalize

Then go to Result printing > Preview the report and print

The reports of the samples generated are given in **Annexures 43.1 and 43.2.**

Report printout:

All the test results should be rechecked by another technician and finally approved by the doctor on duty before printing out.

Note: If there is any discrepancy/invalid result, that is resolved by performing same test of same sample with some other standardized method (by tube method).

ANNEXURE 43.1

Name:	MR No:	Sample Date:
Sex/Age:	IP. No.:	Receiving Date:
Ward/Bed No.:	Lab No:	Report Date:
Referred By:	Dept. Ref No:	OPD/IPD: IPD

Test Report Status: Final

Department of Blood Center

Investigation	Test Result	
Direct Coombs Test (DCT/DAT) (Method: Column Agglutination Technology)	DCT M.R No: 3112 12 (*For color version, see Plate 9*)	

OBSERVATION

Direct Coombs Test (DCT/DAT): Negative

Interpretation of Results

Positive reactions in the microtube are indicated by RBC agglutinates trapped anywhere in the microtube column. Positive reactions can be graded from 1+ to 4+.

A 4+ reaction is indicated by a solid band of RBCs on top in the microtube column.

A 3+ reaction displays agglutinated RBCs in the upper half of the microtube column.

A 2+ reaction is characterized by RBC agglutinates dispersed throughout the length of the microtube column.

A 1+ reaction is indicated by RBC agglutinates mainly in the lower half of the microtube column with some unagglutinated RBCs pelleted at the bottom.

Negative reactions display a pellet of RBCs at the bottom of the microtube column and no agglutinates within the matrix of the microtube column. Mixed-field reactions can also be observed in the microtube column test. These reactions are more commonly encountered during RBC typing procedures, rather than during serum or plasma testing methods, but in either case they are easy to recognize. Antigen positive RBCs, in this case, are completely agglutinated by the specific antisera present and they lie at the top of the microtube column, whereas the remainder of the RBCs that are antigen negative do not agglutinate and pellet at the bottom.

Direct Coombs test is used to detect in vivo sensitization (coating) of red cells with immune antibody (IgG) or the complement generally C3d in cases of hemolytic disease of newborn (HDN), autoimmune hemolytic anemia (AIHA), drug induced red cell sensitization and hemolytic transfusion reactions.

....

Technologist   **Technical Supervisor**   **Consultant Blood Center**

- This report is of the sample received along with test requisition form (TRF) for the patient, the particulars of which are given in the TRF and the report. In case the result does not correlate with the opinion/findings given/inferred in the report, then the patient/referring doctor may check for any sampling error and contact the blood center immediately for reconfirmation by repeating the investigation.
- The blood and other samples received are presumed to be of the patients, the details of which are given on the sample tubes and TRF.
- This report is not valid for medico legal purposes.

ANNEXURE 43.2

Name:	MR No:	Sample Date:
Sex/Age:	IP. No.:	Receiving Date:
Ward/Bed No.:	Lab No:	Report Date:
Referred By:	Dept Ref No:	OPD/IPD: OPD

Test Report Status: Final

Department of Blood Center		
Investigation	**Test Result**	
ICT Coombs Test Indirect (Method: Column Agglutination Technology)	ICT 296971 (*For color version, see Plate 9*)	

OBSERVATION

ICT Coombs Test Indirect: Negative

Interpretation of Results

Positive reactions in the microtube are indicated by RBC agglutinates trapped anywhere in the microtube column.

Positive reactions can be graded from 1+ to 4+.

A 4+ reaction is indicated by a solid band of RBCs on top of the microtube column.

A 3+ reaction displays agglutinated RBCs in the upper half of the microtube column.

A 2+ reaction is characterized by RBC agglutinates dispersed throughout the length of the microtube column.

A 1+ reaction is indicated by RBC agglutinates mainly in the lower half of the microtube column with some unagglutinated RBCs pelleted at the bottom.

Negative reactions display a pellet of RBCs at the bottom of the microtube and no agglutinates within the matrix of the microtube column.

Indirect Coombs test is used to detect presence of incomplete antibodies and complement binding antibodies in the serum after coating on red cells in vitro in compatibility testing for the blood to be transfused, for screening and identification of unexpected antibodies in the serum and for detection of red cell antigens using specific antibodies reacting only in antiglobulin test Fya, Fyb, K, JKa, JKb, etc.

....
Technologist   **Technical Supervisor**   **Consultant Blood Center**

- This report is of the sample received along with Test Requisition Form (TRF) for the patient, the particulars of which are given in the TRF and the report. In case the result does not correlate with the opinion/findings given/inferred in the report, then the patient/referring doctor may check for any sampling error and contact the blood center immediately for reconfirmation by repeating the investigation.
- The blood and other samples received are presumed to be of the patients, the details of which are given on the sample tubes and TRF.
- This report is not valid for medico legal purposes.

METHOD USING SEMIAUTOMATED WORKSTATION

Direct Coombs Test

Materials Required

- Clotted blood sample of the patient
- Ethylenediaminetetraacetic acid (EDTA)/citrate-phosphate-dextrose-adenine (CPDA) blood sample of the patient
- Tabletop centrifuge
- Micropipettes
- Anti-IgG, C3d polyspecific cassette
- Disposable pipette tips
- ORTHO workstation

Procedure

- Prepare 4% suspension of patient's packed red blood cells (RBCs) (1,000 μL normal saline + 50 μL packed cells).
- Take out anti-IgG, C3d polyspecific cassette.
- Label the cassette with patient's name or medical registration (MR) number.
- Open the wells of the cassette.
- Add 10 μL of 4% RBC suspension.
- Centrifuge the card for 5 minutes in ORTHO workstation
- Read and grade the reaction of the result and scan the cassette.
- Upload in HIS and generate the report.

A *positive reaction* is recorded when red cells are retained in or above the column after centrifugation. The reaction is graded.

The Column agglutination test (CAT) card is scanned, and report is generated as given in **Annexure 43.1**.

A negative reaction is recorded (as 0) when a distinct button of cells sedimented to the bottom of direct antiglobulin test (DAT)/DCT is positive in cases of:

- HDN
- AIHA
- Drug-induced red cell sensitization
- Hemolytic transfusion reactions

Indirect Coombs Test

Materials Required

- Clotted blood sample of the patient
- EDTA/CPDA blood sample of the patient
- Tabletop centrifuge
- BLISS

- Micropipettes
- Disposable pipette tips
- ORTHO workstation
- Anti-IgG, C3d polyspecific cassette

Procedure

- Make 4% suspension of pooled "O" cells (washed once in saline) (1,000 μL normal saline + 50 μL pooled "O" packed cells). Otherwise, use commercially available pooled "O" cells.
- Takeout anti-IgG, C3d polyspecific cassette.
- Label the cassette with patient's name or MR number.
- Open the wells of the cassette.
- Add 50 μL of BLISS to each column.
- Add 10 μL of the 4% RBC suspension.
- Add 40 μL of the test serum.
- Incubate for 10 minutes at 37°C in ORTHO workstation incubator.
- Read and grade the reaction of the result, and scan the cassette.
- Upload in HIS, and generate the report as per **Annexure 43.2**.

A *positive reaction* is recorded when red cells are retained in or above the column after centrifugation. The reaction is graded.

A *negative reaction* is recorded (as 0) when a distinct button of cells sediment to the bottom of the column after centrifuge.

Indirect antiglobulin test/indirect Coombs test (IAT/ICT) is used to detect the presence of incomplete antibodies and complement-binding antibodies in the serum, after coating on red cells in vitro in:

- Compatibility testing
- Screening and detection of atypical antibodies in serum
- Detection of red cell antibodies not detected by other techniques (Lea, K, Fya, Fyb, Jka, Jkb, etc.)

Testing for Du Weak Antigen (Semiautomated Method)

SCOPE AND APPLICATION

This standard operating procedure (SOP) describes the method for testing of weak D (D^u) antigen by column technology. If the Rh grouping reaction result is 2+ or 1+, confirm the weak Du antigen status. Such reaction results (2+ or 1+) indicate weak or partial D antigen. This test is also performed on the Rh –ve cases.

RESPONSIBILITY

It is the responsibility of the blood center laboratory technician in the red cell serology laboratory to perform testing for Du weak antigen by column technology.

SAMPLE AND MATERIALS REQUIRED

- Blood sample in ethylenediaminetetraacetic acid (EDTA)
- Diluent [BioVue low-ionic-strength saline (BLISS)] at room temperature
- Micropipettes
- Disposable pipette tips
- Antihuman globulin (AHG) immunoglobulin G (IgG) cassette
- Workstation
- Anti-D [IgG or immunoglobulin M (IgM) + IgG] serum

PROCEDURE

1. Make 4% suspension of red blood cells (RBCs) (1,000 µL normal saline + 50 µL packed red cells).
2. Take out AHG IgG cassette.

3. Label the cassette with patient's name or medical record (MR) number.
4. Open the wells of the AHG IgG cassette. Add 50 µL of BLISS to each column.
5. Add 10 µL of 4% RBC suspension.
6. Add 40 µL of anti-D (IgG or IgM + IgG) serum.
7. Incubate for 10 minutes in workstation.
8. Centrifuge the cassette for 5 minutes in workstation centrifuge.
9. Read and grade the reaction of the result and scan the cassette.
10. Upload in hospital information system (HIS) and generate the report.

DOCUMENTATION

Enter the results in the donor/patient grouping register and requisition form.

Note: 4+ reactions confirm Weak D (D^u) antigen and 3+ to 1+ reactions confirm D variant.

CHAPTER 45

Resolution of ABO Group Discrepancies

SCOPE AND APPLICATION

ABO grouping discordance is defined as either the grading of agglutination reaction in the forward group did not match the expected grading of agglutination in the reverse group, or when the expected agglutination grading is less than grade 3 in the forward group and less than grade 2 in the reverse group, or there are discrepancies between the previous and current test results. Interpretation of ABO grouping should be deferred until the discrepancies are resolved. If an emergency transfusion is needed, transfuse the appropriate O Rh-negative red blood cells (RBCs).

RESPONSIBILITY

It is the responsibility of the blood center laboratory technician in the red cell serology laboratory to resolve the ABO group discrepancies under the supervision of the blood center medical officer.

MATERIALS REQUIRED

- *Equipment*:
    - Tabletop centrifuge
    - Microscope
    - Test tubes
    - Test-tube rack
    - Incubators and refrigerators
- *Sample*:
    - Clotted or anticoagulated whole blood sample
- *Reagent*:
    - Screening panel and/or donor cells
    - Anti-A, anti-B, anti-AB

 – Anti-A$_1$ lectin
 – A$_1$, A$_2$, and B cells

PROCEDURE
General Considerations
1. ABO grouping is not reported.
    a. If the reaction strength is less than grade 3+ in the forward group and grade <2+ in the reverse group
    b. If the previous and current ABO group does not match
    c. If any ABO discrepancy is found
2. *Technical errors that cause false-negative reactions are*:
    a. Failure to interpret or record test results correctly
3. *Technical errors that lead to false-positive reactions are*:
    a. Overcentrifugation
    b. Use of contaminated reagent antibodies, RBCs, or saline
    c. Use of dirty glassware
    d. Misinterpretation or incorrect recording of test results
4. *Problems with RBCs testing (forward type)*:
    a. False positive:
        i. Acquired antigens (B, A)
        ii. Polyagglutination
        iii. B (A) phenomenon
        iv. Post-transfusion/transplantation of different blood group
        v. Direct antiglobulin test (DAT)-positive samples/autoantibodies (auto-Abs)
        vi. Abs to dyes in typing reagents
    b. False negative:
        i. Reduced antigen expression [e.g., acute myeloid leukemia (AML)]
        ii. A subgroup (A$_3$, Ax)
5. *Problems associated with the serum grouping (reverse grouping)*:
    a. False positive:
        i. Small fibrin clots
        ii. Rouleaux patients with abnormally high serum levels
        iii. Proteins or who have received plasma expanders
        iv. Antibodies other than anti-A or anti-B
        v. Antibodies to the chemical constituents of the diluent used to preserve the reverse cells
        vi. Bone marrow transplant from an ABO nonidentical donor
        vii. Very weak or negative reactions from patients with immunodeficiency due to disease, therapy, low immunoglobulin levels, elderly patients, or patients receiving large amounts of intravenous (IV) fluids

      viii. Unexpected reactions when a patient receives a sufficient volume of blood components containing plasma of an ABO group other than their own

  b. False negative

      i. Negative or weak reactions to specimens in infants aged 4–6 months

      ii. Very weak or negative reactions in immunocompromised patients due to disease, treatment, low immunoglobulin levels, elderly patients, or patients receiving large amounts of IV fluids

RESOLVING ABO DISCREPANCIES

In the event of discrepancies, the following important factors should be considered:

- Age of patient
- Diagnosis
- History of transfusion
- Samples and methods used for testing

1. The next course of action is to always repeat ABO group testing since washed red cells can reduce false-positive results associated with rouleaux or autoantibodies and to validate the technique.

2. Recheck the suitability of sample, e.g., samples contaminated with IV fluids can cause weak reactions in the reverse grouping. If the sample is hemolyzed, interpretation cannot be made because it is difficult to see weak reactions or if a hemolyzing antibody is present. In these situations, it is best to use fresh, unhemolyzed specimens so that proper interpretation can be made. *If the identity or the quality of the sample is questionable, collect a new sample and repeat the test.*

3. *If discrepancies persist:*

  a. If the patient appears to be group A, test RBCs with anti-A_1 lectin and serum with A_2 cells. If the patients are negative with the lectin, they are of the subgroup A_2, and if the serum is negative for A_2 cells, this indicates that the serum has anti-A_1.

    ■ This type of discrepancy is most commonly seen.

    ■ Test with additional A_2 cells to confirm specificity to anti-A_1.

  b. Incubate at room temperature (RT) for 30 minutes to detect weakened antibodies or antigens. It is frequently needed in elderly patients. Incubation at 4°C can also be done but must run autocontrol. Cold antibodies are frequently encountered in tests performed at 4°C.

    c. Test the serum against group O adult, group O cord, and a patient autocontrol (patient serum plus patient cells) to determine if cold-reactive antibodies are interfering.

    d. Patient and reagent RBCs are washed several times.

    e. Obtain a new sample.

4. Identify if the problem is in forward grouping or reverse grouping. *Consider the following:*

    o ABO reactions are usually strong. Assume that a weak reaction is suspicious.

    o The problems in reverse grouping are more common.

    o There may be multiple problems; e.g., a weak subgroup of A can have anti-A_1 in serum.

The various possibilities are as follows:

1. Forward grouping has expected positive weak (<3+) or missing reaction(s).
2. Forward grouping has unexpected or extra reaction(s).
3. Reverse grouping has expected positive weak (<2+) or missing reaction(s).
4. Reverse grouping has an unexpected or extra reaction(s).

1. *Forward grouping has expected positive weak (<3+) or missing reaction(s):* When the forward cell typing shows weak reaction but matches the reaction in the reverse grouping, the various possibilities considered are as follows:

- Newborns
- Elderly patients
- Subgroups of A or B
- Suppression in H substrate production
- Depression of antigen production associated with disease
- Presence of two cell populations (chimeras or in patients receiving high amount of type compatible blood)

    a. Determine if the recipient has been transfused with nongroup-specific RBC components in the last 3 months (or history of transplantation).

    b. Check for cloudiness of the supernatant in the anti-A and/or anti-B tubes. Read the ABO tubes microscopically checking for mixed-field reaction(s).

    c. If a mixed-field reaction is noticed and the recipient has been transfused with nongroup-specific RBC components in the last 3 months

    d. Perform an ABO grouping on a pretransfusion sample collected before the transfusion of nongroup-specific donor unit(s), if available.

e. If a pretransfusion specimen is not available and the discrepancy is still not resolved, a report should be sent stating "ABO blood group cannot be determined at this time." If blood components are required, group O cellular and group AB plasma components should be transfused.

f. Record ABO group performed on both samples.

g. Report the ABO group performed on the pretransfusion sample.

h. When a recipient has been transfused with nongroup-specific blood, group-specific blood may not be compatible due to passive ABO antibodies. In these cases, nongroup-specific, group-compatible blood should be crossmatched until no anti-A and/or anti-B are detected by indirect antiglobulin test (IAT) crossmatch.

i. If mixed-field agglutination is present and the recipient has not been transfused in the last 3 months, review the diagnosis. *The possible causes are as follows*:
   - Recent transfusion from a nongroup-specific donor
   - ABO grouping from recipients who have received an allogenic bone marrow or hematopoietic stem cell transplant can give mixed-field results during the transplant period. Mixed-field reactions will remain indefinitely in some recipients.
   - Fetomaternal hemorrhage
   - Weak subgroups (e.g., A3); other subgroups of A or B may not react as mixed field with anti-A and/or anti-B.
   - Altered expression of A and/or B antigens due to disease when the previous ABO grouping does not agree with the current grouping and the recipient diagnosis suggests a reason for the change.
   - Polyagglutinating RBCs such as Tn-activated cells. The reverse grouping fails to confirm the cell grouping.
   - *Twin*: Chimerism (very rare)

j. If there is no mixed-field agglutination, wash the recipient's cells twice and repeat the forward grouping with the washed cell suspension.
   - If additional washing resolves the discrepancy, it may be due to excess blood group substances in the recipient's serum or plasma that neutralize anti-A or anti-B (e.g., mucin-producing adenocarcinoma).
   - If the discrepancy is not resolved, a report "ABO grouping cannot be determined at this time" should be submitted. If blood components are required, group O RBCs and group AB plasma components should be transfused.

2. *Forward grouping has unexpected or extra reaction(s) with anti-A and/or anti-B*:
   a. Repeat the blood grouping after washing the RBCs twice. Use saline warmed to 37°C to wash the cells in case cold-reactive agglutinin is suspected.
   b. Resuspend the cells to make 3% suspension.
   c. Repeat the ABO grouping with 3% washed cells suspension.
   d. Record that the second ABO grouping has been done on a 3% washed cell suspension (and, if applicable, with saline warmed to 37°C).
      This will resolve the discrepancy if it is due to the following:
      o Strong cold autoagglutinin (if washed with 37°C saline)
      o Rouleaux
      o Wharton's jelly
      o Artifactual—fibrin, other debris
      o Presence of anticoagulant (anticomplementary)
   e. Consider acquired B antigen if the problem persists and recipient appears to belong to group AB.
      Acquired B antigen is usually seen in patients with diseases of the lower intestinal tract:
      o Carcinoma of colon or rectum
      o Intestinal obstruction
      o Gram-negative septicemia
      In such cases, RBCs agglutinate with anti-A and anti-B but the reaction with anti-B is very weak. To resolve the issue of acquired B antigen, the following steps are taken:
      o Antigen types the recipient cells using anti-A1 lectin. Acquired B antigen RBCs type as A1.
      o Prepare acidic anti-A and anti-B reagents:
        ▪ Add one drop of 0.1 N HCl to four drops of commercial anti-A.
        ▪ Check the pH value.
        ▪ Adjust to pH 4.5 by adding 0.1 N HCl or anti-A.
      o Repeat grouping with acidic (pH < 6.0) anti-A and anti-B. Extra reaction in the forward grouping should be resolved if acquired B antigen.
      o Set up an autocontrol. The autocontrol shall be negative to confirm the presence of an acquired B antigen as the anti-B present in the patient's serum does not react with autologous cells.
      o Presence of A and B antigens in saliva is tested. If the patient is secretor, antigen A is present but the antigen B is absent.

○ If acquired B antigen has been ruled out or if the recipient does not appear to be group AB, try repeating the ABO group using one of the following methods:
- Antisera from a different manufacturer
- Monoclonal antisera
- Eluted recipient cells

f. If the discrepancy is still not resolved, a report should be sent stating "ABO group cannot be determined at this time." If blood components are required, group O cellular and group AB plasma components should be transfused.

3. *Reverse grouping with weak or missing reactions*: These discrepancies are a result of the presence of protein or plasma abnormalities and result in the rouleaux or pseudoagglutination.

The following are the causes of weak (i.e., weaker than 2+) or missing reactions in the reverse grouping:

- Neonatal recipients may not develop anti-A and/or anti-B up to 4–6 months of age.
- Be suspicious if the recipient is elderly or immunocompromised, e.g., hypogammaglobulinemia or agammaglobulinemia.
- Recipient may have received bone marrow or bone marrow transplant.
- Hematopoietic stem cell transplant (e.g., recipient of group A after receiving a group "O" transplant, will type as group O in the forward grouping but may not have an anti-A). In this case, follow the transfusion protocol of the facility where the transplant occurred.

The following enhancement method(s) are performed in such cases.
Enhancement method #1: (Add more serum/plasma)
- Add two additional drops of recipient serum or plasma to the A_1 and B cell tubes.
- Mix and centrifuge for optimal time. Resuspend, read macroscopically, grade, and record results.
- If the reaction is not enhanced to at least 2+, increase the incubation time to 30 minutes at RT. Mix and centrifuge for optimal time. Resuspend and read macroscopically.
- Grade and record results. If the reaction(s) is enhanced to at least 2+.
- Record the enhancement method on the request form (i.e., four drops of serum/plasma). Confirm the ABO of donor units.
- Interpret the ABO group.
- If the reaction is still weaker than 2+, do not discard the tubes (A_1 and B cells) and proceed with enhancement method #2.

Enhancement method #2: (Incubation at 40°C).
- Set up an autocontrol and antibody screen cells.
- Label tubes appropriately with recipient name, auto, and screen cells.
- Add two drops of serum or plasma to all tubes. If using the A_1 and B tubes from enhancement method #1 that contain four drops of serum or plasma, four drops of serum or plasma are added to the autocontrol and antibody screen cell tubes.
- Add one drop of the appropriate cell suspension to each tube.
- Mix
- Incubate the tubes for A_1, B, autocontrol, and antibody screen cells for 15 minutes at 40°C.
- Centrifuge for optimal time after incubation, resuspend the cells, read macroscopically, grade, and record results.
  a. If the autocontrol and screen cells are negative and the expected reactions with A_1 and/or B cells are enhanced to at least 2+ (i.e., forward agrees with reverse grouping):
     - Indicate the enhancement method on the request form (i.e., 40°C incubation).
     - Confirm the ABO of donor units.
     - Interpret the ABO groups.
  b. If the autocontrol, A_1, B, and all screen cells are positive and the diagnosis is viral or *Mycoplasma* pneumonia or cold agglutinin disease, suspect an auto-anti-I.

  Note: Many normal individuals have an auto-anti-I that react at 40°C but rarely at RT (22°C), and not usually above 15°C.

Repeat the reverse grouping at 37°C:
- If the expected reaction(s) with A_1 and/or B cells is ≥2+ at 37°C, the ABO discrepancy is resolved.
- If the reaction(s) with A_1 and/or B cells at 37°C is weak or 1+ and/or the ABO discrepancy still exists: Repeat the reverse grouping using cold autoadsorbed serum or plasma.
- If the discrepancy is still not resolved, a report should be sent stating "ABO cannot be determined at this time." If blood components are required, group O cellular and group AB plasma components should be transfused.
  c. If extra reactions are observed in the reverse grouping and one or more of the screen cells (autocontrol is negative)
     Perform antibody identification of cold-reactive antibodies if the antibody identification demonstrates a specific cold-reactive alloantibody (e.g., anti-M, - Le^a, -Le^b, -Pi, -N), repeat the reverse grouping at 37°C. If the expected

reaction(s) with A_1 and/or B cells is 2+ or stronger at 37°C, and the discrepancy is resolved, interpret the ABO group.

If the expected reaction(s) with A_1 and/or B cells is weaker than 2+ at 37°C, repeat the reverse grouping using A_1 and B cells that are lacking the antigen to the identified antibody (37°C not necessary). Reverse-grouping cells lacking the antigen may be selected by antigen typing group A and B donor units with the corresponding commercial antisera.

Note: ABO group should not be reported when expected positive reactions with A_1 and/or B cells are weak or 1+ by saline replacement or prewarm technique. If the discrepancy is still not resolved, submit a report stating "ABO cannot be determined at this time." If blood components are required, red blood of group O and plasma of group AB should be transfused.

4. *Reverse grouping with unexpected or extra reactions*: If the reverse grouping has an unexpected or extra reaction(s) with A_1 and/or B cells, suspect:
   - Rouleaux
   - Cold-reactive autoantibodies
   - Anti-A_1
   - Irregular cold alloantibodies: Anti-M, -N, -Pi, -Le^a, etc.
     i. If the recipient's forward group suggests groups A or AB with an unexpected reaction in the reverse group with A_1 cells, the most likely cause of a discrepancy in the reverse group is anti-A_1; therefore, it should be investigated first.
     a. Type the recipient's red cells with anti-A1 lectin.
     b. If the reaction is positive with anti-A_1 lectin, the recipient is group A1 and cannot have anti-A_1. Proceed to set up an autocontrol and antibody screen cells.
     c. If the reaction is negative with anti-A1 lectin, set up the following by saline RT method: Setting up $3A_1$ and $3A_2$ cells will provide an acceptable level of probability that the antibody is anti-A_1 should all A_1 cells and no A_2 cells react.
     d. Label tubes with recipient name, auto, and name of the screen cell, as appropriate.
        - Add two drops of serum or plasma to all tubes.
        - Add one drop of the appropriate ($3A_1$ and $3A_2$ cells, autocontrol and antibody screen cells) cell suspension to each tube.
        - Mix and incubate for 30 minutes at RT.
        - After incubation, centrifuge for optimal time, resuspend, and read macroscopically.
        - Grade and record results.

ii. If anti-A_1 has not been identified (auto is negative and one or more screen cells are positive), suspect a cold alloantibody. Perform antibody identification of cold-reactive antibodies. If the antibody identification demonstrates a specific cold-reactive alloantibody (e.g., anti-M, -Le^a, -Le^b, -Pi, -N), repeat the reverse grouping at 37°C. If the expected reaction(s) with A_1 and/or B cells is 2+ or stronger at 37°C, and the discrepancy is resolved, interpret the ABO group.

iii. If the expected reaction(s) with A_1 and/or B cells is weaker than 2+ at 37°C, repeat the reverse grouping using A_1 and B cells that are lacking the antigen to the identified antibody (37°C not necessary). Reverse grouping cells lacking the antigen may be selected by antigen typing group A and B donor units with the corresponding commercial antisera.

Note: ABO group should not be reported when expected positive reactions with A_1 and/or B cells are weak or 1+ by saline replacement or prewarm technique. If the discrepancy is still not resolved, a report should be sent stating "ABO grouping cannot be determined at this time." If blood components are required, group O cellular and group AB plasma components should be transfused.

The flowchart for resolving ABO discrepancies is given in **Annexure 45.1** and examples of ABO discrepancies and their possible resolution are given in **Annexure 45.2**. Nowadays, molecular blood group typing is used for the genetically exact definition of blood group variants (e.g., RhD and ABO) and to reveal the original genotypes in multitransfused samples, or antibody-masked RBCs.

ANNEXURE 45.1: RESOLVING ABO DISCREPANCIES FLOWCHART

Perform clerical check. Check patient history, age, medications, and diagnosis. Check for technical problems—repeat testing.

Unexpected negative		Unexpected positive	
Reverse	**Forward**	**Reverse**	**Forward**
Incubate at room temperature for 15–30 minutes		Preform antibody screen w/ auto-control	Wash cells w/warm saline and repeat testing
Incubate at 4°C for 15–30 minutes (Include auto-control)	All cells positive	A_1+ (Unexpected) Screen-Auto / Screen-Auto	Resolved? / Unresolved?
Subgroup of Aw/Anti-A_1/Test RBCs w/ A_1 lectin	Increase serum cell ratio / Switch to different anti-serum / Rouleaux saline replacement / Auto-antibody Cold auto-adsorption prewarm	Alloantibody Panel to ID	Rouleaux Wharton's jelly Cold agglutinin / Mixed field Reactions? Transfusion or HPC Transplant / Cells +/all antisera? Polyagglutinable cells Verify w/ Control and Lectin
Repeat grouping w/A_2 cells	Read microscopically	Repeat reverse grouping and antigen Negative RBCs	Check by acquired B "Autologous" anti-B Acidified anti-B / Switch to monoclonal reagents
	Treat RBCs with enzyme		
	Absorption/Elution secretor studies		

If discrepancy remains

(HPC: hematopoietic progenitor cell; RBC: red blood cell)

ANNEXURE 45.2: ABO DISCREPANCIES AND POSSIBLE RESOLUTION

Patient	Forward grouping		Reverse grouping			Autocontrol	Possible cause	Resolution
	Anti-A	Anti-B	A₁ cells	B cells	"O" cells			
1.	0	0	0	0	0	0	Group O newborn; elderly patient; very low immunoglobulin levels	Incubate tests at 4°C, check the age of patient
2.	4+	4+	2+	2+	2+	2+	Rouleaux; cold autoantibody	Wash RBCs and repeat testing test for cold antibodies
3.	4+	0	1+	4+	0	0	Probable A₂ subgroup with anti-A₁	Test with anti-A₁ lectin, test serum with additional A₁, A₂ and O cells and anti-H lectin and A₂ cells
4.	4+	4+	1+	0	0	0	Probable A₂B subgroup with anti-A₁	Test with anti-A₁ lectin, test serum with additional A₁, A₂ and O cells
5.	0	0	4+	4+	4+	0	Probable Oh (Bombay)	Test with anti-H lectin may send to reference lab for confirmation
6.	4+	2+	0	4+	0	0	Group A with acquired B phenotype	Check history for lower GIT problem or septicemia; test with acidified anti-B serum. Test serum with autologous cells
7.	0	4+	4+	1+	1+	1+	Group B with cold antibody	Test for cold antibodies and identify if appropriate
8.	4+	4+	2+	0	2+	0	Group AB with alloantibody	Test for cold antibodies and identify if appropriate
9.	4+	0	0	4+	3+	0	A1 with potent anti-H	Confirm A₁ with anti-A₁ lectin test additional A₂, O, A₁ cells and Oh if available
10.	0	0	2+	4+	0	0	A subgroup probably Ax with anti-A₁	Perform saliva studies or absorption

(GIT: gastrointestinal tract; RBC: red blood cell)

CHAPTER 46

Collection of Blood Sample for Grouping/Crossmatching

SCOPE AND APPLICATION

The prime objective of this standard operating procedure (SOP) is to describe how to collect blood samples from patients for blood grouping and crossmatching. Further, it aims at developing a clear communication between the clinician and the blood center in ensuring a safe blood transfusion.

RESPONSIBILITY

It is the responsibility of the clinician in-charge/resident medical officer (RMO) and the staff nurse on duty in indoor patient department of the hospital.

MATERIALS REQUIRED

- *Equipment*:
    - Disposable 5 mL syringe with needle (0.55 × 25 mm)
    - Tourniquet
    - Spirit wipes
    - Gauze sponges
    - Vacutainers

These tubes (vacutainers) are designed to be filled with a predetermined volume of blood by vacuum. The rubber stoppers are color coded according to the additives contained in the tubes. The purple **(Fig. 1)** and red **(Fig. 2)** top vacutainers are used to collect blood center samples.

Purple Top	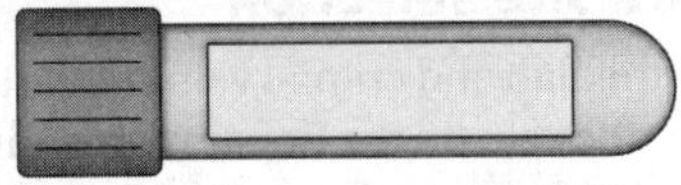
Additive	EDTA
Mode of action	Forms calcium salts to remove calcium
Uses	Hematology (CBC) and Blood Center (Crossmatch); requires *full draw*—invert eight times to prevent clotting and platelet clumping

FIG. 1: Purple top vacutainer. (*For color version, see Plate 9*)

(CBC: complete blood count; EDTA: ethylenediaminetetraacetic acid)

Red top	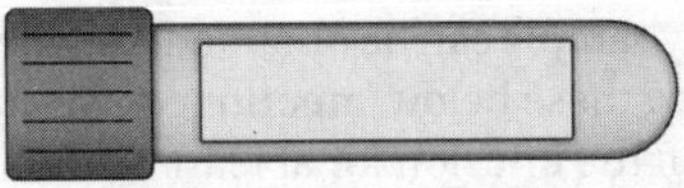
Additive	None
Mode of action	Blood clots, and the serum is separated by centrifugation
Uses	Blood chemistries, immunology and serology, Blood Center (crossmatch)

FIG. 2: Red top vacutainer. (*For color version, see Plate 9*)

REQUIREMENTS FOR BLOOD SAMPLE COLLECTION

Patient Relations and Identification

The phlebotomist's role requires a professional, courteous, and understanding demeanor in all the patient interactions. Introduce yourself, greet the patients, and identify the patients and inform them of the procedure to be performed. Effective communication—both verbal and nonverbal—is essential.

It is essential to identify patient correctly. If the patient can answer, ask for their full name. Ask the patient to provide additional information, such as surname and date of birth, and use the request as a reference.

If possible, chat with the patient during the process to make the patient feel comfortable and focus less on the procedure. Always thank the patient and apologize politely when you are done.

Venipuncture Site Selection

The large, thick median and cranial veins of the arm are most commonly used, but the basilic vein on the dorsum of the arm or dorsal veins in the hand are also suitable for venipuncture. Foot veins are a last resort due to the high potential for complications.

Avoid the following sites when collecting blood samples:

- *Extensive scarring from burns and surgery*: It is difficult to puncture the scar tissue and take a blood sample.
- *The upper extremity on the side of a previous mastectomy*: Lymphedema may affect the test results.
- *Hematoma*: Can cause false test results. Collect samples distal to the hematoma if no other site is available.
- *Intravenous (IV) therapy/blood transfusions*: Fluids may dilute the sample, so collect from the opposite arm if possible. Otherwise, a satisfactory sample can be obtained from below the site of IV therapy by following these below-mentioned steps:
    - Turn off the infusion for at least 2 minutes before venipuncture.
    - Apply the tourniquet below the IV site. Choose a different vein than one with the IV.
- Perform a venipuncture. Take 5 mL of blood and discard before cannula/fistula/heparin lock—hospitals have special policies regarding these devices. In general, blood should not be taken from an arm with a fistula or cannula without consulting the physician.
- *Edematous extremities*: Accumulation of tissue fluid alters test results.

PROCEDURE

Vein Selection

- Palpate and trace the veins with the index finger. Arteries are the most elastic, thick-walled, and pulsating. Thrombosed veins are inelastic, feel like a cord, and roll easily.
- If superficial veins are not immediately visible, massage the arm from the wrist to the elbow, patting the area with the index and middle fingers; a warm, moist washcloth can be placed on the area for 5 minutes to force blood into the veins or lower the extremity over the bedside to allow the veins to fill.

Performing a Venipuncture

- Approach the patient in a friendly and calm manner. He needs to make himself comfortable and get the patient's cooperation.
- Identify the patient correctly.

- Fill out the blood/components correctly in the requisition form.
- Check for allergies to antiseptics, adhesives, or latex by checking wristbands and asking patient questions.
- Position the patient. (The patient should sit in a chair, lie down, or sit up in bed.) Hyperextend the patient's arm.
- Apply the tourniquet 3–4 inches above the selected puncture site. Do not let it stick too tightly or leave it on for >2 minutes.
- Patient should make a fist without hand pumping.
- Select the venipuncture site.
- Prepare the patient's arm with a spirit swab. Cleanse in a circular fashion, starting at the center and working outward. Allow to air dry.
- Grasp the patient's arm firmly with your thumb and pull the skin to secure the vein. The needle should form an angle of 15–30° with the surface of the arm as shown in **Fig. 3**. Quickly insert the needle through the skin and into the lumen of the vein. Avoid injury and excessive probing to collect the blood samples for testing.
- Once the blood sample has been drawn into the syringe, remove the tourniquet.
- Remove the needle from the patient's arm with a quick and backward motion.
- Once the needle is out of the arm, pinch the gauze and apply enough pressure to avoid hematoma formation.
- Place 2 mL of blood sample in the purple top vacutainer and 2 mL in the red top vacutainer.
- Invert the tube with the purple top eight times to mix the blood with ethylenediaminetetraacetic acid (EDTA) to prevent clotting and platelet clumping.
- Label the vacutainer at the patient's bedside.
- Dispose of used materials/supplies in designated containers.
- Immediately send the blood sample to the blood center after properly completing the protocol.

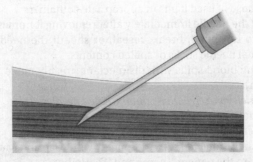

FIG. 3: Needle angle. (*For color version, see Plate 10*)

SAFETY PRECAUTIONS DURING BLOOD SAMPLING

Prevention of Hematoma

- Puncture the uppermost wall of the vein only.
- Before taking out the needle, release the tourniquet.
- Use large superficial veins.
- Ensure that the needle is fully pierced through the uppermost wall of the vein. (Partial penetration can leak blood into the soft tissue surrounding the vein.)
- Apply pressure to the venipuncture site.

Prevention of Hemolysis

- Gently mix the blood sample vacutainer with red top containing anticoagulant eight times.
- Do not draw blood from a hematoma.
- When using a needle and syringe, do not pull back on the plunger too hard.
- Avoid sample frothing.
- Make sure that the venipuncture site is dry.
- Avoid probing or traumatic venipuncture.

Safety and Infection Control

Because of contact between sick patients and their specimens, it is important to follow safety and infection control procedures.

Protect Yourself

- *Practice universal precautions*:
  - Wear gloves and a lab coat or gown when handling blood/body fluids.
  - Change gloves between patients or when soiled with blood.
  - Wash your hands with antiseptic/detergent or disinfect with alcohol.
  - Dispose of used items in appropriate containers.
- Discard the needle immediately after removing it from the patient's vein. Do not bend, break, reseal, or sheath the needle to avoid accidental needle sticks or spilled contents.
- Clean the blood spills with disinfectant (freshly made 10% bleach solution).
- *If you prick yourself with a contaminated needle*:
  - Remove your gloves and dispose of them properly.
  - Squeeze the puncture site to encourage bleeding.
  - Wash the affected area thoroughly with soap and water.
  - Record the patient's name and ID number.
  - Follow institutional guidelines for treatment and follow-up.

Note: Prophylactic use of Tab zidovudine after needle stick injury on exposure to HIV-infected patients has been shown to be effective (about 79%) in preventing seroconversion.

Protect the Patient
- Keep blood collection equipment away from patients, especially children and psychiatric patients.
- Practice good hygiene to protect patients. If gloves are worn, change them between patients and wash hands frequently.
- Always wear a clean lab coat or gown.

TROUBLESHOOTING GUIDELINES

If an Incomplete Collection or No Blood is Obtained
- Reposition the needle as it may not be in the lumen. Move it forward (**Fig. 4**).
- Or you may be penetrating too far, so move backward (**Fig. 5**).
- Adjust the angle as the bevel may touch the vein wall (**Fig. 6**).
- Release the tourniquet. It may obstruct blood flow.
- Try another sample tube. It may not have vacuum.
- Refix the vein. The vein may roll away from the needle tip or puncture site.

If Blood Stops Flowing into the Tube
- The vein may be collapsed (**Fig. 7**). Reattach the tourniquet to increase venous filling. If this does not work, remove the needle, place your hand over the puncture site, and try again.
- The needle may have been pulled out of the vein when the vacutainer is attached for sample collection. Hold the equipment firmly and place fingers against the patient's arm, use the flange as a lever to pull out, and insert the vacutainer.

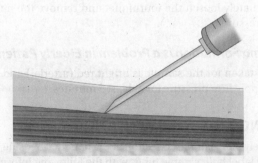

FIG. 4: Needle not in the lumen of the vein. (*For color version, see Plate 10*)

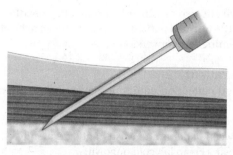

FIG. 5: Needle penetrated too far. (*For color version, see Plate 10*)

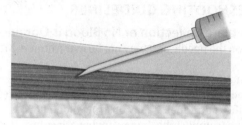

FIG. 6: Bevel touching the vein wall. (*For color version, see Plate 11*)

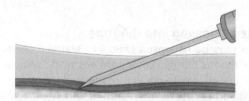

FIG. 7: Collapsed vein. (*For color version, see Plate 11*)

Problems Other than an Incomplete Collection

- A hematoma forms under the skin near the puncture site (**Fig. 8**). Immediately loosen the tourniquet and remove the needle. Apply firm pressure.

Hematoma Formation is a Problem in Elderly Patients

The blood taken for the sample is bright red (arterial) and not venous (**Fig. 9**). Apply firm pressure for at least 5 minutes.

LABELING AND DOCUMENTATION

Immediately after sample collection at the patient's bedside, clearly and accurately label both sample tubes with the following information:

- Patient's first name and last name
- Age and gender

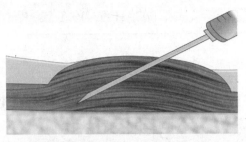

FIG. 8: Hematoma under the skin. (*For color version, see Plate 11*)

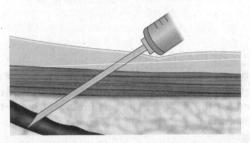

FIG. 9: Bright red (arterial) blood being drawn. (*For color version, see Plate 11*)

- Outpatient department (OPD) number
- Inpatient department (IPD) number
- Ward name
- Admission date
- Signature of the staff drawing the sample and date

Patient names and other details must be verified against patient records and invoices. For unconscious patients, have a family member or another staff member identify the patient.

Do not label sample tubes before taking blood samples. This is because there is a risk of putting the patient's blood into the wrong tube.

A fresh sample is essential to ensure that the patient does not receive incompatible blood.

For newborns up to 4 months, please also send a sample from the mother.

The requisition form must be completed and signed by the attending physician/RMO. All information requested in the request form must be completed accurately and legibly.

CHAPTER 47

Transfusion of Right Blood to Right Patient

SCOPE AND APPLICATION

The prime objective of this standard operating procedure (SOP) is to minimize the risk of a patient receiving a wrong blood/blood component unit and to provide the guidelines for monitoring the patient during the blood transfusion so as to identify the reaction, if any, at the earliest for proper management.

RESPONSIBILITY

It is the responsibility of the staff nurse on duty and consultant in charge/resident medical officer (RMO) to provide right blood to right patient once the blood unit has been received from the blood center.

MATERIALS REQUIRED

The following are needed for administering the blood/blood component:
- Blood/blood component unit
- Sterile blood administration set with filter/pressure line with filter (in case of newborns)
- Tourniquet
- Spirit wipes
- Gauze sponges

PROCEDURAL ISSUES

1. *Getting blood from blood center*: The blood/blood components are processed for the patients on receipt of the properly filled and signed requisition form for blood and blood components **(Annexure 47.1)** from the consultant doctor. Incomplete forms are not to be

entertained. The blood center must provide the following while issuing the unit:

- Patient's details on the crossmatch label and compatibility report
- Patient's ABO and Rh group
- Unique donation no. (unit no.)
- Blood group of the blood unit
- Blood transfusion record/adverse transfusion reaction form **(Annexure 47.2)**

If all the information on the various documents as stated above and the blood/blood component unit correlate, the blood/blood component unit is issued after getting receipt thereof from the person receiving the unit.

2. *Informed consent*: Clinicians are responsible for explaining and obtaining informed consent **(Annexure 47.3)** prior to transfusion and for explaining to the patient or legal guardian the reason for the transfusion as well as the benefits expected, risks, and alternatives as outlined in the consent form. The patient or legal guardian must sign the consent form. This form must be appropriately dated and witnessed.

3. *Checking the blood unit*: Blood unit should always be checked for signs of deterioration:
   - Upon arrival at the ward or upon arrival at the operating room
   - Pretransfusion, if it is not used immediately

Signs of discoloration or leakage are the only indications that the blood is contaminated with bacteria, which can cause serious or fatal reactions during transfusions.

The presence of the following signs/evidence, as shown in **Fig. 1**, *should be checked*:

- Evidence of hemolysis in plasma indicates that the blood has been contaminated, allowed to freeze, or become too warm.
- Evidence of hemolysis in the line between the red blood cells and plasma.
- Signs of contamination, such as red blood cells, will change color and become darker or purple/black.
- Bacterial contamination due to citrate use by proliferating bacteria or blood clots that may indicate that the blood was not mixed properly with the anticoagulant at the time of blood collection.
- Evidence that the blood unit has been leaked or opened.

Do not transfuse if the blood unit is visibly abnormal, damaged, or has been (or may have been) out of the refrigerator for >30 minutes.

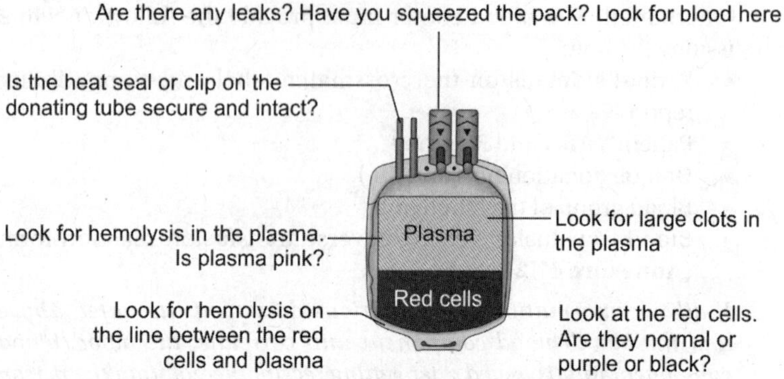

FIG. 1: Various signs of deterioration to be looked for. (***For color version, see Plate 12***)

4. *Storing and transporting of blood or blood component prior to transfusion*: Transfusions of whole blood, red blood cells, and thawed fresh frozen plasma should be started within 30 minutes of removal from the refrigerator following preparation at the transfusion center. If transfusion cannot be started within this time, it should be stored in an approved blood center refrigerator at a temperature between 2 and 6°C. An upper limit of 6°C is essential to minimize the growth of bacterial contamination in blood centers.

The lower limit of 2°C is important to prevent hemolysis, which can lead to life-threatening bleeding problems and renal failure. If your ward or operating room does not have a suitable refrigerator to store blood, the blood components should not be released from the blood centers until immediately prior to transfusion.

It is important that blood is kept within a temperature range of 2–8°C during transport. A system should be installed to monitor the temperature during transportation. This can be accomplished with a blood transport container.

All unused/residual blood products must be safely disposed of according to guidelines of biomedical waste.

5. *Pretransfusion patient and blood unit identification*: A final check at the patient's bedside is the last chance to detect identification errors and prevent potentially fatal incompatible transfusions.

Before starting of blood transfusion, two staff members (one of whom must be a doctor or staff nurse) must ensure the following:
- The patient's complete identity
- The blood units, compatibility reports, and crossmatch labels
- Examine the blood pack for signs of hemolysis or leakage from the pack.

*This is done using the format specified in **Annexure 47.4**. Any discrepancies mean that the blood should not be transfused and that the blood center should be notified.*

6. *Time limit for initiation of transfusion* **(Table 1)**: Blood and its products are at risk of bacterial growth and loss of function once they are removed from the correct storage conditions.

7. *Warming blood: Do not heat the blood in a bowl of hot water as it can cause life-threatening red blood cell hemolysis.* Blood should only be warmed in a blood warmer and warmed blood is mostly needed in the following:
   - *Large-volume rapid transfusion:*
     - Adults: >50 mL/kg/h
     - Children: >15 mL/kg/h
   - Infant exchange transfusion
   - Patients with clinically significant cold agglutinin.

8. *Pharmaceuticals and blood components:*
   - Do not add drugs or fluids other than saline (sodium chloride 0.9%) to blood components.
   - Separate intravenous (IV) line is a must when an IV fluid other than normal saline needs to be administered concurrently with blood components.

9. *Monitoring of transfused patient:* It is important to record baseline observations and monitor patients during and after transfusion to detect adverse events as early as possible according to *blood transfusion record/reaction form in **Annexure 47.2**.* This allows you to quickly take potentially life-saving measures.

Before starting a blood transfusion, it is important to:
- Encourage patients to contact their nurse or doctor immediately if they experience reactions such as shivering, flushing, pain, or shortness of breath or when they begin to feel anxious.
- Make sure that the patient is in direct observation.

Table 1: Time limits for transfusion.		
	Start transfusion	**Complete transfusion**
Whole blood/packed RBC	Within 30 minutes of removing blood unit from the refrigerator	Within 4 hours
Platelet concentrates	Immediately	Within 20 minutes
FFP and cryoprecipitate	As soon as possible	Within 20 minutes
(FFP: fresh frozen plasma; RBC: red blood cell)		

Start transfusion at a rate of 20 mL/h for the first 15 minutes. Severe reactions are most common during the first 15 minutes of transfusion. All patients, especially unconscious patients, must be monitored during this period and for the first 15 minutes of each subsequent unit as most ABO incompatibilities occur in the first 15 minutes.

- If no reaction is noticed after the first 15 minutes, take and record a second set of vital signs.
- Increase the infusion rate based on recipient hemodynamics.
- Transfuse over 2 hours if hemodynamically stable.
- Transfuse over 4 hours if hemodynamically unstable.

This time limit is empirical and based on the time it takes for the blood bag to reach room temperature. Since blood is an excellent culture media, storing blood units at room temperature for a long period of time can lead to bacterial growth. If the recipient's medical condition requires long-term blood transfusions, request blood aliquots from the blood center and administer for at least 4 hours each.

Monitor the patient for each unit of blood transfused:
- Before starting a blood transfusion
- As soon as the transfusion is started
- 15 minutes after the start of transfusion
- At least every 30 minutes during transfusion
- After the transfusion is complete
- 4 hours after transfusion completion

10. *At each of these stages, the staff nurse records the following vital information regarding the patient's blood administration*:
- General appearance of the patient
- Temperature
- Pulse
- Blood pressure
- Respiratory rate
- Fluid balance:
    - Oral and IV fluid intake
    - Urinary output

Records:
- Transfusion start time
- Completion time of transfusion
- Volume and type of all transfused products
- A unique donation ID for all transfused products
- Adverse effects if any

Transfusion of each unit of the blood or blood component must be completed within 4 hours after the blood unit is punctured. If the unit is not transfused within 4 hours, discontinue its use and dispose of the remainder in the biomedical waste system.

Once the transfusion is complete, take a full set of vital signs, document on the blood administration record/reaction form, and discontinue the blood tubing. Used blood bag and IV tubing are disposed of in the red biohazard bag (blood bags and tubing are the exception to the hazardous waste rule and are considered hazardous waste).

11. *Transfusion reactions*: If a patient appears to be experiencing an adverse reaction, the following immediate steps are taken:
    - Stop the transfusion
    - Maintain IV patency with normal saline
    - Check all blood component(s) labels, forms, and patient identification for errors
    - Notify a patient's physician if necessary
    - Treat reaction
    - Notify the blood center; submit workup specimens and report forms

    If a transfusion reaction is suspected, do not discard the blood pack and infusion set. Return the blood bag, administration set, and 5 mL of a patient's posttransfusion blood [ethylenediaminetetraacetic acid (EDTA) and clotted] in a sterile tube and patient's post-transfusion sample of urine to the blood center for testing.

    Submit monthly report of all blood transfusion reactions online to National Institute of Biologicals, Ministry of Health and Family Welfare, Government of India for monitoring under Haemovigilance Programme of India (HvPI) and a copy of the report is also submitted to State Blood Transfusion Council.

    Record the clinical details and actions taken in the patient's case notes.

DON'TS FOR BLOOD TRANSFUSION

- Do not use blood from unlicensed blood centers.
- Do not delay starting transfusions.
- Do not warm the blood.
- Do not use routine transfusion premedication.
- Do not transfuse blood unit for >4 hours.
- Do not leave the patients unattended.
- Do not add any medication to blood bag.
- Discard blood when not used.
- Do not ask for all the blood bags at once.
- Do not use an unmonitored refrigerator for storage.
- Do not use the same transfusion set for multiple blood units.

- Do not wet outlet port of blood.
- Do not store platelets in the refrigerator.
- Do not get complacent when verifying the identity of the patient.
- Do not insist on immediate or directed donations from close relatives.

It is important to document the reason for the transfusion in the patient's case report before administering blood components. If later on, the patient has a potentially transfusion-related problem, the record should identify who ordered the component and why. This information is also useful when conducting audits of blood transfusion operations. A record in the patient's case note is your best defense in the event of future medical legal issues.

The following information should be recorded in the patient record:
- Whether the patient and/or family are informed of the proposed transfusion therapy
- Reason for blood transfusion
- Signature of the prescribing physician
- *Pretransfusion checks of*:
  - Patient identity
  - Blood unit
  - The signature of the person performing the pretransfusion identification
- *Blood transfusion*:
  - Type and volume of each transfused product
  - A unique donation ID of each unit transfused
  - Blood group of each unit transfused
  - Start time of each blood unit
  - Signature of person administering the blood component
  - Patient monitoring before, during, and after the transfusion
- Any transfusion reaction.

ANNEXURE 47.1

REQUISITION FORM FOR BLOOD/BLOOD COMPONENTS
(To be filled by the Requsitioning Department)

Date:................. Received on:.............. At:.........

Request No.:.................. Signature:..................

Place patient ID label and write below:

Patient Details	**Patient's Name**:........................ **MR No**:......................
	IP No.:............... **Age**:.................. **Sex**:...........................
	Father's/Husband's Name:............... **Address**:.................
	Ward/Department:............ **Consultant In-Charge**:.............

Clinical diagnosis with short history: ....

Is the patient newborn? ☐ Yes ☐ No

Hb (g/dL): .... Platelet count: ....PT/PTT:.................

Previous History of:

Any Transfusion : ☐ Yes ☐ No   Blood Group, if known ☐

Any Reaction   : ☐ Yes ☐ No   Antibodies (if any) detected earlier:..........................

Allergy   : ☐ Yes ☐ No

In Case of Females: No. of Pregnancies:............................

Still Birth/Miscarriage:.........................

Hemolytic Disease of New Born:...............

BLOOD OR BLOOD COMPONENTS REQUIRED (Number of Units)							
Whole Blood (WB)	Packed RBCs (PRBC)	Platelet Conc. (RANDOM)	Single Donor Platelet Apheresis (SDP)	Fresh Frozen Plasma (FFP)	Cryopre-cipitate (Cryo ppt.)	Others	

Indication for Transfusion:...

Type of Request: ☐ Routine   ☐ Urgent

Required on:...................:... Time:.................AM/PM

Donors provided: ☐ Yes ☐ No

Specimen collection and labeled by: ....

Sign and ID No.: .... **Date**: .... **Time**: ....

Certified that the blood samples and details in the requisition form are correct. I have explained the necessity of Blood Transfusion or any procedure and the risk associated with it to the patient/relatives. The informed consent for this has been taken from patient/relative.

....
Name of the Doctor I/C & ID No.   **Consultant Blood Center**

CONSENT FOR INVESTIGATIONS (RAPID METHOD)

I am fully aware that the fresh whole blood is needed for my patient's treatment urgently, it has to be tested for infectious diseases like HIV, HCV, VDRL, HBsAg, MP, by Rapid method which have slightly lower sensitivity and may miss such infection, if present in the donor even after testing. Keeping in view the requirement, I am prepared to take the risk involved for endangering the patient to such infections.

Signature of the Attending Physician: ....

Name of Doctor (Assuming Responsibility): ....

Date and Time: .... **Signature:** ....

Emp. ID: ....

PLEASE READ INSTRUCTIONS OVERLEAF

Instructions

1. Send 2 mL blood in **Purple Top vacutainer and 4 mL blood in Red Top vacutainer with the requisition form; These must be labeled with the following information**:
   a. Patient's name and Family name
   b. Age and Sex
   c. MR. No.
   d. IP No.
   e. Patient's ward
   f. Date
   g. Signature of the staff taking the sample
2. In case of new born baby up to 4 months old, send the mother's sample also.
3. All requests must accompany replacement donors.
4. The requisition form will not be accepted if it is not signed or any section is left blank.
5. Blood and its components must be taken when required for definite use, normally once issued it will not be taken back.
6. Cross matched blood will be kept reserve for 72 hours only.
7. Blood must be used as soon as received.
8. Blood will be issued after about 2 hours of receiving the requisition and blood sample.
9. Please ensure appropriate and rational use of blood.

FOR THE USE OF BLOOD CENTER

S. No.	Unit No.	Blood Group	Segment No.	Date of Expiry	Crossmatch Method	Crossmatch Report	Date and Time of Crossmatching	Name and Signature of Technologist	Remarks
1									
2									
3									
4									
5									
6									
7									
8									
9									
10									
11									
12									
13									
14									

ANNEXURE 47.2

BLOOD TRANSFUSION RECORD/ADVERSE TRANSFUSION REACTION FORM

(Return the form duly completed after completion of Transfusion)

Place patient ID label and write below:

Patient details	Name:	Age:	Sex	IPD No.:
	MR No.:	Ward:	Ward/Bed No.:	
	Clinical diagnosis:		Patient's Blood Group:	

Type of blood/Blood component to be transfused:............................

Volume:............mL   Date and time of issue:..............................

Blood/Blood component Unit No.:..

Blood unit Segment No. (Only in case of Whole blood/PRBCs):............

Blood Group: ....

Date of expiry of blood/Blood component:...................................

How long Blood/Blood component unit was out of Refrigerator:...........

Whether Blood has been warmed?   ☐ Yes   ☐ No

Whether pretransfusion check form filled?   ☐ Yes   ☐ No

If filled, Names of two checkers: 1st.................... 2nd....................

Clerical Check (please tick)

Patient ID correct: ☐ Yes   ☐ No

Blood pack correct: ☐ Yes   ☐ No

Blood transfusion record correct: ☐ Yes   ☐ No

Time and date of start of transfusion:.....................................

Rate of transfusion: (i) During 1st 15 minutes: ....drops/minutes

(ii) After 15 minutes:...............drops/minute

Observation during Transfusion:

Period of observation	Vital signs				
	Time	Temp	Respiration	BP	Pulse
Pretransfusion					
During 1st 15 minutes					
After next 30 minutes					
After next 30 minutes					
After next 30 minutes					
After next 30 minutes					
After next 30 minutes					
After next 30 minutes					
After next 30 minutes					
After next 30 minutes					
After 4 hours of completion of blood transfusion					

Date and Time of Completion of Transfusion: ....

Name, Signature and ID of Staff Nurse: ....

Name, Signature and ID of Doctor: ....

(1) The transfusion rate for blood components depends on the clinical context, age and cardiac status of the patient. In stable, nonbleeding adult patients typical administration durations are:

S. No.	Blood Product	Start Transfusion	Complete Transfusion
1	PRBCs (200–300 mL)	Within 30 minutes of removal from storage area	*Within 4 hours*
2	FFP (170–250 mL)	Within 30 minutes of removal from storage area	Within 20 minutes
3	Platelets (50–70 mL)	Immediately	Within 20 minutes
4	SDP 300 mL	Immediately	Within 30–60 minutes
5	Cryoprecipitates (15–25 mL)	Immediately	Within 3–15 minutes transfuse as rapidly as tolerated

(2) Mix components thoroughly by inversion and transfuse through BT set incorporating a standard 170–200 μm filter to remove clots and aggregates.

(3) Rate of transfusion during the first 15 minutes should be slower than the prescribed rate.

(4) Observe closely (particularly during first 15–30 minutes) for the most common acute complications associated

(5) Platelets should always be run through a NEW blood administration set; otherwise the platelets will become trapped in the used filter.

(6) BT set must be changed at least every 2–4 units.

(7) Number of drops per minutes $= \dfrac{\text{Total volume to be transfused}}{\text{Time in minutes}} \times$

drop factor (drop factor for PRBCs = 15, and for other component = 20)

For Transfusion-related Adverse Reaction Notification

(To be filled by RMO)

Observations prior to transfusion	Temp:......°C	Pulse: /min	BP:... / ...mm Hg	RR:.../min
Observations at time of reaction	Temp:......°C	Pulse: /min	BP:... / ...mm Hg	RR:.../min
Time adverse reaction noticed:	Volume transfused:.......... mL			

Please tick relevant symptoms and signs listed below and provide details:

Type of Adverse Reaction	Symptoms	Signs
Mild	☐ Itching ☐ Fever	Localized: ☐ Urticaria ☐ Rash ☐ Temperature increase of 1–1.5°C
Moderate	☐ Anxiety ☐ Itching ☐ Palpitation ☐ Mild dyspnea ☐ Headache	☐ Flushing ☐ Urticaria ☐ Rigors ☐ Temperature rise >1.5°C ☐ Restless ☐ Tachycardia

Severe	☐ Anxiety	☐ Rigors
	☐ Chest pain	☐ Temperature rise (Rise >1.5°C)
	☐ Respiratory distress/ Shortness of breath	☐ Restlessness
	☐ Pain: Chest/Flank/ Abdominal/Infusion site/Other	☐ Hypotension (Fall of ≥20% in Systolic BP)
		☐ Tachycardia (Rise of ≥20% in heart rate)
	☐ Headache	☐ Hemoglobinuria (Red colored urine)
	☐ Dyspnea	☐ Unexplained bleeding (DIC)

Patient under anesthesia: Yes/No

Chest X-ray changes:

Comments/other signs and symptoms:

....
Name, Signature and ID of Doctor

Instructions:

1. In case of no-reaction, send this form duly completed along with empty blood bag. No sample is required.
2. In case of reaction, staff on duty should inform the RMO and start symptomatic treatment.
3. For Mild Reaction:
   a. Slow the transfusion rate.
   b. Administer antihistamine IM (e.g., chlorpheniramine 0.1 mg/kg or equivalent).
   c. If no clinical improvement within 30 minutes or if the condition worsens, treat as moderate reaction.
4. For Moderate Reaction:
   a. Stop the transfusion. Replace the infusion set and keep the IV line open with normal saline.

b. RMO should notify the consultant for the adverse reaction of patient and the blood center immediately.

c. Send the blood unit with infusion set, clotted and EDTA blood samples from the vein opposite infusion site to the blood center and urine for hemolysis to the lab.

d. Administer antihistamine IM/Paracetamol IM/Corticosteroids and bronchodilators as advised by the consultant.

e. If no clinical improvement within 15 minutes or if the condition worsens, treat as severe reaction.

5. For Severe Reaction:

a. In addition to that described under moderate reaction, infuse normal saline to maintain BP.

b. Maintain airway and give flow oxygen by mask.

c. Send blood samples for PBF, Blood counts, Serum bilirubin, Coagulation screening, Urea, Creatinine, Electrolytes and tests as advised by the consultant.

d. Get the chest X-ray done.

e. Further treatment be continued as per the advice of the Consultant depending upon the condition of the patient.

ANNEXURE 47.3

INFORMED CONSENT: TRANSFUSION OF BLOOD/ BLOOD COMPONENTS

> Place patient identification label or write below:
> Name:_____
> MR Number:_____ IP Number:___
> Age/DOB:_____ Sex:_____

My/My patient's Doctor .... has explained that I/my patient have the medical condition ...., for which I/my patient need a blood transfusion. The chances for my/my patient's improvement or recovery will be significantly helped by receiving blood/blood components such as Packed red blood cells, Fresh frozen plasma, Platelets or cryo-precipitates by transfusions. My/My Patient's medical condition requires the following blood product/s.

(DOCTOR TO INDICATE COMPONENTS)

☐ Packed Red Blood Cells (PRBCs)	☐ Random Donor Platelets (RDP)
☐ Fresh Frozen Plasma (FFP)	☐ Single Donor Platelets (SDP)
☐ Cryoprecipitates	

A transfusion is necessary to replace a part of my/my patient's blood and is given to either:

- To replace red blood cells to treat or prevent anemia, improve oxygen transport and relieve symptoms of dizziness, tiredness or shortness of breath or
- To give platelets to help stopping or prevent bleeding or
- To give fresh plasma product to stop, treat or prevent bleeding.

Transfusions are given via cannulae (needle in your vein) or via a central line into my/my patient's vein. During transfusion I/my patient will be closely watched for any possible reactions. I/My patient will also be regularly checked as to whether I/my patient may need another blood transfusion.

I understand that by refusing blood transfusion deemed medically necessary by my Doctor, my/my patient's medical condition will result in delayed recovery or worsen to the extent of putting myself/ my patient at the risk of dying ....

I understand that although the blood/blood products to be administered have been prepared and tested in accordance with the mandatory provisions under The Drugs and Cosmetics Act 1940 and Rules 1945 as amended from time to time yet, there is still a very small (one in a thousand) chance that the blood/blood products will be incompatible with my/my patient's body and a transfusion reaction (Hemolytic Transfusion Reaction) can occur. Although transfusion reactions can be treated successfully, I understand that on very rare occasions they can be fatal (one in two hundred fifty thousand transfusions). I understand that mild reactions like itching, rash, fever and headaches to blood/blood products are more common but can be treated and may not require the transfusion to be stopped. I understand that even with testing by the most up-to-date methods, there is a small chance that blood/the blood products may contain virus/Prions that will enter my/my patient's system and may not be recognized as an infection for many months or years. Even with proper testing, my/my patient's chances of contracting viral Hepatitis may be approximately 30 in every 1 million transfusions or of contracting HIV in three of 1 million transfusions and of contracting bacterial infections in one of one million transfusions. Reactions like respiratory distress (shortness of breath) or lung injury, infection as a result of exposure to blood borne micro-organisms and possible effects on the immune system, which may decrease the body's ability to fight infection are rare.

In some situations, there may be other choices to a blood transfusion and these include—fluid replacement with saline or other artificial compounds and/or iron supplements. I understand that in some instances, it may be possible to collect my/my patient's own blood lost during surgery (intraoperative blood salvage) or shortly after surgery (postoperative blood salvage) or my/my patient's own blood can be used to prepare platelet gel, autologous conditioned plasma, or bone marrow aspirate concentrate. **The Doctor has discussed these with me and I understand that these choices are not suitable for me/my patient.**

I have been given the patient education material regarding blood transfusion.

I was able to ask questions and raise concerns with the doctor about my/my patient's condition, the proposed procedure and its risks, and my/my patient's treatment options. My questions and concerns have been discussed and answered to my satisfaction. I have been given no guarantee or assurance as to the results that may be obtained. All blanks on this form were filled in before I signed. On the basis of the above statements, I give my consent by appending my signatures on this informed consent form to administer blood/blood products for myself/for my patient for the number of units on the date and time as per details mentioned below:

S. No.	Date and Time	Blood/Blood Components	No. of Units	Patient's/Surrogate's (along with relation) Name and Signature	Doctor's Signature

Name of Patient:......................................

Signatures of Patient:...........................

Date and Time:.....................................

Name of Surrogate:...............................

Signatures of Surrogate:.........................

Date and Time:.....................................

(Consent of surrogate is to be obtained only when the patient is not in a condition to sign)

Relation to Patient:............ **Reason for Surrogate Consent:**............

Name of Witness:..................... **Signatures of Witness:**......................

(I) **I have explained to the patient/surrogate all the above points in the "INFORMED CONSENT: TRANSFUSION OF BLOOD/BLOOD COMPONENTS" form and I am of the opinion that the patient/surrogate has understood the information.**

(II) **Emergent/Life Threatening Circumstances**

Informed Consent was not obtained because of a life threatening/emergent medical condition. I have not provided the patient with information sufficient to be considered as Informed Consent and I have proceeded with ordering blood/blood components to be administered in sufficient quantity to alter, improve or reverse a life threatening/emergent medical conditions.

Note: *Please strike out whichever is not applicable*

Name of Doctor: ....   **Designation:** ....

Signature: ....   **Date and Time:** ....

Name of the Institution

LOGO

Date:...............

Place patient identification label or write below:

Name:

MR Number:_____ IP Number:_____

Age/DOB:_____ Sex:_____

ANNEXURE 47.4

PRE-TRANSFUSION CHECKS

Ward/Dept:................. Bed No:.................

Check for →	Must match what is on the →	Patient's Medical Record File	Patient's Wrist Band	Blood Unit Label-Primary Label on the Component	Compatibility Label on the Blood/Component Unit	Compatibility Report	Blood/Blood Component Unit
Physician's Order							
Patient's First and Last Name							
Patient's MR No.							
Patient's ABO/Rh							
Donor's ABO/Rh							
Expiry Date and Time of Blood/Blood Component							
Type of Component Ordered for Transfusion							
Blood/Blood Unit No. and Segment No.							
Must look for							
Pack Integrity							
Presence of Large Blood Clots							
Evidence of Hemolysis in the Plasma or at the Interface of Red Cells and Plasma							

Name of S/N: ....   **Sign:** ....   **ID No.:** ....
(1st checker)

Name of the Doctor: ....   **Sign:** ....   **ID No.:** ....
(2nd checker)

Note:

- Before beginning the transfusion, it is extremely important to correctly identify the patient and the Blood product. A registered Staff Nurse and a second Doctor must carry out the pretransfusion checks.
- The pretransfusion checks must be carried out at the bed side of the patient.
- Utilize the format given above while carrying out the pretransfusion checks.
- Inform the Blood Center immediately of any discrepancy. Do not start the transfusion until the discrepancy is resolved.
- To complete the process of pretransfusion checks, both the Checkers must sign at the appropriate place on the format.

CHAPTER 48

Workup of Transfusion Reaction

SCOPE AND APPLICATION

A transfusion reaction is defined as an adverse event that occurs during or after a transfusion of blood or blood components.

Blood transfusions can be helpful and lifesaving when used with care and according to clear instructions. In spite of precautions and preventive measures, adverse reactions do occur and sometimes prove fatal. Therefore, blood replacement therapy requires a considerable level of expertise to maximize recipient protection. Recognizing potential adverse effects can help prevent their occurrence and aid clinical management.

This standard operating procedure (SOP) describes the workup of a transfusion reaction.

RESPONSIBILITY

It is the responsibility of the blood center technician to accept the blood/component implicated in the transfusion reaction, which is returned from the ward/operation theater (OT). It is the duty of the same technician to ensure that there is documented evidence of the nature of reaction either on the transfusion record/adverse reaction form or on a separate letter addressed to blood center, along with the post-transfusion blood sample [both ethylenediaminetetraacetic acid (EDTA) and clotted], residual blood unit and urine specimen, if necessary. The direct antiglobulin test (DAT) should be performed on the post-transfusion EDTA sample immediately on receipt before refrigeration. The blood unit and samples should be preserved properly for detailed investigations.

CLASSIFICATION OF TRANSFUSION REACTIONS

The transfusion reactions are classified into acute reactions (**Annexure 48.1**), which occur during or within 24 hours of transfusion, and delayed reactions, which occur after 24 hours (**Annexure 48.2**).

MATERIALS REQUIRED

- *Equipment*:
    - Refrigerator to store samples and reagents at 2–6°C
    - Tabletop centrifuge
    - Microcentrifuge [for column agglutination technology (CAT) cards]
    - Micropipettes
    - Microscope
    - Disposable pipette tips
    - Incubator
- *Specimen*:
    - Blood/component bag returned room ward/OT
    - Patient's pretransfusion blood sample (clotted)
    - Patient's post-transfusion blood sample (EDTA and clotted)
    - Patient's post-transfusion urine sample
- *Reagents*:
    - Anti-A, anti-B, anti-AB, anti-D, anti-H, and anti-A1 lectin antisera
    - Group A, B, and O pooled cells
    - Three-cell panel for screening of atypical antibodies
    - CAT cards
    - Papain-cysteine/22% bovine albumin
    - Antihuman globulin reagent [anti-immunoglobulin G (IgG) anti-C3d] and anti-IgG
    - IgG-sensitized control cells
    - 0.9% saline
    - Low-ionic-strength saline (LISS) solution
    - Distilled water
- *Glassware*:
    - Serum tubes
    - Coombs tubes (for patient grouping only)
    - Microtubes
    - Pasteur pipettes
    - Glass slides
    - Small funnel
    - 20 mL test tubes
    - 5 mL pipette

- *Miscellaneous*:
  - − Disposal box
  - − Two plastic beakers
  - − Test tubes (5 and 10 mL)
  - − Test tube rack
  - − Disposable micro tips

WORKUP OF ACUTE ADVERSE TRANSFUSION REACTION LESS THAN 24 HOURS

1. Suspect adverse transfusion reactions by the presence of combination of the following signs and symptoms:
   - i. *Inflammatory*:
     - a. Fever/chills
     - b. Skin color changes
     - c. Pain at infusion site
   - ii. *Allergic*:
     - a. Itching
     - b. Urticaria
     - c. Rash
     - d. Anaphylaxis
   - iii. *Circulatory*:
     - a. Blood pressure changes
     - b. Shock
     - c. Hemoglobinemia/hemoglobinuria
   - iv. *Pulmonary*:
     - a. Dyspnea, orthopnea, wheezing
     - b. Full respiratory failure
   - v. *Coagulation*:
     - a. Unexplained increase in bleeding
     - b. Disseminated intravascular coagulation (DIC)
   - vi. *Psychological*:
     - a. Anxiety
     - b. Restlessness
     - c. Sense of unease or impending "doom"

   The adverse transfusion reactions can be mild, moderate, and severe.
2. *General philosophy*:
   - i. Assume that all suspected reactions are hemolytic and work to disprove your reaction.
   - ii. Predict a high index of suspicion which is much better than a low index.
   - iii. This assumption is wrong most of the time. But wrong once, when saved lives, is right.

    iv. Anyone (nursing staff, perfusionists, resident medical officer, and physician) involved in blood transfusion initiates the transfusion reaction workup.

3. *Responsibilities of staff at bedside:*
   i. Stop the blood transfusion immediately.
   ii. Keep the intravenous (IV) line open with normal saline.
   iii. Perform clerical check on blood unit, transfusion reaction form, medical record, and wristband to make sure that the right blood/ component unit is transfused to the right patient. This is done by anyone who has suspected the adverse transfusion reaction. Physician in charge of the patient is informed.
   iv. Record the symptoms in the adverse reaction form.
   v. The physician in charge evaluates the patient, treats as needed, and orders the workup of suspected adverse blood transfusion reaction following SOPs. Blood center/transfusion service physician is consulted for guidance regarding further evaluation and treatment.

4. *Responsibilities of blood center staff:*
   i. Primary testing (ABO blood grouping) is performed by the technician.
   ii. The report is submitted by the technician to the blood center/ blood transfusion service physician.
   iii. Additional tests as required by the blood center/blood transfusion service physician are also performed by the technician.
   iv. The physician in charge of the patient is informed immediately about the hemolysis, bacterial contamination, and other adverse events related to the transfusion.
   v. The final report for the adverse transfusion reaction is generated including interpretation of the transfusion reaction and recommendation for future transfusion.

The responsibilities of staff at bedside and the blood center staff are shown in **Annexure 48.3**.

5. *Basic testing of a post-transfusion reaction sample:*
   A. *Clerical check:* Clerical check is performed by the laboratory technician to see that the information on post-transfusion sample, transfusion documentation, and blood unit (when available) matches or not.

       In case of discrepancy, notify the physician in charge of patient to take necessary steps to prevent another adverse reaction. Secondary testing is performed only if requested by the physician.

   B. *Hemolysis check:*
   a. The blood unit received back is visually inspected for the color (dark color is suspicious of a bacterial contamination unit), clots, or aggregates.

b. Visible hemoglobinemia is checked by the presence of pink-red color in the supernatant after centrifuging the EDTA post-transfusion sample, which is compared with the pretransfusion as little as 2.5–5 mL of hemolysis anywhere in the body. The EDTA sample is preferred for detecting visible hemoglobinemia because it can also be used for DAT.

If no hemolysis is detected, rule out nonhemolytic causes of adverse blood transfusion reactions. But if present, hemolysis should be confirmed on the freshly redrawn sample if requested by the physician.

C. *DAT: Refer to Chapter 33 for details of DAT. This is done with polyspecific method (IgG + C3d).*

Interpretation:

a. If DAT is positive, results should be compared with DAT results of a pretransfusion sample.

b. *Positive DAT*: It does prove an acute hemolytic reaction since it can be positive in hospitalized patients, autoantibodies, drugs, and patients who have been administered Rh immunoglobulin (RhIG)/intravenous immunoglobulin (IVIg). Such cases require *elute testing*. When testing the eluate, make sure that reagent A1 cells and B cells are included. This will identify passively acquired anti-A1 or anti-B as IVIg may contain blood group antibodies which cause a positive DAT and hemolysis.

c. It should be noted that negative DAT does not negate the occurrence of an acute hemolytic reaction. This can happen in case of a patient who had brisk hemolysis of donor cells (especially when ABO-incompatible blood is transfused). DAT, when done with the tube method, is also negative in patients having a small amount of residual donor red blood cells (RBCs) (<10% circulating RBCs), and in such cases, DAT done with the column agglutination method helps.

D. *Repeat ABO/Rh testing:*

a. This testing is performed on pre- and post-transfusion samples. This is done to check that right blood has been issued to right patient.

b. It also rules out for any technical errors in performing ABO/Rh grouping. In case of any discrepancy, the test is performed with a freshly redrawn sample.

Basic testing of post-transfusion reaction sample has been summarized in **Annexure 48.4**.

The physician is notified about taking necessary steps to prevent another reaction in case another patient is involved. Secondary testing is performed only if requested by the physician.

6. *Secondary testing of pretransfusion and post-transfusion reaction samples:* Secondary testing may be considered on the basis of results of the basic hemolysis test of the post-transfusion sample in the following situations:
   A. Hemolysis in basic testing
   B. No hemolysis in basic testing
   A. *Hemolysis in basic testing:*
      i. *The pretransfusion sample is tested for hemolysis:*
         a. If hemolysis is present, it can be due to a nonimmune mechanism.
         b. If no hemolysis is present, the following tests are required to be performed:
            • Repeat hemolysis test with the post-transfusion sample
            • Three-cell panel antibody screening
            • Repeat crossmatch
            • Antigen typing of blood unit
         If any of the above tests is positive, repeat testing on the pretransfusion sample.
      ii. *DAT testing:*
         a. DAT is done on a pretransfusion sample and is positive or negative. Repeat the following tests on the post-transfusion sample:
            • Three-cell panel antibody screen
            • Crossmatching
            • If any of the above is positive, repeat testing of the pretransfusion sample.
         b. DAT is positive with the pre- or post-transfusion sample. The following tests need to be performed:
            • DAT with IgG, C3D, and elute on sample with stronger reactivity
            • Baseline and follow-up testing
            • Plasma hemoglobin (Hb)
            • *Hb lactate dehydrogenase (LDH):* This is a marker for hemolysis but not specific for intravascular hemolysis. Its rise confirms the intravascular hemolysis but not diagnostic.
            • *Total and direct bilirubin:* Both the levels rise to the maximum level and return to normal within 24 hours if liver is normal.
            • Haptoglobin
            • *Urine Hb:* It is not as sensitive as hemoglobinemia for intravascular hemolysis. It is only useful if testing for plasma Hb is delayed or doubtful.

    iii. Repeat ABO testing on a pretransfusion sample:
        a. Determine for any clerical, collection, procedural error.
        b. Take necessary steps to prevent any other adverse reaction in case any other patient is involved.

B. *No hemolysis in basic testing*:
  1. The following additional tests for suspected respiratory reactions are performed:
    a. Culture sensitivity of the blood component
    b. Serum IgA levels
    c. Anti-IgA if serum IgA is not detectable
    d. X-ray chest for transfusion-related acute lung injury (TRALI) when required
    e. Human leukocyte antigen (HLA) and human neutrophil antigen (HNA) antibody screening. If the donor is positive, white blood cell (WBC) antigen typing of the patient
    f. Brain natriuretic peptide (BNP)
    g. Arterial blood gases (ABG)
    Serum IgA and anti-IgA are done in cases of severe allergic reactions.
  2. Additional testing for suspected septic reactions is done only when suggested by clinical findings, e.g.:
    a. Temperature >102°F
    b. Temperature rise greater than expected (2°F or 3°F)
    c. Severe rigors
    d. Signs for septic shock-type findings (marked hypotension, gastrointestinal complaints, later findings of multiorgan failure, DIC, etc.)
    In such cases, the following tests are done for both the patients and blood component transfused:
      • Both aerobic and anaerobic blood culture of patient
      • Consider for culture of IV fluids used
      • Gram stain and culture of blood component

Secondary testing of pretransfusion and post-transfusion samples has been summarized in **Annexure 48.5**.

DELAYED TRANSFUSION REACTION MORE THAN 24 HOURS

The workup of the delayed transfusion reactions (**Annexure 48.6**) is described as follows:
- Delayed hemolytic reaction
- Transfusion-associated graft-versus-host disease (TA-GvHD)
- Post-transfusion purpura (PTP)
- Iron overload

Delayed Hemolytic Reaction

Delayed hemolytic reaction is seen in patients who have been previously sensitized by transfusion, pregnancy, or transplant and in whom an antibody is detectable by standard pretransfusion techniques. The signs and symptoms are usually mild. An unexpected decrease in Hb or hematocrit following transfusion should be investigated. The following testing is done whenever a patient is suspected for a delayed hemolytic reaction after 24 hours.

- *DAT:*
  - If negative, in case ongoing hemolysis is not suspected, no further testing is required.
  - If positive or ongoing suspicion of hemolysis even if DAT is negative, perform *elution* test which if positive, antigen typing of unit transfused if available and even this can be done from the blood sample of the segment of blood unit. Antigen typing of the pretransfusion sample of the patient is also repeated.
- *Other markers of hemolysis* such as LDH, total and direct bilirubin, and haptoglobin are performed.

No further testing is recommended in case the *elution test* is negative.

The workup of a delayed hemolytic reaction is summarized in **Annexure 48.7**. Usually no treatment is given but if the patient has hypotension and oliguria, treat the patient as acute intravascular hemolysis.

Transfusion-Associated Graft-Versus-Host Disease

This is a complication of blood component therapy or bone marrow transplantation. It is due to proliferation of T-cell lymphocytes derived from donor blood. Usually, such patients have a history of blood transfusion from the relatives. The symptoms appear 3–30 days after the transfusion. Gamma irradiation of blood components is the best current therapy to prevent the TA-GvHD.

Post-transfusion Purpura

Post-transfusion purpura is a rare complication after transfusion of platelet concentrates. There is rapid onset of thrombocytopenia due to anamnestic reaction of platelet alloantibody. Six hourly platelet count is tested and treated with antigenic negative blood for transfusion. High dose of steroids, IVIg, and plasma exchange are the treatment modalities.

Iron Overload

Iron overload is seen in cases of congenital hemolytic anemia, aplastic anemia, and chronic renal failure who require repeated transfusion support as a part of treatment. Each unit of RBCs contains 225 mg of iron which is accumulated and affects the function of heart, liver, and endocrine glands.

- Prophylactic or therapeutic phlebotomy
- Subcutaneous infusion of Deferoxamine (DFO)—an iron-chelating agent
- Hypertransfusing units rich in neocytes (young RBCs) have also been shown to reduce the frequency of transfusion.

ANNEXURE 48.1

ACUTE REACTIONS <24 HOURS

Reaction	Frequency	Usual cause	Prevention
Hemolytic transfusion reaction	Uncommon	ABO incompatibility	Proper identification of the patient from sample collection to blood administration, proper labeling of samples and products is essential. Prevention of nonimmune hemolysis requires adherence to proper handling, storage, and administration of blood components
Febrile nonhemolytic transfusion reaction	Common	Cytokines, anti-leukocyte antibody	A proportion of patients who have febrile reactions will have similar reactions to subsequent transfusions. Many are prevented by leukocyte filtration (either bedside or prestorage)
Allergic transfusion reaction	Uncommon	Antibodies to plasma proteins	In case of history of experiencing repeated urticarial reactions, give an antihistamine such as chlorpheniramine 0.1 mg/kg IM or IV 30 minutes before commencing the transfusion, where possible
Anaphylaxis transfusion reaction	Uncommon	Antibodies to IgA	Patients with anti-IgA antibodies require special blood components such as washed red blood cells and plasma products prepared from IgA-deficient donors. Manage further transfusion in consultation with the hematologist-on-call

Continued

Continued

Reaction	Frequency	Usual cause	Prevention
Transfusion-related lung injury (TRALI)	Rare	Antibodies to leukocytes	• Firstly, there should be a clear indication for the transfusion. Screening of the donors for the presence of HLA antibodies is expensive and time-consuming. Earlier detection may lead to early diagnosis, treatment, and prevention • Recently, the method for prevention of transfusion-related acute lung injury using riboflavin and light has been patented. This prevents the formation of bioactive substances in a pathogen-inactivated blood component. The steps include illuminating the blood component with light at a sufficient energy so that an alloxazine photosensitizer present in the blood component may be photolyzed to inactivate any pathogens which may be present, preventing the formation of bioactive substances in the pathogen inactivated blood component and storing the pathogen-inactivated blood component
Marked fever with septic shock	Rare	Bacterial contamination	Inspect blood components prior to transfusion. Bacterial contamination and other abnormalities can be detected by visual inspection in some of the units (clots, clumps, or abnormal color). Maintaining appropriate cold storage of red cells in a monitored blood center refrigerator is important. Transfusions should not proceed beyond the recommended infusion time (4 hours)

Continued

Continued

Reaction	Frequency	Usual cause	Prevention
Congestive heart failure	Common	Volume overload	• Packed cells should be given slowly over 4 hours. The usual rate of transfusion is about 200 mL/h. In a patient at risk, the rate of 100 mL/h or less is appropriate • Diuretics should be given at the start of the transfusion and only one or two units of concentrated red cells should be transfused in any 24-hour period • Blood transfusion should be given during the daytime. Overnight transfusion should be avoided. Wherever possible, packed cell should be used instead of whole blood
Hypocalcemia	Uncommon	Citrate toxicity	The anticoagulant citrate is usually metabolized to bicarbonate following blood transfusion. Therefore, the prophylactic use of calcium salts, such as calcium chloride, is not recommended. Their use should only be restricted in cases of clinical or biochemical evidence of reduced ionized calcium
Hypothermia	Uncommon	Rapid infusion of cold blood	Appropriately maintained blood warmers should be used during massive or exchange transfusion. Additional measures include warming of other intravenous fluids and the use of devices to maintain patient body temperature
Hyperkalemia	Uncommon	Red cell storage	Fresh blood <7 days old is used

ANNEXURE 48.2

DELAYED REACTIONS >24 HOURS

Reaction	Frequency	Usual cause	Prevention
Hemolytic	Uncommon	Development of a red cell antibody	An antibody screen is performed as part of pretransfusion testing. When an antibody is detected, it is identified and appropriate antigen negative blood is provided. Sometimes, antibodies fall below detectable limits and may not be detected by pretransfusion testing. However, some reactions are due to rare antigens (i.e., anti-Jk^a blood group antibodies) that are very difficult to detect during pretransfusion testing
Transfusion-associated graft-versus-host disease (TA-GvHD)	Rare	Engraftment of transfused functional lymphocytes	It is prevented by gamma irradiation of cellular blood components given to patients at risk to stop the proliferation of transfused lymphocytes. Alternately leukocyte depletion of blood components is done
Post-transfusion purpura (PTP)	Rare	Antiplatelet antibodies	Leukocyte reduction of blood components to levels <10^6/ unit reduces the likelihood of alloimmunization. This can be achieved through the use of prestorage or bedside leukocyte-reducing blood products

Continued

Continued

Reaction	Frequency	Usual cause	Prevention
Iron overload	The transfusion-dependent patients accumulate iron over a period of time since there is no physiological mechanism to eliminate iron	Multiple transfusions	Iron-binding agents, such as deferoxamine, are widely used to minimize the accumulation of iron in these patients. The aim is to keep serum ferritin levels at <2,000 µg/L
Transfusion transmitted diseases	1 in 10,000 transfused units	For example, human immunodeficiency virus (HIV), hepatitis, variant Creutzfeldt-Jakob disease (vCJD)	*The single most effective way of protecting patients against both known and unrecognized blood-borne infections is to avoid the use of blood components or tissues unless there is a well-founded reason.* Donor selection criteria and subsequent screening of all donations are designed to prevent disease transmission, but these do not completely eliminate the hazards. Blood or blood product should be released for transfusion until these and all other nationally required tests are shown to be negative

ANNEXURE 48.3

RESPONSIBILITIES OF STAFF AT BEDSIDE AND BLOOD CENTER STAFF IN INITIAL WORKUP FOR ADVERSE TRANSFUSION REACTION

Bedside of patient	Blood center/blood transfusion service
• Bedside of patient • Nurse and physician responsibilities	• Blood center/blood transfusion service • Lab. technologist/medical officer • Responsibilities

Nurse	Physician	Technologist	Transfusion service physician
• Stop the transfusion • Keep the IV line open with normal saline • Perform clerical checks on blood unit, transfusion adverse reaction form, medical record and wrist band • Inform the physician	• Evaluate the patient and treat as needed • Order for transfusion adverse reaction workup, inform the blood center and follow SOPs • Consult with blood center physician for guidance for further evaluation and treatment	• Perform primary testing on post-transfusion sample • Report findings to blood center physician • Perform additional testing as per orders of blood center physician	• Evaluate initial reaction workup • Order additional testing if needed • Report to patient physician immediately if hemolysis, bacterial contamination or other serious adverse event related to transfusion suspected • Generate final report including interpretation of transfusion reaction and recommendation for future transfusion

ANNEXURE 48.4

BASIC TESTING FOR POST-TRANSFUSION REACTION SAMPLE

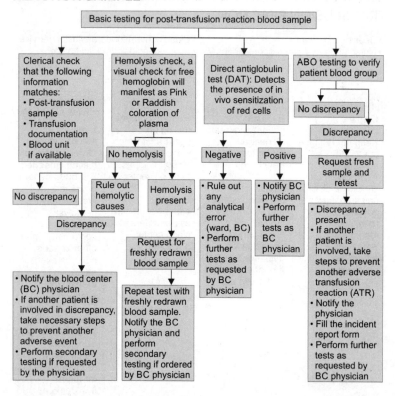

ANNEXURE 48.5

SECONDARY TESTING OF THE POST-TRANSFUSION AND PRETRANSFUSION REACTION SAMPLES

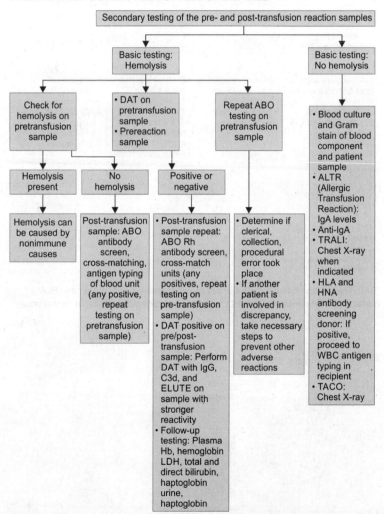

(ALTR: allergic transfusion reaction; DAT: direct antiglobulin test; HLA: human leukocyte antigen; HNA: human neutrophil antigen; LDH: lactate dehydrogenase; TACO: transfusion-associated circulatory overload; WBC: white blood cell)

ANNEXURE 48.6

WORKUP OF DELAYED TRANSFUSION REACTIONS

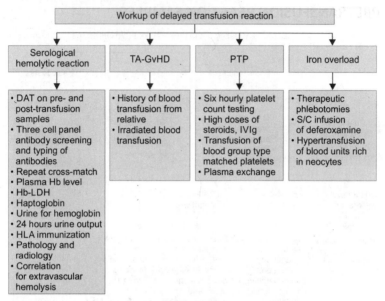

Workup of delayed transfusion reaction			
Serological hemolytic reaction	**TA-GvHD**	**PTP**	**Iron overload**
• DAT on pre- and post-transfusion samples • Three cell panel antibody screening and typing of antibodies • Repeat cross-match • Plasma Hb level • Hb-LDH • Haptoglobin • Urine for hemoglobin • 24 hours urine output • HLA immunization • Pathology and radiology • Correlation for extravascular hemolysis	• History of blood transfusion from relative • Irradiated blood transfusion	• Six hourly platelet count testing • High doses of steroids, IVIg • Transfusion of blood group type matched platelets • Plasma exchange	• Therapeutic phlebotomies • S/C infusion of deferoxamine • Hypertransfusion of blood units rich in neocytes

(DAT: direct antiglobulin test; Hb-LDH: hemoglobin-lactate dehydrogenase; HLA: human leukocyte antigen; TA-GvHD: transfusion-associated graft-versus-host disease)

ANNEXURE 48.7

DELAYED TRANSFUSION HEMOLYTIC REACTION

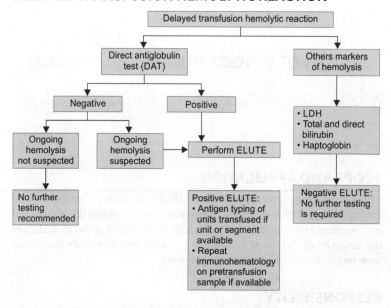

CHAPTER 49

Return of Blood/Blood Components

SCOPE AND APPLICATION

This standard operating procedure (SOP) describes the process of return of issued blood/blood components after leaving the controlled temperature environment and entry into inventory in order to maintain the integrity of the blood/blood components and to ensure that these may be safely issued for future transfusion.

RESPONSIBILITY

It is the responsibility of the technical supervisor and laboratory technicians to decide as to whether the returned blood/blood components should be taken back into the inventory or discarded as per defined policy guidelines.

MATERIALS REQUIRED

- Issue register
- Thermometer
- Master record for blood (stock register)

POLICY GUIDELINES

- Blood/blood components shall be returned immediately to the blood center if the decision is made not to transfuse.
  - The blood/blood components that have been out of controlled temperature longer than 30 minutes shall not be taken back into the inventory and shall be discarded as per biomedical waste handling rules.

- The acceptable temperature ranges for components are:
    o Packed red blood cells: 1–10°C
    o Platelets: 20–24°C
    o Thawed plasma: 1–10°C
    o Thawed cryoprecipitate: 20–24°C
- All seals of blood/blood components shall be intact on visual inspection when entered into the inventory.
- The whole blood/blood component unit is discarded if:
    - The blood unit has been out of refrigerator/controlled temperature for longer than 30 minutes, or
    - If the seal is broken, or
    - There is any sign that the unit has been opened, or
    - There is any sign of hemolysis, or
    - If the temperature of the unit is over +10°C.

PROCEDURE

1. Document the date and time of the return of blood/blood components to the blood center. Ensure that time out of controlled temperature has not exceeded 30 minutes.
2. Inspect the blood/blood components visually and document them.
3. Ensure that the temperature meets the quality requirement as defined.
4. Blood/blood components meeting the above criteria may only be taken back into the inventory.
5. Document the final status and the reason for final disposition/discard of the blood/blood components.

DOCUMENTATION

Make entries in the issue register and master blood stock register regarding the date and time of return and observations on the above.

Problems and Troubleshooting in Blood Centers

INTRODUCTION

The role of the blood center is very crucial as the blood and its components are undeniably essential to saving lives. Doctors as well as medical technologists working in blood centers are of paramount importance. They should be knowledgeable in all the four stages of blood center processes: Donation, screening, inventory, and preparation of blood and its components to be issued for the patients in order to maintain safety in blood transfusion by supplying right blood to right patients. At the same time, they should also be able to identify the problems at each stage of the blood center process and should be able to troubleshoot the problems. The problems and how to troubleshoot those can be grouped area-wise.

DONOR AREA

Problems

The various problems encountered in the blood donation area are as follows:

- *Proper identification of donor:* In some instances, impersonation is done by the donor; hence, the donor should show some identification proof to identify him/her.
- Undercollection of blood
- Clotting of blood in blood bags
- Prolonged collection time, i.e., time of start of collection to completion of phlebotomy
- Microbial contamination of blood units
- Wrong labeling of blood bags
- Adverse blood donor reactions

Troubleshooting

Undercollection of Blood

- Ensure proper selection of lager and good caliber vein, i.e., median cubital and cephalic veins.
- The needle may not be positioned in the lumen. Therefore, change the position of the needle by moving it forward or move backward in case the needle has penetrated too far.
- The bevel of the needle may be against the wall of the vein and requires adjustment in the angle of the needle.
- Loosen the tourniquet if it is obstructing the blood flow.
- Resecure and tighten the tourniquet to increase the venous filling if the vein has collapsed.

Clotting of Blood in Blood Bags

Frequent gentle mixing of the blood during donation at regular intervals with the anticoagulant/preservative in the bag is critical to avoiding blood clots and can be performed manually or with a mechanical mixing device.

Prolonged Collection Time

Blood donation should complete in 8–10 minutes. Blood donation units are not suitable for component separation in case donation is collected in more time.

Microbial Contamination of Blood Bags

During phlebotomy, divert 20 mL of the initial flow of blood which contains skin particles and bacteria to the diversion pouch. This minimizes the level of bacterial skin contaminants in the blood collection bags. Blood collected in the diversion pouch is used for mandatory investigations and also any other investigation required.

Wrong Labeling of Blood Bags

- Any blood unit or component should be identified with two to three identifiers such as:
    - Blood unique identification number
    - Segment number of the bag
    - Blood group and Rh type (if done)

    The same should be recorded in all documents, i.e., donor form, donor register, component register, blood grouping, transfusion transmitted infection (TTI) screening, and master records which can be traced.

- *Blood unit unique identification number:* The primary bag used for blood collection, all attached satellite bags, sample tubes, and the donor registration form must be labeled with a unique identification number along with the year [preferably for fresh frozen plasma (FFP) and cryo products] which should be robust sticker labels with preprinted serial numbers. This must be done carefully by the phlebotomist before starting the donation and after verifying the identity of the donors with the donor questionnaire and informed consent form. The collected blood and its components, and blood samples used for testing, can be traced back to the original donor registration record.
- Record the details in the donor register with the same unique identification number.

Adverse Blood Donor Reactions

Majority of the donors tolerate the process of blood donation, but adverse donor reactions do occur. These have been covered in the Chapter 10 on blood collection and counseling during blood donation. However, they should be able to identify the following high-risk donors to prevent donor reactions.

- First-time donor
- Donor who has not slept
- Anxious donor
- Donor with a previous history of reaction during donation

SEROLOGY

ABO and Rh blood group and compatibility testing are the main tests performed in the serological laboratory of the blood center. The correctness of the blood groups and compatibility is of utmost importance in providing and ensuring safe blood transfusions to the recipients. Therefore, blood center technology specialists must be knowledgeable in all aspects of blood banking—routine and specialized tests, including problem-solving.

Problems

The problems in the serology section may be related to:

- Blood group discrepancies
- Incompatible crossmatch

Blood Group Discrepancies

Refer to Chapter 45 on "Resolution of ABO Group Discrepancies."

Incompatible Crossmatch

This can be due to:
- Preanalytical errors
- Analytical errors
- Postanalytical errors

Preanalytical Errors

These are the major errors in diagnostic test results and are subdivided into two categories:

1. *Pre-preanalytical*: This is undertaken outside the blood center and not under the control of blood center personnel. This involves the following:
   a. Test requisition
   b. Patient identification
   c. Sample identification
   d. Sample collection
2. *"True" preanalytical*: This involves the following steps required for preparation of sample for analysis in the blood center.
   a. Specimen accessioning and processing
   b. Centrifugation
   c. Aliquotting

Troubleshooting:
- Continuous phlebotomy training and education for all the personnel for reduction of preanalytical errors.
- Use of appropriate technology, e.g., barcodes, radiofrequency identification, and wristbands, for right patient identification.
- Choose appropriate products for proper sample collection, e.g., closed blood collection system using vacutainers.
- Follow standard guidelines and manufacturer's recommendations for venous blood specimen collection guidelines for correct order of draw and for proper draw volume to ensure proper additive-to-blood ratios, respectively.
- Proper written standard operating procedure (SOP) for each procedure, e.g., identification of patient, collection of blood sample, and transportation of specimens, reduces the heterogeneity in the process and streamlines the blood center workflow.
- Validate any new instrument or procedure before switching to a new product or procedure.
- Keep a record of preanalytical errors observed, monitor, and take corrective measures.

Analytical Errors

- Procedural
- Not adding reagents
- Not following SOPs

Troubleshooting:

- Proper written SOP for every procedure to scale back the heterogeneity in process and streamline the blood center workflow.
- Internal quality control (QC) procedures must be followed.
- Participate in external quality assessment programs.
- Certification/accreditation by professional bodies
- Adopt the practice of keeping a record of the errors at all stages of analysis and then devising corrective strategies for prevention of errors.

Postanalytical Errors

- Issuing wrong blood/blood component
- Wrong patient identification
- Delay in transfusion
- Nonmaintenance of cold chain before transfusion

Troubleshooting:

- The blood/blood component unit must only be issued after verification of the blood unit, compatibility, and patient details. A piece of the integral tubing with at least one numbered segment should remain attached with the blood bag being issued.
- Each unit of blood should be visually inspected before issue and should not be issued if there is any evidence of hemolysis, leakage, or suspicion of microbial contamination.
- It is vital to make the final identity check at the bedside of the patient as per SOP. It should be undertaken independently by two staff members, at least one of whom should be a doctor, and the patient's identity is checked with blood unit, compatibility label, and patient's record.
- The blood center should have a policy for acceptance of blood units returned within half an hour when the cold chain has not been broken.
- The time limits for transfusion of blood/blood components should be adhered to as given in **Table 1**.

Blood, once issued, should not be taken back in blood center after 30 minutes, especially when the cold chain is broken.

Table 1: Time limits for transfusion.		
Name of blood/blood component	**Start transfusion**	**Complete transfusion**
Whole blood/PRBCs	Within 30 minutes of removing from refrigerator	Within 4 hours
Platelet concentrate	Immediately	Within 20 minutes
Fresh frozen plasma	Within 30 minutes	Within 20 minutes
(PRBC: packed red blood cell)		

SCREENING OF TRANSFUSION TRANSMISSIBLE DISEASES

Screening of donor blood for TTIs is a part of a blood safety and available strategy. As per provisions in Schedule F (Part XII B) of Drugs and Cosmetics Act 1940 and Rules, 1945, it is mandatory to screen all blood units for human immunodeficiency virus (HIV) 1 and 2, hepatitis B, hepatitis C, venereal disease research laboratory (VDRL), and malaria. The main types of assay used for blood screening are enzyme immunoassays (EIAs), chemiluminescent immunoassays (CLIAs), hemagglutination assays (HAs)/particle agglutination (PA) assays, rapid/simple single-use assays (rapid tests), and nucleic acid amplification technology (NAAT) assays. A highly sensitive and specific assay should be selected for blood screening to detect all possible infected donations while minimizing wastage due to false-positive results. Donations with reactive or indeterminate test results should be discarded using methods under standard safety precautions.

The *problems* which lead to erroneous results are:
- Preanalytical errors
- Analytical errors
These are the same as have been described in Serology above.

Troubleshooting

Troubleshooting is also the same as described under *Serology* section. But in addition, the following steps are also required to be undertaken.
1. Include internal kit controls in the run. At times, a calibrator is provided by the manufacturer; the same is also included.

2. Include external positive samples from the laboratory, either pooled or single, diluted or undiluted, to monitor quality in testing procedure.

3. Use Levey–Jennings (LJ) control chart to know the systematic variation and random variation in results and aberrant results.

Trend: Results change gradually in either direction indicating slowly changing parameters due to deteriorating reagents and slowly faltering equipment.

Shift: Results fall abruptly/sharply on one side of the mean indicating a major change has occurred.

Interpretation of Shift and Trends

Shift: Control values of six consecutive runs fall on one side of mean. The possible causes are:
- Switching to new lots of Kits
- New reagents
- Changes in incubation temperature
- New technical hand

Trend: Six consecutive points distributed in one general direction. The possible causes are:
- Deterioration of reagents
- Deterioration of light source
- Gradual deterioration of calibration
- Slowly faltering equipment.

Random Variation: It is evidenced by observance of one result significantly different from other results without any pattern and can be due to:
- Transcription errors
- Sample mix up
- Poor pipette precision
- Lack of maintenance and calibration
- Poor technique
- Sudden change of staff/Kit
- Lack of periodic training and following SOPs

BLOOD COMPONENT AREA

The whole blood is separated into different blood components, namely packed red blood cell (PRBC) concentrate, platelet concentrate, FFP, and cryoprecipitate. These components are used for different indications, thereby maximizing the utility of one whole blood unit and allowing the specific component to be transfused to the patient avoiding the use of the unnecessary component. Blood/blood components need different storage conditions and temperature requirements for therapeutic efficacy. The components are separated by centrifugation of whole blood units because of different specific gravities of the various blood components.

The problems in separating blood into quality blood components conforming to requirements of Drugs and Cosmetics Act 1940 and Rules 1945 and their troubleshooting are as follows:
- Technical problems
- Blood bag problems

Technical Problems

The various technical problems encountered during component preparation are:
- Rupture of blood bag in refrigerated centrifuge
- Component yield is not constant; proper relative centrifugal force (RCF), acceleration, deceleration, and time are required to be programmed either by taking the manufacturer's instructions or by trial and error method.
- Choking of the filter during leukofiltration
- Red blood cells (RBCs) in FFP/platelets
- Wrong labeling of blood components
- Variations in laboratory procedures and practices
- Equipment failure
- Quality management and quality assurance systems are lacking.
- Lack of trained personnel

Troubleshooting
- Proper balancing and packing of cups ensure consistent yield and good interface.
- Blood bags are weighed out to a maximum tolerance of 5 g.
- Ensure facing the broad side of the bags outside the wall of the cup.
- The blood bags must sit firmly in the cups to avoid any folds as folds lead to the formation of nests (accumulation of cells) evading the sedimentation process, thereby leading to poor results.
- Correct speed and time of centrifugation dictate yield and prevent cell injury.
- Look for any abnormal vibrations of the centrifuge.
- Gentle handling of centrifuged blood bags prevents mixing at the interface.

- The staff must be well qualified, oriented, motivated, and experienced in component preparation.
- Strict adherence to working SOP
- SOPs for labeling must be in place and adhered to.
- The various blood components must be stored at required temperature.
- All equipment and instruments should be maintained, calibrated, and validated at set intervals as per a planned schedule to ensure that it provides reliable results.
- Adhering to good quality control measures to prevent testing/procedural errors.

Blood Bags Problems

The common problems related to blood bags for component preparation are:
- Under-/overcollection of blood units
- Clotting in blood units
- Hemolysis of blood units
- Leakage of blood unit bags and tubing

Troubleshooting

- An uninterrupted flow of blood. The blood unit is not suitable for component separation in case donation is collected in >8 minutes.
- Collection of the correct volume of donor blood maintaining an accurate anticoagulant blood ratio.
- Adequate mixing of anticoagulant and blood is to be ensured by using automatic mixing.
- A clean aseptic site of venipuncture is a must to avoid contamination of blood with skin bacteria.
- Under-/overweight, hemolyzed, TTI reactive, and leaking blood units as well as blood units containing blood clots are identified and rejected in-house before component separation.
- Use good quality triple and quadruple blood bags.

SUMMARY

The numerous problems in all the different sections of the blood center are particularly associated with procedures, blood center staff, and equipment. To prevent errors, the following below-mentioned strategies need to be implemented:
- Periodical staff training, retraining, and competency assessment
- Describing the significance of SOPs and blood transfusion process flow in the institution's month-to-month induction program for doctors and nurses, including newcomers

- Maintenance of error register and its daily evaluation by blood center medical officers
- Appointment and training of transfusion nurses, including operations theater complex and emergency department
- Induction of automation in blood center crossmatch laboratory for compatibility testing

It is of paramount importance that the blood center equipment is maintained, calibrated, and validated at set intervals as per requirements of Drugs and Cosmetics Act 1940 and Rules 1945 to make sure that it provides reliable results. The quality management system in the blood center also helps in the identification of any errors which must be corrected to ensure safe blood for all the recipients. Participation in an external quality assurance program, besides evaluation in overall performance and accuracy in blood center testing, provides additional confidence to the blood center.

Anti-human Immunodeficiency Virus 1/2 Testing

SCOPE AND APPLICATION

Anti-human immunodeficiency virus (anti-HIV)-1/2 antibody testing is mandatory on all blood samples of blood units before being released for transfusion. If the number of blood units is small, a rapid test kit is used, and if the number of blood units is large, an enzyme-linked immunosorbent assay (ELISA) method is used.

RESPONSIBILITY

Blood center technicians working in the transfusion transmitted infection (TTI) laboratory are responsible for conducting tests under the supervision of the technical supervisor, and the results are approved by the medical officer.

RAPID TEST KIT METHOD

Materials Required

- HIV-1 and 2 test devices
- Kit package inserts
- Disposable sample dropper
- Buffer solution
- Clotted/ethylenediaminetetraacetic acid (EDTA) blood sample

Procedure

Principle

The HIV-1/2 kit contains a membrane strip with a region of test band 1 containing recombinant HIV-1 capture antigens (gp41, gp120) and test band 2 region containing HIV-2 recombinant capture antigens (gp36).

Recombinant HIV-1/2 antigen (gp41, gp120, and gp36)-colloidal gold conjugates and the specimen sample move chromatographically along the membrane to the test region (T) to form an antigen–antibody–antigen gold particle complex with a high degree of sensitivity and specificity. The formation of this complex results in the appearance of a visible line in the test region(T). The test device has letters 1, 2, and C as test line 1 (HIV-1), test line 2 (HIV-2), and control lines, respectively. Both the test and control lines in the result windows are not visible before applying the sample. Control lines are used to control the procedure. The control line will appear if the test procedure has been performed correctly and the control line test reagents are working.

Storage

Store the test kit in a sealed pouch at 2–40°C until the expiration date. The test device is sensitive to both humidity and heat. Remove the test device from the foil pouch and start testing immediately.

Method

Important: Check the actual volumes and procedure instructions provided with the test kit. This may vary from lot-to-lot number.

1. Bring all the reagents and samples to room temperature (RT) before starting the test.
2. Remove the test device from its pouch and place it on a flat dry surface.
3. Slowly pour 25 µL of serum/plasma into the sample window and let it soak.
4. Add two drops of assay buffer to the same sample window.
5. Read results within 20 minutes.

Note: Reagent addition procedures must be followed strictly to avoid conflicting results.

Validation

The performance of HIV-1/2 rapid test is evaluated by National Institute of Biologicals (NIB) Noida with positive and negative samples as per their protocol. The sensitivity and specificity of the test are ≥99.5 and ≥98.0%, respectively.

Interpretation

- If two lines, control and T-1, are displayed, the sample is reactive for antibodies to HIV-1.
- If two lines are displayed, one for control and one for T-2, the sample is reactive for antibodies to HIV-2.

- If all three lines, control, T-1, and T-2, are displayed, the sample is reactive for antibodies to HIV-1 and 2.
- If the control line does not appear, the test is invalid; repeat the test with a new card.
- If only the control line is visible, the sample is negative for HIV antibodies.

ELISA METHOD

Materials Required

- Reagent kit
- Micropipettes and disposable pipette tips
- Timer
- ELISA reader
- ELISA washer
- Incubator 37°C
- Vortex mixer
- Glassware
- Distilled water

Procedure

Principle

Human serum or plasma is diluted in specimen diluent and incubated with HIV-1, HIV-2 proteins coated on microplate wells. If the HIV antibodies are present in the test sample, it will bind to the proteins coated on the microwells. After washing away unbound analyte, horseradish peroxidase conjugated to anti-human immunoglobulin G (IgG) antibody is added. Enzyme conjugate binds through the antigen–antibody complex if present. Unbound analyte is washed away, and a substrate solution is added. Color develops in proportion to the amount of HIV antibodies present in the sample. At the end of the incubation, stop the reaction by adding stop solution. The reaction is read by ELISA reader.

Method

Anti-HIV antibody testing is performed according to the manufacturer's kit insert instructions. Use the negative, positive, and cutoff controls for each series of determinations to validate the results.

1. Remove reagents from the fridge 30 minutes prior to testing. Mix the reagents gently by inverting the vials without foaming.
2. Bring the samples to RT before testing.

3. Carefully establish the sample distribution and identification plan.
4. Prepare the dilute washing solution.
5. Take the carrier tray and the strips out of the protective pouch.
6. Apply directly, without prior washing of the plate, and in succession:
    a. 25 μL of the diluents in each well
    b. 75 μL of the negative control serum in well A1
    c. 75 μL of cutoff control serum in wells B1, C1, and D1
    d. 75 μL of positive control serum in well E1
    e. 75 μL of specimen 1 in well F1
    f. 75 μL of specimen 2 in well G1, etc.
7. Incubate the microplate at 37°C for 30 ± 5 minutes.
8. Remove the seal and wash five times with the buffer ensuring a soak time of about 30 seconds between each cycle.
9. Invert the plate and tap on a clean paper towel to remove excess wash buffer.
10. Add 100 μL of conjugate solution in each well.
11. Incubate the microplate at 37°C for 30 ± 5 minutes.
12. Remove the seal and wash five times with the buffer ensuring a soak time of about 30 seconds between each cycle.
13. Add 80 μL of substrate solution after reconstituting in each well.
14. Incubate the microplate at RT for 30 ± 5 minutes in a dark place.
15. Add 100 μL of stop solution.
16. Read absorbance at 450–620 nm within 4–30 minutes in ELISA reader.

Calculation and Interpretation of Results

The presence or absence of antibodies to HIV-1 and/or HIV-2 is determined by comparing the absorbance measured for each sample to a calculated cutoff absorbance.
- Calculate the mean absorbance of the cutoff control serum.
- Calculate the cutoff value obtained from the ratio of 10 to the mean of the cutoff control serum.

Assay Validation
- The absorbance of the negative control serum should be <70% of the cutoff value.
- The mean absorbance of cutoff control sera should be >0.80.

Interpretation of Results
Negative: Samples with absorbance value below the cutoff value

Positive: Samples with absorbance values greater than or equal to the cutoff value

Samples with absorbance value just below the cutoff value (CO-10% < OD < C < O) should be interpreted with caution.

Record the results in a bloodstock register along with a printout.

Hepatitis B Surface Antigen Testing

SCOPE AND APPLICATION

Hepatitis B surface antigen (HBsAg) is a mandatory test for screening blood units prior to transfusion. This is done for samples from all donor units. Testing is performed by either rapid kit or enzyme-linked immunosorbent assay (ELISA) method.

RESPONSIBILITY

It is the responsibility of the blood center technician under the supervision of a medical officer to carry out the test.

RAPID KIT METHOD

Materials Required

- Test device
- Package insert
- Clotted blood sample
- Pipette

Procedure

Principle

The HbsAg test cassette contains a membrane strip precoated with a mouse monoclonal hepatitis B surface antibody (anti-HBs) capture antibody in the test band region. Mouse monoclonal anti-HBs colloidal gold conjugate and the serum mitigate chromatographically along the membrane to the test (T) region forming a visible line as the antibody–antigen gold particle complex forms. The HBsAg test cassette has letters T and C for "test line" and "control line," respectively, on the surface of the cassette. Both the test and the control lines in the result window are not visible before applying the sample. The control line is displayed whenever the test procedure has been performed properly and the control line reagents are functioning.

Storage

Store the test kit at 2–40°C in the sealed pouch until expiration date.

Method

Important: Check the actual volumes and instructions provided with the test kit. This may vary per batch number.

1. Bring the sealed pouch and serum to room temperature.
2. Remove the test device from the pouch.
3. Write the patient's name or identification number on the examination card.
4. Add 60 µL of serum/plasma sample into the sample window and allow to soak in.
5. Read the results within 20 minutes.

Note: It is important that the background is clear before the results are read. Do not read the results after >30 minutes.

Validation

- The performance of HBsAg rapid test has been evaluated by the National Institute of Biologicals (NIB) India with positive and negative samples as per its protocol.
- The sensitivity and specificity of the test are ≥99.0% and ≥98.0%, respectively.

Interpretation

Reactive: One distinct pink-colored line in the test (T) region and a pink-colored line in the control (C) region.

Nonreactive: Only one pink-colored line in the control (C) region. No apparent line in the test (T) region.

Invalid: A total absence of color in either region or no colored line in the control (C) region is an indication of procedural error and/or test reagent deterioration due to improper storage.

Record the results in bloodstock register.

ELISA METHOD

Materials Required

- ELISA reader
- ELISA washer
- Incubator
- Micropipettes and disposable tips
- Timer
- Disposable gloves
- Disposal container with sodium hypochlorite
- Absorbent tissue
- Distilled water
- 1 mol/L sulfuric acid
- Hepatitis kit

Procedure

Principle

In the monoclonal enzyme immunoassay (EIA) procedures, microplate wells coated with monoclonal anti-HBs are incubated with serum or plasma and anti-HBs peroxidase (horseradish) (anti-HBs-HRPO) conjugate in one-step assay. During the incubation period, HBsAg, if present, is bound to the conjugate (anti-HBs-HRPO). Unbound material is aspirated and washed away. On the addition of substrate, color develops in proportion to the amount of HBsAg which is bound. The enzyme reaction is stopped by the addition of stop solution.

Method

1. Carry out the test as per the manufacturer's instructions given in the package insert by the manufacturer.
2. Remove reagents from the fridge 30 minutes prior to testing. Mix the reagents gently by inverting the vials without foaming.
3. Bring reagents and samples to room temperature before testing.
4. Arrange all donor unit test tube samples, apheresis samples, serially in an ascending order in a test tube rack. Add the required number of internal kit controls and external lab controls.
5. Discard all disposable tips into hypochlorite solution.
6. Place the tray in front of the test tube rack.
7. Arrange the samples so that well A1, B1, C1, and D1 are negative controls, and E1 is positive control, and thereafter samples to be tested are arranged from F1 onward.

8. Add 100 µL of controls and samples to the corresponding wells.
9. Add 50 µL of conjugate to the wells.
10. Mix the plate gently and cover with a seal.
11. Incubate at 37°C for 30 minutes.
12. Remove the seal and wash five times with the buffer ensuring soak time of about 30 seconds between each cycle.
13. Invert the plate and tap on a clean paper towel to remove excess wash buffer.
14. Dispense 100 µL substrate/chromogen to each well.
15. Cover the plate with a sealer and incubate at 37°C for 30 minutes.
16. Add 100 µL of stop solution to each well. On adding this, the pink color of the substrate disappears or turns from blue to yellow (for positive samples).
17. Remove moisture from bottom of the plate and read optical density (OD) at 450 nm using a plate reader within 4–30 minutes of stopping the reaction.

Validation and Interpretation

- Cutoff OD is automatically calculated by the ELISA reader. Calculate the cutoff value by adding 0.050 to the mean absorbance (NCx) of the negative control

$$Cutoff = NCx + 0.050$$

- All the values of the negative controls should be ≤0.080 unit of OD.
- The positive control value (OD) should be ≥1.000.
- The test must be redone if all control values are out of these norms.
- Check the printout carefully for absorbance value.
- Divide the sample absorbance by the cutoff value to find out the ratio of the OD of the sample to the cutoff value.
  - *Positive*: Ratio absorbance/cutoff ≥1.0
  - *Negative*: Ratio absorbance/cutoff <0.080
  - *Equivocal*: Ratio absorbance/cutoff ≥0.9 < 1.0
- Equivocal results are reanalyzed.
- Paste the printout in the HBsAg register and record the results in a bloodstock register.

CHAPTER 53

Hepatitis C Virus Antibodies Testing

SCOPE AND APPLICATION

Hepatitis C virus antibody (anti-HCV) testing is a mandatory pretransfusion test for all blood units. This test can be performed using the rapid kit method or the enzyme-linked immunosorbent assay (ELISA) method.

RESPONSIBILITY

It is the responsibility of the blood center technician under the supervision of the medical officer to carry out the test.

RAPID CARD METHOD

Materials Required

- *Test kit*—The components of the test kit are:
  - HCV device
  - Buffer solution
  - Protein A conjugate
  - Sample dropper
- Clotted/ethylenediaminetetraacetic acid (EDTA) blood sample

Procedure

Principle

Hepatitis C virus is a rapid, visual, sensitive, and qualitative in vitro test for the detection of antibodies to HCV in human serum/plasma. It was developed using modified HCV antigens that represent the immunodominant regions of HCV antigens. The device (immunofiltration membrane) contains two test points "T" and a built-in quality control point "C" that constantly develops color during the testing to ensure proper functioning of the device. The T line is precoated with recombinant HCV antigen (core, NS3, NS4, and NA5), and the C line is precoated with a control line antibody conjugated with colloidal gold. Samples and the reagents pass through the membrane and are absorbed onto the underlined absorbent pad. If HCV antibodies are present in serum/plasma, they will bind to the immobilized antigen. Unbound serum/plasma proteins are removed during washing steps. Addition of the protein A conjugate binds to the Fc portion of the antibody, resulting in a distinct burgundy T line against the white background of the test area.

Method

Important: Check the actual volumes and procedure steps provided with the test kit; this can differ from lot-to-lot number.

1. Bring all the reagents and samples to room temperature (RT) before beginning the test.
2. Place the required number of HCV test devices at the working area.
3. Cut open the pouch and take out the device for performing the test.
4. Write the sample ID number to be tested on the device.
5. Add 25 µL drops of serum/plasma into the sample window.
6. Add two drops of buffer solution.
7. Read the results after 20 minutes.

Note: It is important to allow each solution to soak in the test device before adding the next solution.

Validation

This test includes a quality control line "C" that produces a constant burgundy line throughout the test to ensure that the kit reagents are working properly and the procedure is being used correctly.

This assay has only been validated with serum/plasma from individual patients/donors and not pools of serum/plasma or other bodily fluids.

The performance of the HCV rapid test has been evaluated by the National Institute of Biologicals (NIB) India on positive and negative samples according to protocol. The sensitivity and specificity of the test exceed 99.0% and 98.0%, respectively.

- If only one line appears in control area "C," this indicates that the sample is not reactive to HCV antibodies.
- The two lines seen in test area "T" and control area "C" indicate that the sample is reactive to antibodies against HCV.

Record the results in a blood log.

ELISA METHOD

Materials Required

- ELISA reader
- ELISA washer
- Micro shaker
- Incubator
- Micropipettes and disposable tips
- Timer
- Disposable gloves
- Disposable container with sodium hypochlorite solution
- Absorbent tissue
- Distilled water
- 1 mol/L sulfuric acid
- Test kit

Procedure

Principle

This test is based on the principle that microwells are coated with recombinant HCV-encoded antigens as a solid phase. If HCV antibodies are present, they can be bound to a solid phase and detected by complementary anti-human immunoglobulin G (IgG) coupled to an enzyme (which can act on a chromogenic substrate). The substrate is added to the bound complex, and the presence of antibody is detected by the development of a colored end product.

Method

The anti-HCV ELISA test is performed according to the kit manufacturer's instructions. For details on kit procedures and interpretation of results, please refer to the package insert of the kit used. Remove the reagents from the refrigerator 30 minutes before testing. Gently mix the reagents by inverting the vial without foaming.

1. Bring samples to RT before testing.
2. Prepare wash buffer solution as per pack insert.
3. Prepare the substrate solution as per pack insert.
4. Discard all disposable tips in a container with hypochlorite solution.
5. Prepare the record (plate map) identifying the placement of controls, calibrators, and specimens in the microwells. Arrange the assay control/calibrator so that well A1 is the reagent blank. As per configuration of the software, arrange all the controls and calibrators.
   a. Reagent blank—A1
   b. Negative calibrator—B1

    c. Negative calibrator—C1

    d. Negative calibrator—D1

    e. Positive control—E1

    f. Positive control—F1

6. Add 200 μL of specimen diluents to all wells, including A1.
7. Add 20 μL of the controls, calibrators, and specimens to the appropriate wells.
8. Mix the plate gently and cover with a seal.
9. Incubate at 37°C for 60 ± 5 minutes.
10. Remove the seal and wash five times.
11. Invert the plate and tap on a clean paper towel to remove excess wash buffer.
12. Dispense 200 μL conjugate to all wells.
13. Cover the plate with sealer and incubate at 37°C for 60 ± 5 minutes.
14. Remove the seal and wash five times.
15. Prepare substrate 10 minutes prior to use and add 200 μL of substrate solution to all the wells, including A1.
16. Incubate at RT in the dark for 30 minutes.
17. Add 50 μL of 4N sulfuric acid to all wells, including A1, and mix.
18. Read absorbance at 450–620 nm within 60 minutes in ELISA reader.

Calculation and Interpretation of Results

- Individual negative calibrator values must be ≤0.120 and ≥−0.005.
- A plate is considered valid if the blank value is ≥0.020.
- Plates are considered valid if both positive control values are ≥0.800.
- Calculate the cutoff by adding 0.600 to the mean absorbance (NCx) of the negative control.

$$\text{Cutoff} = NCx + 0.600$$

Interpretation of Results

Negative: Samples with absorbance value below the cutoff value

Positive: Samples with absorbance values equal to or greater than the cutoff value

    Samples with absorbance values <−0.025 should be retested in a single well.

    Paste the printout into the HCV register and record the results in a bloodstock register.

Venereal Disease Research Laboratory (VDRL) Testing

SCOPE AND APPLICATION

Venereal disease research laboratory (VDRL) testing for screening of syphilis is mandatory for each blood unit before it is transfused. This can be done by either rapid kit or enzyme-linked immunosorbent assay (ELISA) method.

RESPONSIBILITY

Technicians working in the transfusion transmitted infection (TTI) laboratory are responsible for performing tests under the supervision of technical supervisor and medical officers.

RAPID KIT METHOD

Materials Required

- Test device kit [store in the sealed pouch or closed canister either at room temperature (RT) or refrigerated (2–40°C) conditions]
- Disposable specimen droppers
- Pipette and its tips
- Package insert
- Serum/plasma sample

Procedure

Principle

The rapid syphilis test is based on the principle of immuno-chromatography. The device contains a strip padded with dried gold conjugate containing recombinant *Treponema pallidum* (TP) antigen. The nitrocellulose membranes are immobilized with recombinant TP antigen in the "T" region of the test line and another protein in the "C" region of the control line. As the test sample flows through the test membrane assembly, the recombinant *Treponema* antigen-colloidal-gold conjugate forms a complex with *Treponema*-specific antibodies when present in the sample. This complex continues to migrate across the membrane, where it is immobilized by the recombinant TP antigen coated on the membrane, forming a pink/purple line in the test line region "T," indicating that the sample is positive for syphilis and antibodies against TP are present.

If the sample does not contain TP antibodies, a pink/purple line will not appear in the test line region "T," indicating that a negative result for syphilis and specimen does not contain antibodies against TP. Unreacted conjugates and unbound complexes migrate along the membrane with mouse immunoglobulin G (IgG) gold conjugate and are then immobilized by a goat anti-mouse antibody coated on the control region of the membrane assembly, forming a pink/purple band. Control bands help to validate tests.

Method

Important: Check the actual volumes and instructions provided with the test kit. This may vary from lot-to-lot number.

1. Remove the test strip from the protective pouch and bring the test strip to RT (15–30°C) before starting the test.
2. Label the test strip with patient or sample ID.
3. Using the pipette provided with the kit, add 60 μL (two drops) of serum sample to the sample well and ensure that there are no air bubbles. Avoid overflow.
4. Read the results in 15 minutes. Do not read the results after 20 minutes. Before reading the results, it is important that the background is clear.

Validation

These kits are pre-validated by the manufacturers with claim of 100% sensitivity and specificity.

Interpretations

Positive: Distinct pink/purple band in addition to pink/purple band in control (C). The positive result should be confirmed by other confirmatory tests.

Negative: Only pink/purple bands are visible in the control (C) region. No apparent band on the test (T) region.

Invalid: No color in either region, no colored lines. Control area (C) is an indicator of procedural error and/or test reagent deterioration. Repeat the test with a new kit.

Details of the test performed daily are entered in a register:
- Date of test
- The name of the kit used
- Kit lot number and expiration date
- Initials of the performing technician

The results of blood units tested are then recorded in the master record for blood and its components.

ELISA (SYPHILIS ENZYME IMMUNOASSAY II TOTAL ANTIBODY)

Materials Required
- ELISA reader
- ELISA washer
- Micropipettes and disposable tips
- Timer
- Disposable gloves
- Waste container with sodium hypochlorite solution
- Absorbent tissue
- Distilled water
- *Kit*: Plate [12 strips of 8 wells coated with TP antigens, wash solution, negative control (NC), positive control, conjugate, substrate, and stop solution]
- Serum or plasma can be used

Procedure

Principle

Syphilis enzyme immunoassay (EIA) II total antibody uses three recombinant antigens in a sandwich test to produce a test that is both highly specific and sensitive. The antigens will detect TP-specific IgG, immunoglobulin M (IgM), and immunoglobulin A (IgA), enabling the test to detect antibodies during all stages of infection.

Method

Syphilis EIA II total antibody test is carried out as per the kit manufacturer's instructions. The details of the kit procedure and interpretation of results are as per the pack insert of the kit in use. The kit is stored at 2–8°C.

The samples should be stored at 2–8°C if the testing is to be carried out within 7 days or stored at −20°C for a longer period.

Remove reagents from the fridge 30 minutes prior to testing. Mix the reagents gently by inverting the vials without foaming.

1. Bring samples to RT before testing.
2. Dilute wash buffer 1 in 20 with distilled water prior to use.
3. Discard all disposable tips in a container with hypochlorite solution.
4. Arrange the samples so that wells 1A, 1B, and 1C are NCs, 1D and 1E are positive controls, and thereafter samples to be tested are arranged.
5. Dispense 50 μL of the controls as well as undiluted samples in the corresponding wells.
6. Add 50 μL of conjugate to the wells.
7. Mix the plate gently and cover with a seal.
8. Incubate at 37°C for 30 minutes.
9. Remove the seal and wash five times with the buffer ensuring a soak time of about 30 seconds between each cycle.
10. Invert the plate and tap on a clean paper towel to remove excess wash buffer.
11. Dispense 50 μL of substrate/chromogen to each well.
12. Cover the plate with a sealer and incubate at 37°C for 30 minutes.
13. Add 50 μL of stop solution to each well. Blue color will change to yellow.
14. Remove moisture from bottom of the plate and read optical density (OD) at 450 nm using a plate reader within 30 minutes of stopping the reaction.

Validation

The OD of each NC should be 0.080 or less. If any of the control values is above the value, the reading is ignored, and the remaining two are used to calculate the limits.

The OD of each positive control should be $\geq 1,000$.

Cutoff Value

It is calculated from the mean NC value plus 0.100.

i.e.,
$$\frac{\text{negative control (NC)}1 + NC2 + NC3 + 1.000}{3}$$

INTERPRETATION

Specimens with an OD below the cutoff value are considered negative for total syphilis EIA II antibodies.

Results just below the cutoff value (CO-10%) should be interpreted with caution and retesting of the samples is recommended.

Specimens with an OD equal to or greater than the cutoff value are considered positive for total syphilis EIA II antibodies.

Immunodiagnostic Assay (Chemiluminescence) of Viral Markers and Syphilis

SCOPE AND APPLICATION

This standard operating procedure (SOP) explains the operation of VITROS ECiQ Immunodiagnostic (Chemiluminescence) System for screening of the serum/plasma for various analytes [human immunodeficiency virus (HIV) 1 and 2, hepatitis B surface antigen (HBsAg), hepatitis B core antigen (anti-HBc), hepatitis C antibody (anti-HCV), and syphilis].

RESPONSIBILITY

It is the responsibility of the technical supervisor and laboratory technicians to operate VITROS ECiQ Immunodiagnostic (Chemiluminescence) System to screen serum/plasma for transfusion transmissible infections.

EQUIPMENT AND MATERIALS REQUIRED

- *Equipment*:
  - VITROS ECiQ Immunodiagnostic System
  - Benchtop centrifuge
  - Incubator
- *Materials*:
  - Gloves
  - Micropipettes (5–50, 20–200, and 100–1,000 μL)
  - Micro sample cups
  - VITROS Versatips
  - Eppendorf Tubes
  - Vacutainers
  - Micro tips

- *Sample*:
  - Human serum/plasma
- *Reagents*:
  - VITROS ECiQ Reagent Pack for various analytes, calibrators, and controls
  - VITROS ECiQ signal reagent (SR)
  - VITROS ECiQ universal wash reagent (UWR)
- *Miscellaneous*:
  - Radioimmunoassay (RIA) tubes
  - Worksheet
  - Tissue paper gauze
  - Gauze

PROCEDURE

General

1. Check the room temperature and and maintain the temperature at 25°C.
2. Check the UPS.
3. Switch on the VITROS ECiQ Immunodiagnostic System by pressing the main switch and hold it for about 10–15 seconds.
4. Wait for the instrument to get ready after initialization.
5. Do the daily maintenance as per the chart.
6. Empty the solid waste container.
7. Switch off the vacuum and pressure switch.
8. Disconnect and open the liquid waste bottle cap and empty the same.
9. Disconnect and change the UWR bottle or fill the UWR, if required.
10. Switch on the vacuum and pressure switch.
11. Remove the outdated and empty reagent packs and SR packs.
12. Inspect the universal sample tray for cleanliness.
13. Remove the reagent packs, calibrators, controls, and SR packs as per the requirement from the refrigerator.
14. Centrifuge the samples at 5,000 rpm for 8 minutes or at 3,500 rpm for 15 minutes.

Loading of Reagent Pack

1. Remove the reagent pack from the sealed pouch and load the pack as follows.
2. Reagent pack may be loaded at any time during the operation except when the system is in diagnostic mode or in the initialization process.

3. Check the light-emitting diode (LED) at the autoload station, and it should be green before loading the pack. If it is yellow, do not try to load the reagent pack.
4. Open the outer load door and place the reagent pack into the autoload station on the reagent pack shuttle.
5. Close the outer load door.
6. The reagent pack shall be taken into the system automatically by the reagent pack shuttle, and the inventory shall be determined by the system automatically.
7. While loading the reagent pack in the system for the first time or while loading the new lot of reagent pack, the magnetic card is supplied with the calibrator pack. Protocol card and reagent lot calibration card shall be scanned to upload the information.
    a. Protocol cards are normally scanned once per assay.
    b. Reagent lot calibration card must be scanned when a new lot of reagent is loaded.
    c. While loading, check that both the reagent lot and the calibrator lot are the same. It is not possible to calibrate the reagent lot with another lot of calibrator.

Loading of Signal Reagent (SR)

1. Remove the SR pack from the sealed pouch.
2. SR pack may be loaded at any time during the operation.
3. Open the SR pack load door and place the SR pack and confirm the same by clicking on the "Action" icon and pressing return.
4. The system automatically rotates the SR pack from the load position to the in-use position when the in-use pack is empty.
5. **Do not load either empty or previously used or partially used SR pack.**

Verifying the Onboard Reagent Inventory

1. Check the inventory of the reagent pack, SR and UWR by pressing on the "Reagent Management" icon.
2. The reagent pack inventory may be obtained by pressing on the "well count" icon.
3. The SR and UWR inventory may be obtained by pressing on the "view supplies" icon.

Calibration of the Assay

1. Check for sufficient volume of fluid in a calibration container. If less, transfer to cups as necessary.

2. Check for any bubbles in the calibrator. If so, do centrifuge the same or transfer to the cups.
3. Place the calibrator container in the universal sample tray and load the tips.
4. Place the sample tray in the sample supply.
5. Press the "sample programming" icon in the main menu.
6. Enter the tray number using keyboard and press enter.
7. Enter the calibrator ID in the box and press enter.
8. Touch the "Cal" icon. The assay to be calibrated shall be automatically selected.
9. Touch "Save/Next" icon.
10. For the next calibrator, enter the calibrator ID in the box and press enter.
11. Touch the "Cal" icon and then touch "Save/Next" icon.
12. Press the "sampling on" icon, and the sampling shall be carried out by aspirating the sample and will be loaded on the wells.
13. After sampling is completed, press the "sampling off" icon.
14. Wait until the calibration process is completed.
15. If the calibration is successful, proceed for the calibration verification using specific control fluids.
16. If the calibration is unsuccessful, identify the root cause of the issue, rectify the same, and redo the calibration process.

Programming of Controls

1. After successful calibration, do calibration verification using specific control fluids.
2. Reconstitute the VITROS assay-specific control with the required volume of distilled water (injection grade) as specified in the instruction for use manual and leave the vial undisturbed for about 10 minutes.
3. Mix the reconstituted controls and transfer to the cups as required.
4. Place the cups with control fluid in the universal sample tray and load the tips.
5. Place the sample tray in the sample supply.
6. Press the "sample programming" icon in the main menu.
7. Enter the tray number using keyboard and press enter.
8. Enter the control ID in the box and press enter.
9. Touch the "control" icon and select the assay to be processed.
10. Touch "Save/Next" icon.
11. For the next control sample, enter the control ID in the box and press enter.
12. Touch the "control" icon and then touch "Save/Next".

13. Press the "sampling on" icon. Now the sampling shall be carried out by aspirating the control sample and load on to the wells.
14. After completion of process, check the obtained results and compare with the expected results. The obtained results should be within ±2 standard deviation (SD).
15. If the obtained results exceed ±2 SD, check the reconstituted stability of the control and onboard stability of the reagent pack.
16. Repeat the same with fresh control and fresh reagent pack.
17. If not satisfactory, do recalibration.

Programming of Samples

1. Check for sufficient sample (serum/plasma) in the sample container. If less, transfer the sample to the sample cups as necessary.
2. Check for any clot, fibrin particles, or bubbles in the sample. If so, recentrifuge the same or transfer to the cups.
3. Place the serum or plasma samples in the universal sample tray and load the tips.
4. Place the sample tray in the sample supply.
5. Press the "sample programming" icon in the main menu.
6. Enter the tray number using keyboard and press enter.
7. Enter the sample ID in the box and press enter.
8. Select the tests to be carried out by touching the assays or panels to be processed for that sample.
9. Touch "Save/Next" icon.
10. For the next sample, enter the sample ID in the box and select the test as mentioned above.
11. Press the "sampling on" icon. Now the sampling shall be carried out by aspirating the sample and loading on to the wells.
12. For batch programming, enter the tray number and press enter.
13. Select the assays or panels to be processed.
14. Touch "batch save" icon.
15. In the new screen, enter the sample ID and then touch OK or save.
16. Press the "sampling on" icon.

Reviewing the Results

1. Press the "results review" icon on the main menu.
2. Press "monitor results" for viewing the results continuously.
3. For viewing the results specifically, press "Edit or Verify results" icon and enter the sample ID or patient name in the search criteria menu.

4. Press start. The prompt line indicates the number of records on the fixed disk that match the search criteria. If only one record matches the search criteria, record is displayed on the screen.

5. If multiple result records match, touch start again to begin displaying the records one at a time, starting with the oldest record on file.

6. To view the "status of the sample and the time required to complete the assay," touch "View Sample Status" icon.

7. In the new window, the sample ID along with the time for completion of the assay will be shown.

8. Select the sample ID and then touch "View Sample Details" icon in the bottom row.

9. In the new window, the status of the assay process will be shown.

10. To view the results, touch "Edit/Review" icon in the bottom row.

11. In the new window, the results will be shown.

12. Select the sample ID and then touch edit patient data for editing patient demographics if any.

13. For printing out the results, press laboratory or patient and press return.

CALCULATION AND INTERPRETATION OF RESULTS

For VITROS HIV combo, HBsAg ES, and anti-HCV, the results are calculated as a normalized signal relative to the cutoff value (signal/cutoff or S/C).

During the calibration process, a lot-specific parameter, encoded on the lot calibration card, is used to determine a valid stored cutoff value for the VITROS ECiQ System.

$$\text{Result} = \frac{\text{Signal for test sample}}{\text{Signal at the cutoff (cutoff value)}}$$

Patient sample results will be displayed with a "Negative," "Borderline," or "Reactive" label.

Result S/C	<0.90	≥0.90 and <1.0	≥1.00
Result interpretation	Negative	Borderline	Reactive

A sample found borderline or reactive should be retested in duplicate to verify its status. Before retesting, the sample is centrifuged to ensure freedom from cells, cellular debris, or fibrin. If results on repeat testing are <0.90 for both replicates, the sample is considered negative. If either duplicate retest result is ≥0.90, the sample should be tested by supplemental tests to confirm the result. A repeatedly reactive sample confirmed by supplemental tests should be considered as "positive." In case of repeatedly borderline results, analysis of follow-up samples is recommended.

In VITROS, Syphilis Treponema pallidum agglutination (TPA) assay, the result is interpreted based on the signal relative to the cutoff value (signal/cutoff, S/C) as follows:

Result S/C	<0.80	≥0.80 and <1.2	≥1.20
Result interpretation	Negative	Borderline	Reactive

The VITROS anti-HBc (*Anti-hepatitis B core antigen*) is intended for the in vitro qualitative detection of total antibody [immunoglobulin G (IgG) and immunoglobulin M (IgM)] to total anti-HBc in human serum and plasma [ethylenediaminetetraacetic acid (EDTA) and citrate], based on competitive immunoassay.

Results are calculated as a signal relative to the cutoff value (signal/ cutoff, S/C).

Result S/C	<1.0	≥1.00 and <1.2	≥1.20 to <4.8	≥4.8
Result text	Reactive	Borderline	Negative	Retest

Rare patient samples occur that give high result ratios beyond the normal negative population and which may be negative or positive for anti-HBc. The results of these samples are flagged "Retest?" These samples should be diluted 1 in 20 in High Sample Diluent B and retested. The results of the diluted sample do not require correction for the dilution factor. Interpret the obtained results with the diluted sample as mentioned above.

Precautions

- Serum is the recommended specimen for infectious disease screening.
- Do not use turbid specimens. Turbidity in specimens may affect test results.
- Samples should be thoroughly separated from all cellular materials. Failure to do so may lead to an erroneous result.
- Results from citrate plasma samples will be proportionally lower due to dilution by the liquid anticoagulant.
- The results from this or any other screening test should be used and interpreted only in the context of the overall clinical picture.

NAT Screening of Hepatitis C, Hepatitis B, and Human Immunodeficiency Viruses

SCOPE AND APPLICATION

The Drug and Cosmetics Act, 1940 and Rules 1945 mandate third-generation serological assays for screening blood donors for hepatitis B virus (HBV), hepatitis C virus (HCV), and human immunodeficiency virus (HIV). Serological assays (immunoassays), rapid tests, enzyme-linked immunosorbent assay (ELISA), and chemiluminescence detect antibodies to viruses or viral antigens. Screened seronegative blood donations are at risk for transfusion transmission infections (TTIs) because of the "window period" (WP) between the donor's exposure to the virus and the production of antibodies to the virus.

Additionally, for HBV, the occult HBV infection (OBI) represents the risk and outcome of TTIs.

The risk of infection in donated blood is missed by the immunoassay testing due to low viral load during this period. These undetected WP infections are responsible for most TTIs. The blood samples of groups (such as thalassemia, sickle cell anemia, and hemophilia) requiring repeated blood transfusions have low viral load, and therefore, such samples require highly sensitive assays for detection of viral loads to ensure safe blood transfusion. Nucleic Acid Amplification (NAT) reduces this WP, thereby offering blood centers a much higher sensitivity for detecting such viral infections. NAT testing, the most advanced technology for direct testing of viral nucleic acid in whole blood and plasma samples, has been approved by the World Health Organization (WHO). NAT has been shown to reduce the WP for HBV to 10.34 days, HCV to 1.34 days, and HIV to 2.93 days. Therefore, all blood units collected and screened as negative by chemiluminescence are further screened by NAT test. The blood units screened as negative by the NAT test are issued for transfusion to add safety in blood transfusion.

Nucleic acid amplification testing is extremely sensitive and specific for viral nucleic acids. This is based on the amplification of specific sequences in viral ribonucleic acid (RNA) or deoxyribonucleic acid (DNA) and detects them earlier than the serological screening methods.

RESPONSIBILITY

The blood center laboratory technician working in the laboratory is responsible for the collection of fresh blood sample in K2 ethylene-diaminetetraacetic acid (EDTA) tube and perform the test. The results are compiled and validated by the medical officer in charge at the blood center.

SAMPLES AND MATERIALS REQUIRED

- Blood donor samples in K2 EDTA tubes
- Cooling centrifuge
- Pipette 1,000 μL
- Pipette 200 μL
- Powder-free gloves
- Biosafety cabinet L2
- Extraction machine
- Amplification machine [real-time polymerase chain reaction (PCR)]
- Mini centrifuge

PROCEDURE

Principle

NATSpert ID TripleH detection test is a qualitative in vitro diagnostic test, based on real-time PCR technology, for the detection and discrimi-nation of HCV-specific RNA, HIV-specific RNA, and HBV-specific DNA. The assay does not discriminate between HIV-1 Group M RNA, HIV-1 Group O RNA, and HIV-2. The assay includes a heterologous amplification system [internal control (IC)] to identify possible PCR inhibition and to confirm the integrity of the reagents of the kit.

Intended Use

The test is based on hydrolysis probe chemistry amplification of specific conserved targets of HIV, HCV, HBV, and IC. The amplified product is detected by the generation of fluorescent signals from target-specific fluorescent probes. Four unique fluorescent dyes are used for HIV, HCV, HBV, and IC targets, thus allowing independent identification of all three viruses. All three HIV targets (HIV-1 Group M RNA, HIV-1 Group O RNA, and HIV-2) are identified using the same dye and thus are not discriminated from each other.

Materials/Reagents for Extraction and Amplification: Disposables

- Sterile filter pipette tips
- 1.5/2 mL centrifuge tubes
- Extraction cartridge with extraction reagents
- Liquid container for waste
- PCR mix cartridge
- Control reagents

Preparation of Sample for NATSpert Real-time Assay

- Clean the work surfaces.
- Clean products such as 5% bleach
- RNAse/DNAse away to reduce the risk of nucleic acid contamination.

Executing the Protocol

1. Switch the instrument on.
2. Instrument will boot to display initial human-machine interface (HMI) screen **(Fig. 1)**.
3. If any one or both sensor/s is/are *red,* then adjust the magnet by using the following tabs till it turns *green:*
   a. Magnet UP: For *upward* movement of magnet
   b. Magnet Dwn: For *downward* movement of magnet
   c. Magnet FF: For *forward* movement of magnet
   d. Magnet Rev.: For *reverse* movement of magnet.

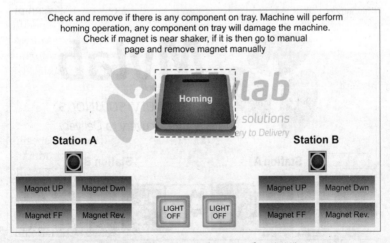

FIG. 1: Compact XL human-machine interface (HMI) screen.

4. Once both sensors are green, start homing by pressing "OK" on HMI touch screen **(Fig. 2)**.
5. During homing instrument will adjust syringe, deck, and magnet to zero position.
6. Home screen will be displayed after homing which contains different parameters and maintenance protocols **(Fig. 3)**.

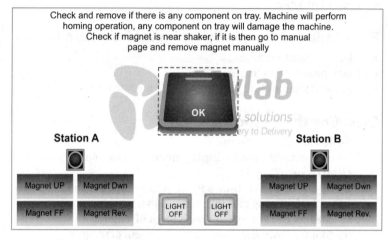

FIG. 2: Compact XL human-machine interface (HMI) ready to start.

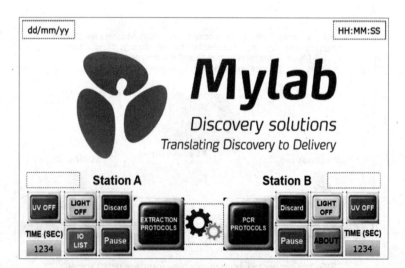

FIG. 3: Compact XL human-machine interface (HMI) main screen.

7. *Different maintenance tabs are as follows*:
   a. UV: Switch ON/OFF UV light
   b. TIME: Set timings in seconds for UV light
   c. DISCARD: Will move deck to center to remove discard bin and to home position after discarding.
   d. PAUSE: To pause run during operation.
   e. FAN ON/OFF: To switch ON/OFF Peltier for cooling of PCR cartridges.
8. Set the work deck on the compact XL as described in the diagram.
9. Load the consumables in the order described in **Figure 4**.
10. Add 1 mL of plasma sample to sample tube.
11. Centrifuge extraction cartridge before setting it on the deck.
12. Keep the sample tube in the indicated slot with 1 mL plasma sample.
13. Make sure that all the consumables, samples, and discard trays are in their right position.
14. During run, current processing will be mentioned on-screen on the left of station annotation.
15. Close the front lid to protect the instrument from environmental contamination.
16. When the protocol is completed, remove the elution tubes. The extracted samples are ready for use in downstream applications or store at –20°C or –70°C until use.

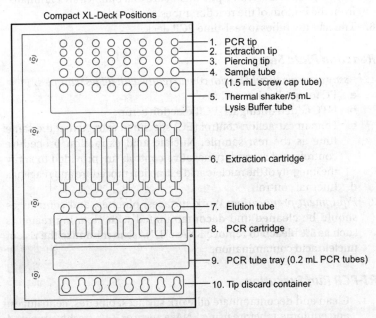

Compact XL-Deck Positions

1. PCR tip
2. Extraction tip
3. Piercing tip
4. Sample tube (1.5 mL screw cap tube)
5. Thermal shaker/5 mL Lysis Buffer tube
6. Extraction cartridge
7. Elution tube
8. PCR cartridge
9. PCR tube tray (0.2 mL PCR tubes)
10. Tip discard container

FIG. 4: Deck positions.

(PCR: polymerase chain reaction)

17. After completion of run, the instrument will discard used tips and return to home position and dehighlight protocol.
18. Now select "PCR" protocol from HMI screen to start dispensing of PCR reagents.
19. After completion of transfer, PCR tubes to real-time PCR instrument for amplification.

Test Controls Run Setup

1. Keep positive control (PC) tubes in the place of RNA sample tubes. Mix PC, HIV-1 and HIV-2.
2. *Negative template control (NTC)*: Use nuclease-free water as assay NTC.
3. Set PCR cartridge.
4. Select "PCR" protocol from HMI screen to start dispensing PCR reagents for control run.
5. Once all processes are complete, remove all used consumables and dispose of them in the biowaste bin. Power off the device. Wipe the deck surface and the fixture surfaces with a soft cloth or tissue paper (lint free) moistened with 70% isopropanol, a mild detergent sodium dodecyl sulfate (SDS).
6. Switch on the UV in between runs for 10 minutes (600 seconds).
7. Cap PCR tubes and short spin. Make sure that bubbles are eliminated from the bottom of the reaction tubes.
8. Transfer the tubes to real-time PCR deck.

Reaction Plate Setup

1. *Assay controls should be run concurrently with all test samples*:
   a. PC for qualitative analysis
   b. NTC added during RT-PCR reaction setup
   c. Human extraction control (EC) specimen extracted at the same time as the test sample. Nucleic acid extraction procedure controls and secondary negative controls are provided to verify the integrity of the nucleic acid extraction procedure and reagents.
   d. Internal control
2. *Equipment preparation*: Work surfaces, pipettes, and centrifuges should be cleaned and decontaminated with cleaning reagents such as 5% bleach to remove RNAse/DNAse to minimize the risk of nucleic acid contamination.

RT-PCR Run Execution

1. Clean and decontaminate all work surfaces, pipettes, centrifuges, and equipment before using RNAse away or 0.1% freshly prepared bleach.

2. Briefly centrifuge the reaction tube strip for 10–15 seconds. After centrifugation, return the reaction tube strip to cold rack. If using a 96-well plate, centrifuge plate for 30 seconds at 500 × g.

3. Power on the QuantStudio 5 PCR instrument and the associated computer.

4. Launch the QuantStudio™ software icon on the computer.

5. Check if the instrument is connected properly with the computer.

6. Click Open. Select Create New Experiment > Template. Navigate to and select the desired file template of triple assay and then click Open.

7. Navigate the experiment workflow by clicking previous or next at the bottom of each page or by using the tabs across the top of the screen.

8. Enter experiment name (mandatory). The experiment name determines the file and name of the experiment.

9. Targets are predefined as reference fluorescent dye as given in **Table 1**.

10. Enter a user name (mandatory).

11. Select plate wells in the plate layout.

12. *In the samples table*: Select the check box of a sample to assign it to the selected well(s). Name the individual well with sample detail.

13. In the samples table, click Add.

14. Click on the sample name to edit. Fill in the sample name/number for the particular sample.

15. Sample details will be loaded.

16. Use clear option to delete a sample from the table.

17. Load a PCR plate or PCR tubes sealed with the appropriate optical sealing tape into the instrument by selecting the Open/Close button on the instrument's touchscreen.

18. To start run, click the "run" option and click on the "start" run button. A window will appear asking to save the file. Assign appropriate file name and date of run. Run data is then saved in a predefined data folder with a .eds file extension.

19. Thermal cyclic parameters **(Table 2)**.

Table 1: Targets predefined.	
Target	**Reporter**
HIV	FAM
HCV	VIC
HBV	NED
IC	Cy5
(HBV: hepatitis B virus; HCV: hepatitis C virus; HIV: human immunodeficiency virus; IC: internal control)	

Table 2: Thermal cyclic parameters.			
Parameters	**Cycles**	**Temperature**	**Time**
RT incubation	Hold	50°C	15 minutes
Enzyme inactivation	Hold	95°C	20 seconds
PCR amplification	45	95°C	5 seconds
		60°C	30 seconds (data collection)
(PCR: polymerase chain reaction; RT: room temperature)			

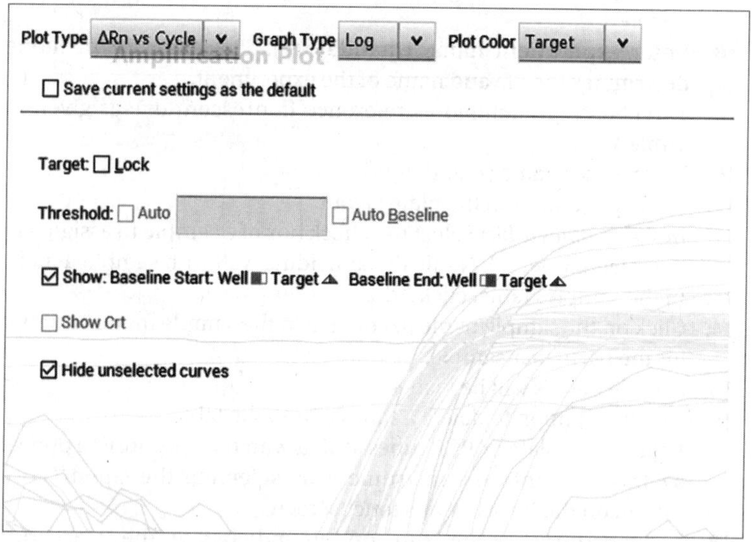

FIG. 5: Window after clicking on plot setting in result tab.

Result Interpretations

1. Fluorescence data should be collected during the 60°C extension step. Save the run after its completion and analyze the collected data.
2. Data analysis and interpretation
3. Save and analyze the data according to the instructions of the software, and the data is interpreted according to guidelines provided in the kit manual.
4. In the results tab, click on plot setting. The following window would open **(Fig. 5)**.
   Click on each target (HIV/HBV/HCV) and set threshold at 0.1.
5. Analysis must be performed separately for each target after setting manual threshold setting at 0.1 for HBV, HCV, and HIV and 0.04 for IC.

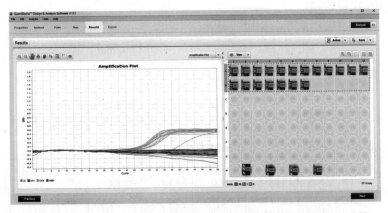

FIG. 6: Polymerase chain reaction (PCR) amplification result in real-time PCR. (***For color version, see Plate 12***)

6. Threshold should be set to fit at the beginning of the exponential phase of the fluorescence curves and above any background signal and negative control.
7. Click on analysis tab. Analyze and save the run.
8. Check the individual sample while selecting the well (**Fig. 6**).

TEST VALIDITY DETERMINATION

Prior to determining clinical sample results, it must be determined that the plate run is valid. For the test to be valid, the controls must show the expected results (**Table 3**).

Qualitative diagnostic test run is invalid:
- If the run has not been completed.
- If any of the control conditions is not met for a valid diagnostic test run.
- If a control within a lot is invalid, the entire lot is invalid and must be repeated.

Result Interpretation

If the test run is valid, interpret the sample result as shown in **Table 4**.
Export results in the export tab:
1. Enter the export file name.
2. Select a file type and format.
3. Click Browse, and navigate to select a folder destination D/: For the exported file.
4. Select open exported files when complete.

Table 3: Expected results for controls.

	HIV	HBV	HCV	Internal control	Interpretation
Threshold must be at 0.1 (Ct values at 0.1 threshold)					
Multiplex positive control	Ct 25–27	Ct 28–30	Ct 25–27	Ct 30–32	Valid
HIV-1 O positive control	Ct 27–30	Undetermined	Undetermined	Undetermined	Valid
HIV-2 positive control	Ct 25–28	Undetermined	Undetermined	Undetermined	Valid
Negative control	Undetermined	Undetermined	Undetermined	Ct 30–32	Valid
No template control	Undetermined	Undetermined	Undetermined	Undetermined	Valid

(Ct: cycle threshold; HBV: hepatitis B virus; HCV: hepatitis C virus; HIV: human immunodeficiency virus)

Table 4: Interpretation of results.

Target	Ct value	Interpretation	Ct value	Interpretation	Ct value	Interpretation
HIV	20–38	Reactive	39–42	Repeat for conformation	43–50	Non-reactive
HCV	20–38	Reactive	39–42	Repeat for conformation	43–50	Non-reactive
HBV	20–38	Reactive	39–40	Repeat for conformation	41–50	Non-reactive
IC	30–37	Valid extraction	38–42	Inhibition: Repeat for conformation	No Ct value	Inhibition: Repeat for conformation

(Ct: cycle threshold; HBC: hepatitis B virus; HCV: hepatitis C virus; HIV: human immunodeficiency virus; IC: internal control)

5. Select auto export to export data automatically after analysis. Select auto export during setup or before starting a run.
6. Select the results to export.

Troubleshooting

When IC fails, the sample is repeated from sample preparation.

Immunochromatographic Test for Malaria (Pan Malaria)

SCOPE AND APPLICATION

Plasmodium screening is a mandatory pretransfusion test for each unit of blood. Standards for blood centers and transfusion services adopted by the National AIDS Control Organisation (NACO) state that all blood units should be tested for malaria parasite using a valid and sensitive antigen test.

RESPONSIBILITY

It is the responsibility of the blood center technician working in a transfusion transmitted infection (TTI) laboratory to perform the test under the supervision of a technical supervisor, and the results are approved by a medical officer.

MATERIALS REQUIRED

- *Test kit*: The components of the kit are:
  - Malaria test device
  - Sample applicator
  - Dropper bottle nozzle and nozzle cap
  - Buffer solution
- Ethylenediaminetetraacetic acid (EDTA) blood sample

PROCEDURE

Principle

The Pan Malaria card is a "sandwich" immunoassay. This method uses a colloidal gold-conjugated anti-pan specific pLDH (parasite lactate dehydrogenase) monoclonal antibody and another anti-pan specific pLDH monoclonal antibody immobilized in a thin line onto a nitrocellulose strip. After adding the test sample to sample well "A," assay buffer is added to buffer well "B." If the sample contains *Plasmodium falciparum/Plasmodium vivax/Plasmodium malariae/Plasmodium ovale*, the colloidal gold conjugate binds to pan specific pLDH in the lysed sample to form a complex. This complex moves through the nitrocellulose strip by capillary action. When the complex meets the immobilized antibody line, it is captured and forms a magenta band, confirming the reactivity test result. Absence of a colored band in the test area indicates a nonreactive test result. To serve as a procedural control, an additional line of anti-mouse antibody has been immobilized on the strip as control. *The test is performed according to the kit manufacturer's instructions.*

Method

1. Bring the complete kit and the specimens to room temperature before testing.
2. Remove the test card from the foil pouch before use. The test should be performed immediately after removing the test card from the foil pouch.
3. Write the donor ID on the test card.
4. Tighten the bottle cap of the buffer solution provided with the kit in clockwise direction to pierce the dropper bottle nozzle.
5. Gently swirl the anticoagulated blood sample to homogenize it before use.
6. Dip the sample applicator (5 μL) into the sample to draw 5 μL of blood sample.
7. Load 5 μL of blood sample into the "sample injection point (S)."
8. Add four drops (110 ± 5 μL) of the buffer in the "buffer port (B)" on the test device.
9. Let the reaction proceed for 20 minutes.
10. Read result after 20 minutes.

INTERPRETATION

- The appearance of two magenta bands, one each in the test (T) and control (C) regions, indicates that the sample is reactive to *P. falciparum/P. vivax/P. malariae/P. ovale.*
- The appearance of a magenta band in the region of control area indicates that the sample is nonreactive to all *Plasmodium* species.
- After the test is completed, if no band is visible on either a transparent background or a completely magenta background, the test is considered invalid and should be repeated with a new card.

Validation

This test has an inbuilt quality control line "C" that develops constantly during the test to ensure proper functioning of the device and reagents and correct use of procedures. This test can detect parasitemia levels of 200 parasites per microliter of blood. The sensitivity and specificity of the test are 100% and 98.08%, respectively.

Record the results in master record of blood and its components.

CHAPTER 58

Quality Control of Blood/Blood Components

SCOPE AND APPLICATION

The primary goal of blood transfusion services is transfusion of a safe unit of blood by ensuring availability of sufficient supply of blood or blood components of high quality with maximum efficacy and minimum risk to both donors and patients. Quality assurance of blood transfusion services is multifaceted and requires a well-organized management scheme with adequate focus on the following areas:

- Personnel and premises
- Standard operating procedures (SOPs)
- Laboratory testing (techniques)
- Reagents
- Equipment
- Documentation

It is important to develop an elaborate quality assurance program and procedures as provided under the Drugs and Cosmetics Act, 1940 and Rules, 1945, Indian Pharmacopoeia, 2022 and National Blood Policy.

RESPONSIBILITY

It is the responsibility of the administration/management to ensure that staff, design, and construction of blood center comply with the requirements as laid down in the Drugs and Cosmetics Act, 1940 and Rules, 1945. Blood center technical staff are responsible for ensuring a high level of safe blood and transfusion practices for blood donors, physicians, patients, and patients' families. Assurance of a quality product includes patient and donor safety, quality control of reagents, monitoring of equipment repair and maintenance, competence of personnel, and testing of a defined number of units of each product for appropriate parameters and hazardous waste management. This goal also includes providing a safe working environment. Proper records are essential to assure product quality and safety. In addition, proper data collection, retrieval, and analysis are also essential for quality monitoring.

Blood center is responsible to develop and practice its own SOPs to meet the specified standards uniformly, monitoring the performance of the task in more effective way, standardizing staff training, reducing the adverse effects on performance in case of change/absence of staff, etc. Technical staff is also responsible for the blood/blood component collection, processing, labeling, storage, distribution, and documentation of blood/blood components.

Technical staff must also ensure that all blood center equipment/instruments is in good working order and that the reagents are stored and used in accordance with manufacturer guidelines and regulatory requirements.

QUALITY CONTROL OF BLOOD AND BLOOD COMPONENTS

Whole Human Blood IP

Quality Requirements

- *Control frequency*: 1% of all blood units, at least 4 units/month
- *Storage*: 2–6°C; for citrate-phosphate-dextrose adenine-1 (CPDA-1), the storage period is 35 days.
- *On expiration date*: Measure hematocrit (HCT), pH, total hemoglobin (Hb), and K^+, and perform sterility testing.
- *Volume*: 350/450 mL ± 10% without anticoagulant, which is 49/63 mL for 350/450 mL blood collection bag, respectively
- *HCT*: 40 ± 5%
- pH >6.5
- K^+ <27 mmol/L
- *Hb*: At least 45 g/unit for 450 mL blood collection bag
- *Leukocyte count*: <5 × 10^6/unit
- *Sterility*: No growth
- All units must be transfusion transmitted infection (TTI) negative, including hepatitis B surface antigen (HBsAg), anti-hepatitis C virus (HCV), anti-human immunodeficiency virus (HIV) 1 and 2, syphilis, and malaria.

Note: Whole human blood is included in IP with its mandatory standards of quality including test for sterility to be performed as per Indian Pharmacopoeia 2022, "in the general notices" however, it does not preclude from employing alternate method of analysis having equivalent accuracy. Therefore, it is suggested that *BACTEC method** described in Chapter 71 can be performed for blood and blood components for ensuring sterility compliance. This method, which is automated and convenient, can be employed after proper validation and prior approval from the State Licensing Authority (SLA).

Packed Red Cells IP

Quality Requirements

- *Control frequency*: 1% of all units, at least 4 units/month. At least 75% of tested packed red cells (PRCs) shall conform to quality control criteria.
- *Storage*: 2–6°C, for CPDA-1 the storage time is 35 days.
- *On expiration date*: Measure HCT, pH, total Hb, and K$^+$, and perform sterility testing.
- *Volume*:
  - 250 mL ± 10% from 450 mL bag (+100 mL additive solution)
  - 150 mL ± 10% from 350 mL bag
- *HCT*:
  - 65–70% when stored in CPDA-1
  - 50–60% when stored in saline-adenine-glucose-mannitol (SAGM)
- pH >6.5
- K$^+$ <78 mmol/L
- *Hb*: Minimum 45 g/unit
- *Leukocyte count*: <5 × 10^6/unit
- *Sterility*: No growth

Saline-washed Red Cells

Quality Requirements

- Within locally specified volume range
- *HCT*: 50–60%
- *Leukocyte count*: <5 × 10^6/unit
- *Total protein content*: <5 mg/unit

Irradiated Red Cells

Irradiated red blood cells (RBCs) are prepared by gamma cell or 25 Gy X-ray irradiation to prevent graft-versus-host disease due to lymphocyte proliferation.

Frozen Packed Red Blood Cells

Cryoprotectants can be added to the packed RBCs for long-term storage between –80 and –196°C.

Quality Requirements

- *Control frequency*: 1% of all units or if made less frequently, then every unit
- *Storage*: –80°C to –196°C
- *Volume*: Within locally specified volume range
- *HCT*: 50–60%
- *Sterility*: No growth

Packed Red Cell Aliquot

This is prepared for transfusion to pediatric patients aseptically.

Red Cells for Infant or Neonate

Quality Requirements

- *Control frequency*: 1% of all units or if made less frequently, every unit
- *Volume*: 55 mL ± 20%
- *HCT*: 50–60%
- *Sterility*: No growth

Red Cells, Pediatric

Quality Requirements

- *Control frequency*: 1% of all units or if made less frequently, every unit
- *Volume*: 120 mL ± 30 mL
- *HCT*: 50–60%
- *Sterility*: No growth

Platelet Concentrates IP

Quality Requirements

- *Control frequency*: Evaluate at least 4 platelet preparations monthly for platelet count, pH value, and plasma volume.
- *Storage*: 20–24°C

Platelet Concentrate [Platelet-rich Plasma (PRP) Method]

- *Volume*: 50–70 mL for all units
- *pH value*: ≥6
- *Platelet count*: ≥3.5/4.5 × 10^{10}/unit from a unit of 350 and 450 mL blood units, respectively
- *White blood cell (WBC) contamination*: ≥0.12 × 10^9/bag

- *RBC contamination*: <0.5 mL/bag
- *Macroscopic appearance*: No visible platelet aggregates
- *Sterility*: No growth

Platelet Concentrates (Buffy Coat Method)

- *Volume*: 50–90 mL for all units
- *pH value*: ≥6
- *Platelet count*: >6 × 10^{10}/unit
- *WBC contamination*: ≥0.12 × 10^9/bag
- *RBC contamination*: <0.5 mL/bag
- *Macroscopic appearance*: No visible platelet aggregates
- *Sterility*: No growth

Pooled Platelets

Prepared by pooling of six units of random donor platelets, preferably ABO or Rh type matched, are pooled into one bag of "pooled platelets."

Quality Requirements

- *Control frequency*: 4 units/month/1% of all units (whichever is more)
- *Storage*: 20–24°C
- *Volume*: >200 mL
- *pH value*: >6 (at the end of permissible storage period)
- *Platelet count*: >2 × 10^{11}/unit
- *WBC contamination*: ≥0.12 × 10^9/bag
- *RBC contamination*: Traces to 5 mL/bag
- *Macroscopic appearance*: No visible platelet aggregates
- *Sterility*: No growth

Platelet yield of the unit:
Calculate the yield of each unit by the following formula:

$$Platelet\ yield = count\ of\ platelet\ of\ unit \times weight\ of\ unit\ in\ g$$
$$(or\ volume\ in\ mL) \times 1{,}000$$

Fresh Frozen Plasma

Quality Requirements

- Every 10 units/week, estimate the volume.
- *Storage*:
  - 24 months at below –30°C
  - 12 months at –25 to –30°C
  - 3 months at –18 to –25°C

- Thawed at temperature between 30 and 37°C and transfused within 24 hours after thawing.
- *Frequency of control*: 4 units/month or 1% of all units (whichever is more)
- *Volume*:
    - 180–220 mL from 350 mL bag
    - 220–300 mL from 450 mL bag
- *Factor VIII*: At least 70 iu/bag
- *Fibrinogen*: 200–400 mg
- No leakage after pressure in plasma extractor, before freezing and after thawing.
- *Macroscopic*: No abnormal color or visible clots.
- *Residual cell*:
    - Red cell: $<6.0 \times 10^9/L$
    - Leukocyte: $<0.1 \times 10^9/L$
    - Platelets: $<50 \times 10^9/L$

Cryoprecipitate

Quality Control

- Assayed on at least 4 bags/month—for factor VIII.
- *Storage*: 24 months at below –30°C
    - 12 months at –25 to –30°C
    - 3 months at –18 to –25°C
- Must be thawed at 37°C and used within 6 hours.

Quality Assurance

- *Volume*: 15–20 mL
- *Factor VIII*: At least 80 iu/bag
- *Fibrinogen*: At least 150 mg/unit
- *Macroscopic*: Homogenous
- *Sterility*: No growth

Single Donor Platelets

Quality Control

- *Control frequency*: 4 units/month/1% of all units (whichever is more)
- *Storage*: Shall be kept up to 5 days between 20 and 24°C with continuous agitation.

Quality Assurance

- *Volume*: >200 mL
- *pH*: ≥6 (at the end of permissible storage period)

- *Platelet count:* >3 × 10^{11}/unit
- *WBC contamination:* <5 × 10^6/bag
- *RBC contamination:* Traces to 5 mL/bag
- *Macroscopic appearance:* No visible platelet aggregates
- *Sterility:* No growth

Note:
- It is difficult to measure the volume of the blood collected in a blood bag. Volume is indirectly determined by weighing the blood bag on a blood collection scale. The factor to convert blood volume to weight is 1.05, i.e., 1 mL of blood = 1.05 g of blood. Therefore, the volume of blood collected in a 350/450 mL blood bag is calculated by the following formula:

$$Total\ weight\ of\ blood\ bag = (volume\ of\ blood \times 1.05) + weight\ of\ empty\ bag$$

- Hb is measured by the cyanmethemoglobin method and is expressed in grams per unit.
- The pH of the blood and its components is measured with a pH meter after the expiration date labeled on the unit.
- The packed cell volume is determined using a micro-HCT centrifuge after thoroughly mixing the sample.
- Total leukocytes, RBCs, and platelet counts are done by recognized methods.
- Factor VIII coagulation activity is usually outsourced to any reputed laboratory.
- Sterility testing is performed according to IP or alternate method.
- Macroscopic inspection of all blood components is performed by the blood center staff prior to processing and issuing for any abnormal appearance, e.g., hemolysis.
- All tests except TTI are performed on expired units in blood centers.

An effective and accurate documentation at each stage forms an important part of quality control that ensures traceability of all blood transfusion activities and is the foundation of good quality management.

CHAPTER 59

Quality Control of Reagents

SCOPE AND APPLICATION

The primary objective of reagent quality control (QC) is to ensure that the diagnostic reagents meet standards and provide reliable and reproducible results. In addition, it must be ensured that the blood and blood components produced are fit for purpose, pose no risk of infection, and contain the required bioactive substances. Quality standards for antisera have been included in the Indian Pharmacopoeia 2018 which are mandatory for their manufacturers. Therefore, the manufacturer's instructions are also important when checking the quality of these reagents.

RESPONSIBILITY

It is the responsibility of Blood Center technicians to ensure that the reagents, including antisera, react as expected on each day of use and that these are stored as per the manufacturer's instructions. It must be ensured that the reagents are from licensed manufacturers and their label bear drug manufacturing license number of manufacturing firm and expiry date.

QUALITY CONTROL OF REAGENTS

Antisera

General Principles for Quality Control

- Examine the entire stocks of antisera/reagents on arrival for their acceptability. QC on their receipt is typically limited to inspection for turbidity, discoloration, or hemolysis, and reagents showing any turbidity and discoloration should not be accepted.
- Ensure that the reagents have a shelf life of at least 1 year and are stored according to manufacturers' instructions.

- Ensure that the reagents are clearly labeled with lot/batch number, date of manufacture, expiration date, and storage conditions.
- Each lot includes positive and negative controls to ensure that reagents are specific and effective.
- Blood centers should maintain uniformity in use of the reagents/kits, which must be of good quality and from a reputed manufacturer. In case of changeover, these should be properly assessed and tested for their quality parameters before switchover.
- Reagents for polyclonal antibodies (human origin) must demonstrate that the product is negative for hepatitis B surface antigen (HBsAg) and nonreactive for human immunodeficiency virus (HIV) antibodies.
- Anti-D reagents, either from two different manufacturers or two different batches of the same manufacturer, should always be available.
- Internal and external QC should be performed to ensure that the tests performed comply with the protocol and that the obtained results are reliable and reproducible.
- Blood centers shall participate in a proficiency testing program conducted by the National Blood Transfusion Council (NBTC).

Frequency of Quality Control Tests

The Drugs and Cosmetics Rules 1945 require that representative samples of the following reagents and/or solutions shall be tested regularly on a scheduled basis by methods described in the standard operating procedures (SOPs) manual to determine their capacity to perform as given in **Table 1**.

Parameters for Quality Control of Antisera

The parameters to be tested for QC of the antisera are given below.

Specificity

It means that the sera react with the corresponding antigen as designed by the manufacturer and fail to react with other antigens. Similarly, reagent red blood cells (RBCs), which are designed to express a specific blood group antigen, are shown to react with antisera of the corresponding specificity. This circularity invites creation of a simple QC system in which demonstration of reactivity of a reagent RBC is linked to demonstration of the specificity of the corresponding antiserum.

Potency

Avidity (reactivity): This is a measure of how quickly the antiserum agglutinates the RBCs. According to IP, below are the minimum

Table 1: Frequency of quality control testing of reagents and solutions.	
Reagents and solutions	**Frequency of testing along with controls**
• Antihuman serum	Each day of use
• Blood grouping serums	Each day of use
• Lectins	Each day of use
• Red cells for serum grouping	Each day of use
• Antibody screening and reverse grouping cells	Each day of use
• Hepatitis test reagents	Each run
• Syphilis serology reagents	Each run
• Enzymes	Each day of use
• HIV-1 and 2 reagents	Each run
• Normal saline (LISS and PBS)	Each day of use
• Bovine albumin	Each day of use
• Column agglutinating cards	Each day of use
(HIV: human immunodeficiency virus; LISS: low-ionic-strength saline; PBS: phosphate-buffered saline)	

requirements for the time taken by anti-A and anti-B sera to show macroscopic agglutination when mixed on a slide with equal volume of a 5.0–10.0% v/v suspension of A_1, A_2, A_2B cells, and B cells.

- *Intensity*: Strength of reaction which is scored as follows—
  - + + + + = Complete agglutination into one or two large clumps
  - + + + = Numerous clumps clearly visible to the naked eye
  - + + = Granularity just visible to the naked eye; very large clumps and unagglutinated corpuscles seen under a microscope
  - + = Not very large clumps; numerous unagglutinated corpuscles
  - (+) = Clumps of 8–12 corpuscles
  - w = Distinct but a very weak reaction with evenly distributed very small clumps of four to six corpuscles
  - ? = Uneven distribution of red blood corpuscles without distinct clumps
  - – = All red blood corpuscles separated and evenly distributed
- *Titer*: An antibody titer is a measurement of how much antibody is present. It is conventionally expressed as the inverse of the greatest dilution level that still gives a positive result. It denotes the strength of the reagent.
- *Stability*: The reagents and antisera are stable for the period of storage and retain their activity as expected on each day of use.

Testing

- *Avidity*
  - **Anti-A**
    Materials required:
    o 20% A cells
    o Glass slide
    o Anti-A serum
    Procedure:
    1. Take one drop of 20% A cells on the slide.
    2. Put one drop of anti-A and start mixing.
    3. At the same time, start the stopwatch.
    4. As soon as agglutination is visible, stop the watch.
    Limit:
    o *15 seconds*: Appearance of clear agglutination
  - **Anti-B**
    Materials required:
    o 20% B cells
    o Glass slide
    o Anti-B serum
    Procedure:
    1. Take one drop of 20% B cells on a slide.
    2. Add one drop of anti-B and start mixing.
    3. At the same time, start the stopwatch.
    4. As soon as agglutination is visible, stop the watch.
    Limit:
    o *15 seconds*: Appearance of clear agglutination
  - **Anti-D**
    Materials required:
    o 20% Rh positive cells
    o Glass slide
    o Anti-D serum
    Procedure:
    1. Take one drop of 20% Rh positive cells on a slide.
    2. Add one drop of anti-D and start mixing.
    3. At the same time, start the stopwatch.
    4. As soon as agglutination is visible, stop the watch.
    Limit:
    o *60 seconds*: Appearance of clear agglutination
  - **Potency of antisera**
    Materials required:
    o Antisera
    o Test cells
    o Test tubes
    o Pasteur pipette

o Centrifuge
o Normal saline

Procedure:

1. According to dilution of antisera (1:1 to 1:512), label the test tubes in a row.
2. Put one drop of saline to all tubes except the first.
3. Add one drop of antisera to tubes 1 and 2 (dilution 1:1).
4. Mix the contents of tube 2 with a clear Pasteur pipette, then transfer one drop of the mixture to tube 3.
5. Continue the same technique through all the tubes and remove one drop from the dilution tube of 1:512 and discard.
6. Add one drop of 5% saline suspension of appropriate RBCs to each tube.
7. Incubate for 5–10 minutes.
   a. For anti-A and anti-B at room temperature
   b. For anti-D at 37°C
8. Centrifuge at 1,000 rpm for 1 minute.
9. Gently resuspend the RBCs and look for agglutination with naked eye.

Result

Aggregation titers are recorded as the reciprocal of the highest dilution showing weak agglutination.

The minimum requirements for quality products of antihuman globulin (AHG) are:

- Anti-immunoglobulin G (IgG) 1:64
- Anti-C3/C4 1:4

The acceptance criteria for titer, specificity, and avidity for anti-A (monoclonal), anti-B (monoclonal), anti-AB (monoclonal), anti-D [immunoglobulin M (IgM)] monoclonal, and anti-D (IgG + IgM) (blend) are shown in **Tables 2 to 6**.

Quality Control of Red Cell Reagents

Red Cells should be prepared daily and free of hemolysis. A minimum pool of three individual cells for each group is required. Each lot of reagent cells (A, B, and O) prepared for serum grouping should be tested to ensure specificity. Acceptance criteria are shown in **Table 7**.

Wash the red cells. The cells are suitable for use if the supernatant is clear and there is no hemolysis.

Quality Control of Red Cell Panel

Commercially available or in-house prepared panels of RBCs should be used. The RBCs should be frozen or stored at 4°C. Commercial RBC

Table 2: Acceptance criteria for titer, specificity, and avidity for anti-A (monoclonal) reagent.

Name of the reagent	Type of the reagent	Physical appearance and color	Type of red cells	Titer	Avidity (time in seconds)	Intensity	Specificity	Reactivity (rouleaux hemolysis prozone)
Anti-A	Monoclonal	Clear, no turbidity, precipitate, particles or gel formation by visual inspection and blue-colored liquid	A_1	≥1:256	3–4	3+	Positive	Absent
			A_2	≥1:128	5–6	2+ to 3+	Positive	
			A_2B	≥1:64	5–6	3+ to 4+	Positive	
			B	–	–	–	Negative	
			O	–	–	–	Negative	

Table 3: Acceptance criteria for titer, specificity, and avidity for anti-B (monoclonal) reagent.

Name of the reagent	Type of the reagent	Physical appearance and color	Type of red cells	Titer	Avidity (time in seconds)	Intensity	Specificity	Reactivity (rouleaux hemolysis prozone)
Anti-B	Monoclonal	Clear, no turbidity, precipitate, particles or gel formation by visual inspection and blue-colored liquid	B	≥1:256	3–4	4+	Positive	Absent
			A_1B	≥1:128	5–6	2+ to 3+	Positive	
			A_1	–	–	–	Negative	
			O	–	–	–	Negative	

Table 4: Acceptance criteria for titer, specificity, and avidity for anti-AB (monoclonal) reagent.

Name of the reagent	Type of the reagent	Physical appearance and color	Type of red cells	Titer	Avidity (time in seconds)	Intensity	Specificity	Reactivity (rouleaux hemolysis prozone)
Anti-A, B	Monoclonal	Clear, no turbidity, precipitate, particles or gel formation by visual inspection and blue-colored liquid	A_1	≥1:256	3–4	4+	Positive	
			B	≥1:256	3–4	4+	Positive	
			A_2	≥1:128	5–6	3+	Positive	Absent
			A_x	–	–	–	Negative	
			O	–	–	–	Negative	

Table 5: Acceptance criteria for titer, specificity, and avidity for anti-D (IgM) monoclonal reagent.

Name of the reagent and type of the reagent	Physical appearance and color	Type of red cells	Titer	Avidity (seconds)	Intensity	Specificity	Reactivity (rouleaux hemolysis prozone)
Anti-D (IgG + IgM) Blend monoclonal	Clear, no turbidity, precipitate, particles or gel formation by visual inspection and colorless liquid	O+ve R_1r (or) R_1R_2	IS: 1:32–1:64	5–10	3+	Positive	Absent
			After 30-minute incubation at **37°C**	–	–	Negative	
			1:128–1:256				
		Rh-negative (IAT)	–				

(IAT: indirect antiglobulin test; IgG: immunoglobulin G; IgM: immunoglobulin M; IS: immediate spin)

Table 6: Acceptance criteria for titer, specificity, and avidity for anti-D (IgG + IgM) (blend).

Name of the reagent and type of the reagent	Physical appearance and color	Type of red cells	Titer	Avidity (seconds)	Intensity	Specificity	Reactivity (rouleaux hemolysis prozone)
Anti-D (IgG + IgM) Blend monoclonal	Clear, no turbidity, precipitate, particles or gel formation by visual inspection and colorless liquid	O+ve	IS: 1:32–1:64	10–20	3+	Positive	Absent
		R₁r (or) R₁R₂	After 30-minute incubation at **37°C** 1:128–1:256	–	–	Negative	
		Rh-negative (IAT)	–				

(IAT: indirect antiglobulin test; IgG: immunoglobulin G; IgM: immunoglobulin M; IS: immediate spin)

Table 7: Acceptance criteria for red cell reagent.

Parameter	Quality requirements	Frequency
Appearance	No hemolysis or turbidity in the supernatant	Daily
Reactivity	Clear reaction with known antisera	Daily

Table 8: Acceptance criteria for antiglobulin reagent.

Parameter	Quality requirement	Frequency of control
Appearance	No precipitate, particles, or gel formation by visual inspection	Each day
Reactivity and specificity	No prozone phenomenon	Each lot
	No hemolysis or agglutination of unsensitized red cells	Each day
	Agglutination of red cells sensitized with anti-D serum	Each day and each new lot/batch

panels should not be used after the expiry date. However, a panel of expired RBC can be used to solve complicated immunohematology cases as per SOP.

Quality Control of Antihuman Globulin Reagent

- One vial of each new batch should be tested for specificity and reactivity using (incomplete anti-Rh) IgG-coated cells.
- Positive and negative controls should be included for each test.
- Absence of nonspecific reactions should be ensured by using nonsensitized A, B, and O cells.
- All negative AHG tests must be confirmed by adding IgG-coated cells in the test. IgG-coated cells should give positive agglutination.

The acceptance criteria for antihuman globulin reagents are shown in **Table 8**.

Quality Control of 22% Bovine Serum Albumin

Reagents should be free of nonspecific agglutinins and should not react with the saline suspension of A, B, and O cells. Reagent should give a positive reaction with Rh (D) positive cells coated with incomplete anti-Rh (D). The acceptance criteria for bovine serum albumin (BSA) are shown in **Table 9**.

Table 9: Quality control of 22% bovine serum albumin (BSA).		
Appearance	No precipitate, particles, or gel formation by visual inspection	Each day
Purity	>98% albumin	Each new lot
Reactivity	No agglutination of unsensitized red cells; no hemolytic activity; no prozone phenomenon	Each new lot
Potency	IgG anti-D should give a titer of 32–64 with "O" pooled red cells/R$_1$R$_1$ cells	Each month
(IgG: immunoglobulin G)		

Table 10: Acceptance criteria for enzyme reagents.		
Parameter	**Quality requirements**	**Frequency of control**
Reactivity	No agglutination or hemolysis using inert AB serum. Agglutination (+++/ C) of cells sensitized with a weak IgM (anti-D)	Each day
Potency	An IgG antibody, preferably anti-D standardized to give a titer of about 32–64 by protease technique, should show the same titer on repeated testing with different batches	Each batch
	The two-stage enzyme titer should at least be equal to the titer obtained with IgG (anti-D) by AHG test	Each batch
(AHG: antihuman globulin; IgG: immunoglobulin G; IgM: immunoglobulin M)		

Quality Control of Enzyme Reagents

- Reagents should provide specific results when using incomplete anti-Rh(D) in positive and negative controls using standard techniques used in each laboratory.
- Standard procedures should be followed for preparation of working reagents.
- Aliquoted enzymes should be stored in a frozen state. Thaw only as much as needed for the day.
- Any unused enzyme should be discarded at the end of each day. Acceptance criteria for enzyme reagents are shown in **Table 10**.

Quality Control of Gel Cards

- Inspect the gel cards for decreased fluid levels, dryness, contamination and discoloration, opened or damaged seals, air bubbles, or artifacts. Gel cards with unacceptable visual appearance are discarded.
- Visually inspect the foil seal on the gel wells. If the foil is punctured, the gels may dry out and become unusable. If there is no fluid on the top of the gel, do not use the well and discard.
- Record the lot number and expiry date of the reagents used in the QC log.
- Follow test procedures as described in the specific package inserts of the gel cards and reagents.
- Controls are included according to quality assurance guidelines.
- Gel cards should be stored at room temperature (18–25°C).
- Test cells are stored at 2–8°C and are used before expiry date.

Quality Control of Hepatitis B Antigen, Anti-HCV, and Anti-HIV-1 and 2 Test

- Kits [enzyme-linked immunosorbent assay (ELISA)/rapid test] approved by the Central Drugs Standard Control Organization (CDSCO) are recommended for usage. Any other recently approved techniques with equal or improved sensitivity can be used.
- Manufacturers' instructions must be adhered to when performing tests.
- Positive and negative controls (kit and in-house) should be run with every lot. The Levey–Jennings chart (L–J chart) should be used and interpreted according to Westgard rules.
- CDSCO-approved rapid test kits are for emergency screening only, in rural areas or any center collecting small volumes or where power and equipment maintenance is a problem.

Note: Documentation of all tests and results is an important part of QC. The following data are documented:

- The date on which the test is run
- The name of the kit used
- Lot number and expiration date of kit
- Technician signatures
- Supervisor's signatures
- Reactive units are segregated from inventory for discard.

CHAPTER 60

Assigning of Identification Numbers to Equipment

SCOPE AND APPLICATION

This standard operating procedure (SOP) describes the process of assigning identification (ID) numbers to all equipment in the blood center in order to have traceability and reference in all related documents.

RESPONSIBILITY

It is the responsibility of technical supervisor to assign ID numbers to all the equipment.

MATERIALS REQUIRED

- Blood center equipment
- Printed stickers
- Writing pen

PROCEDURE

Equipment installed in the blood center shall be assigned unique ID number as per the steps outlined below:

1. The first and second characters shall correspond to two alphabets denoting the name of the equipment.
2. The third character shall be "/" (slash).
3. The fourth and fifth characters shall denote the room in which the equipment is installed. The codes for each room shall be as follows:
   a. *DR*: Donor room
   b. *SL*: Serology laboratory
   c. *TT*: Transfusion transmissible laboratory
   d. *AP*: Apheresis room

    e. *BC*: Blood component preparation room
    f. *QC*: Quality control
    g. *MO*: Medical officer's Room
    h. *BS*: Blood storage room
4. The sixth character shall be "/" (slash).
5. The seventh, eighth, and ninth characters shall be the numerical digits for the serial number of equipment. The first number of the equipment shall be 001, 002, 003, and so on.

    For example, the complete ID number of "donor couch" installed in donor room shall be *DC/DR/001* and blood center refrigerator in blood storage room shall be *BC/BS/001*.

6. All equipment with the same make, design, function/use shall be given separate ID numbers.
7. The ID sticker shall be affixed on the equipment.
8. A list of equipment installed in various rooms shall be prepared, approved by the blood center officer, and displayed in the respective room and updated as and when required.

DOCUMENTATION

The inventory of all the equipment along with their ID numbers is maintained in the stock register.

Calibration and Validation of Equipment

SCOPE AND APPLICATION

This standard operating procedure (SOP) describes the measures that must be taken to ensure the integrity, accuracy, and reliability of measurement data for equipment and instruments used during the collection, testing, and storage of blood/blood components. This SOP applies to all equipment used to control or assess the suitability of starting materials in processing components and final components.

RESPONSIBILITY

The blood center technical supervisor is responsible for the following:
- Planning, scheduling, organizing, and maintaining records of calibration programs for various equipment in the blood center
- Making sure that equipment and instrument are continuously calibrated or removed when not in use
- Training of staff to ensure that they are able to execute performance checks.

DEFINITIONS

Calibration

Calibration is a series of operations that establish the relationship between the values displayed by a gauge and standard under specific conditions.

Performance Checks

The routine checking of an instrument is done to ensure that it is within a specified range of accuracy and precision.

Accuracy

Accuracy is the closeness of agreement between the measurement and the true value of the measurement. Calibration determines the accuracy of an instrument.

Precision (Repeatability)

Precision is the closeness of agreement between successive measurements of a defined procedure repeated several times under prescribed conditions.

Measurement Standard

It is the measuring instrument or material which physically defines the unit of measure or quantity value. Measurement standards used for calibration must be able to trace back to the SI units of standard measurement.

PROCEDURES

Calibration Schedules

- Purchase new equipment or instrument according to specifications.
- Register your newly purchased device in the equipment register before using it.
- Ask the supplier to calibrate new equipment and provide a calibration certificate prior to delivery or after installation.
- Establish a calibration/maintenance schedule for all equipment.

The following should form the basis of the performance check calibration schedules:
- Recommendations from manufacturers
- The history of items by reliability
- Reference standards
- Equipment recalibration based on time intervals

Limits for Calibration, Traceability, and Reference Standards

Reference Standards and Traceability

All measurement standards used to calibrate equipment must be traceable to one of the following national measurement standards:
- Purchase calibrated and certified standards directly. These must be supported by a calibration document or certificate from the supplier stating the date, accuracy (assigned values and units of measurement), traceability, and the conditions under which the

results were obtained. These standards should be recalibrated at specified intervals.

- Indirectly, by preparing an internal working standard calibrated against certified standards. These should be supported by internal test reports and any other supporting documents.
- In the absence of approved external standards, internal standards can be established and calibrated, provided a documented procedure is established and a rationale for assigning values, precision, and units is established. These standards must be supported by the appropriate calibration records listed above.

Calibration Limits

Calibration involves measuring values, comparing them to standard tolerance limits and making adjustments or corrections as necessary.

Compare the calibration results to the meter's specified accuracy limits. If the device to be calibrated is not within limits, readjust and recalibrate until it is within predefined limits. In that case, stop using the equipment.

Limit settings should be based on a combination of:
- Specified at time of purchase
- Recommendations of manufacturers
- Limits set on reference standards

The tolerance limits required for adequate calibration of each piece of equipment should be identified or stated in the appropriate procedures.

Calibration and Performance Check Procedures

Prepare and use documented procedures, based on the instrument manufacturer's written instructions, for the calibration and performance verification of all gauges and measurement standards.

The calibration procedure should include:
- A list of equipment to which the procedure applies
- Calibration points, environmental requirements, and special conditions
- Accuracy limits
- A sequence of calibration procedures
- Data collection instructions with reference to appropriate standard forms. Performance review procedures should follow a similar format.

Labeling

Label all calibrated equipment with the following information:
- Date of last calibration
- Signature of the person who performed the calibration
- Next scheduled calibration date

Label the equipment that are past their calibration date until they are recalibrated.

DOCUMENTATION

Maintain complete records of the calibration and performance checks of all equipment and instruments.

Calibration and performance check test records should include (if applicable):
- Equipment ID number
- Equipment serial number
- Calibration limits
- Date of calibration/performance check
- When the next calibration is due
- Details of adjustments or repairs
- Calibration/performance check results
- Declaration of compliance or details of noncompliances and actions taken
- Signatures/initials of the person who performed the calibration/performance check
- *Record the calibration results before and after each adjustment.*
- Maintain records for calibration and performance check for 5 years.

Corrective Action

- Perform a review if any equipment is out of calibration and needs adjustment. Take corrective action if necessary.
- If the item can be calibrated, it will often continue to be used. If the item cannot be calibrated, do not use it until the situation is resolved. In that case, affix a label stating that the item is under repair and not to be used.
- The supervisor should assess the possible impact of the inaccuracy of the affected measurements on blood/blood component quality. Factors influencing the level of risk include:
  - Critical nature of the measurement
  - Quality control sensitivity to imprecision results
  - Production records and performance test history

Additional quality control tests may be performed to determine if quality is intact. If quality is likely compromised, communicate to management and document reports.

Relocation of Instruments

In case the equipment (especially nonportable) is relocated, recalibrate the equipment. When moving nonportable equipment, the manufacturer's recommendations regarding the need for recalibration should be obtained and considered.

External Calibration Contractors

Make an agreement with the contractors to provide written reports of calibration including:
- Use of standards and references traceable to national standards
- Equipment manufacturer certification/licensing, if any
- Check all certificates or reports provided by an approved external laboratory on receipt.
- Certificates and reports must include the details as mentioned above for documentation.

CHAPTER 62

Temperature Check for Temperature-dependent Equipment

SCOPE AND APPLICATION

All temperature-dependent equipment (TDE) in the blood center are continually monitored to ensure that blood/blood components are stored at mandatory temperature ranges.

The blood center equipment in which blood/blood components are stored must maintain temperatures in the following ranges:

- *Blood center refrigerator*: 2–6°C
- *Deep freezer*: –18°C or colder
- *Platelet incubator*: 20–24°C

RESPONSIBILITY

It is the responsibility of the technical supervisor and laboratory technician of the blood center to monitor all TDE in the blood center to ensure that blood/blood components are stored at mandatory storage conditions.

EQUIPMENT AND MATERIALS

- Refrigerator, freezer, or platelet incubator to be checked
- Refrigerator, freezer, or platelet incubator temperature chart

PROCEDURE

Daily Checking of Continuous Monitored Chart System

1. Temperatures of TDE are documented daily at about the same general time of day.

2. Document the temperature of each TDE on *blood center temperature check* form as per details below and affix on the equipment.

Date	Time	Shift	Temperature	Signature

3. Assess that the temperature recording chart is turning properly and is within the temperature guidelines and is currently at the appropriate day and time on the chart.
4. The person recording the daily temperatures should sign the chart each day when it is checked to verify the proper day/time setting.
5. Ensure continuous power supply.

Weekly Chart Change

1. Temperature charts are changed weekly at about the same general time. Information listed on the back of each chart should include the equipment identification number, the date, time the chart is placed on the equipment, and initials of the person replacing the chart.
2. Completed charts should have the date and time of removal and should be initialed.
3. Weekly charts are paper-clipped together and placed in the file for review.

Procedure for Abnormal Results

Audible Alarm Sounds

The audible alarm for the refrigerator and platelet incubator is set to sound before the upper and lower temperature range is reached. If a refrigerator or freezer temperature reaches unacceptable limits at any time, an alarm sounds in the blood center. When this situation occurs, the following steps should be taken:

- *Compare chart and thermometer readings*: If these are within range, the probable cause is prolonged door opening. Limit entry into the refrigerator or freezer and monitor the temperature, which should begin to return to normal range shortly. The technician noting the alarm and deviation of temperature should sign and make a note on paper chart to reflect the cause of the alarm.

  If the continuous automated monitoring chart system is not operational, temperatures must be recorded and documented every 4 hours to ensure that blood/blood components are being stored at the desired temperature.

- *Temperature of equipment does not return to normal range*: Carefully monitor the temperature of equipment so that blood/blood components remain within an acceptable range. Call the maintenance department for STAT assessment of equipment. If equipment temperature remains the same or continues to increase, blood/blood components must be removed to prevent loss. Red blood cell (RBC) units and reagents should be moved to another monitored refrigerator in the blood center. Frozen components should be placed in insulated boxes with dry ice placed on top of the units. Platelets may be placed in room temperature (RT) platelet shipping boxes for up to 24 hours without agitation.

  Remove blood/blood components when temperatures of equipment approach the following sustained temperatures:
  - Refrigerator: ≥6.0°C
  - Platelets: ≥24°C
  - Fresh frozen plasma (FFP): Above −18°C

Actions If System is Inoperable

- *Power failure*: In the event of a power failure, make sure that auxiliary power is functioning. If this cannot be ascertained, call maintenance. In the event of a complete power equipment failure, other hospital facilities may be called to provide help for storage of blood/blood components. In case of power failure, red cells should be maintained in boxes with bags of wet ice placed on top. FFP should be maintained in boxes with dry ice placed on top of units. Platelets can be maintained in platelet shipping boxes for up to 24 hours without agitation. Reagents should be placed in insulated boxes with bags of wet ice placed on top.
- *Refrigerator/freezer/platelet alarm inoperable*: If blood/blood components are stored under unmonitored conditions, the temperature should be checked every 4 hours and documented on *manual temperature recording log* form. This will document that proper storage temperature was maintained.

When the Refrigerator/Freezer/Incubator is Back in Service

Before blood/blood components and/or reagents are placed back into the TDE after repairs, ensure that the temperature of the equipment remained stable for at least 4–24 hours. Temperature and alarm checks on the TDE must be satisfactorily performed and recorded. Reagents and antisera should be inspected for blood quality concerns and must pass quality control (QC) test before patient blood testing is performed. Reagents and/or antisera that do not pass quality must be discarded.

DOCUMENTATION

Maintain complete record including blood center temperature check forms and temperature charts to document that the blood/blood components were stored at appropriate temperatures.

CHAPTER 63

Equipment Maintenance

SCOPE AND APPLICATION

This standard operating procedure (SOP) applies to regular checking and calibrations of all the instruments and equipment installed in the blood center for ensuring collection, processing, testing, storage, and issue/distribution of blood/blood components as per Drugs and Cosmetics Rules 1945.

RESPONSIBILITY

Blood center technical supervisor and technicians are responsible for ensuring that the equipment is in good working order. The equipment used for the collection, processing, testing, storage, and issue/distribution of blood/blood components should be maintained in a clean and proper manner so that cleaning and maintenance can be done easily. The equipment must be monitored, standardized, and calibrated in accordance with SOPs prepared, taking into account the equipment manufacturers' recommendations and the provisions of the Drugs and Cosmetics Rules 1945.

The SOPs for all equipment defining all maintenance requirements (e.g., routine/preventive), regardless of whether performed by an internal or external agency, should be written. The prepared maintenance schedule for all equipment includes the following:

- Preventive maintenance
- Routine maintenance
- Additional maintenance
- Calibration

All equipment need preventive maintenance including cleaning, regular calibration, and periodic verification of performance accuracy. This is either conducted by the own biomedical department or manufacturer's engineer under maintenance contract or any National

Accreditation Board for Testing and Calibration Laboratories (NABL)—certified vendor with authoritative scope for the required parameters to be validated with their calibrated/validated instruments having valid master traceability. The maintenance plan as given by the manufacturer of the equipment should be adhered to.

PROCEDURES

General Guidelines

1. All the equipment must comply with the specifications.
2. Processing/producing quality components requires maintenance, periodical servicing, and fault repairing.
3. Each equipment must have a logbook.
4. The frequency of testing any equipment is determined by:
   a. Type of equipment
   b. Malfunctioning
   c. Provisions of Drugs and Cosmetics Rules 1945
   d. Review of past quality control records

Equipment Maintenance

Equipment used to collect, process, test, store and distribute blood/blood components should be kept clean and tidily arranged for easy cleaning and maintenance. In accordance with regulatory requirements, the equipment must be regularly monitored, standardized, and calibrated according to the criteria given in **Table 1**.

Table 1: Schedule of observation, standardization, and calibration of equipments.			
Equipment	**Performance**	**Frequency**	**Frequency of calibration**
Temperature recorder	Compare against thermometer	Daily	As often as necessary
Refrigerated centrifuge	Observe speed and temperature	Each day of use	As often as necessary
Hematocrit centrifuge	–	–	Standardize before initial use, after repair or adjustments, and annually

Continued

Continued

Equipment	Performance	Frequency	Frequency of calibration
General lab centrifuge	–	–	Tachometer, every 6 months
Automated blood typing	Observe controls for correct results	Each day of use	–
Hemoglobi-nometer	Standardize against cyanmethemoglobin	Each day of use	–
Refractometer or urinometer	Standardize against distilled water	Each day of use	–
Blood container weighing device	Standardize against container of known weight	Each day of use	As often as necessary
Water bath	Observe temperature	Each day of use	As often as necessary
Rh view box	Observe temperature	Each day of use	As often as necessary
Autoclave	Observe temperature	Each time of use	As often as necessary
Serologic rotators	Observe controls for correct results	Each day of use	As often as necessary
Laboratory thermometers	–	–	Before initial use
Electronic thermometers	–	Monthly	–
Blood agitator	Observe weight of the first container of blood filled for correct results	Each day of use	Standardize with container of known mass or volume before initial use and after repairs or adjustments
Standard certified weight(s)	–	–	Once a year

Continued

Continued

Equipment	Performance	Frequency	Frequency of calibration
Equipment for transfusion-transmitted infection (TTI) laboratory such as ELISA plate reader if enzyme-linked immunosorbent assay (ELISA) is used or chemiluminescence immunoassay (CLIA) or enzyme-linked fluorescence assay (ELFA)	–	Each run Each day of use	Once a year
Micropipettes if ELISA is used	–	–	Once a year

Important Equipment Maintenance Guidelines

Centrifuge for Gel Cards

No internal part of the centrifuge is to be lubricated or oiled.

Time	Activity	Carried out by	Method
As required	Cleaning	Laboratory technician	Clean the tub, lid, outer housing, and surface of centrifuge head with a lint-free cloth moistened with 70% ethyl alcohol after switching off and removing the power cord. Clean inside of the cardholder in the same way. Allow the machine to dry
As required	Decontamination	Laboratory technician	In case of contamination, the machine should be decontaminated immediately. *Never use cleaning agent containing chloride or ammonium*

Continued

Continued

Time	Activity	Carried out by	Method
Weekly	Checking the mobility of the ID cardholder	Laboratory technician/ tech support	The ID cardholders are checked for ease of movement and the full 90° swivel angle. If it does not fall back into its original position or the movement is stiff, contact in-house biomedical team or company engineer
Weekly	Inspecting the seal and lid	Laboratory technician/ technical support	Seal and lid are safety components. Check for any damage, e.g., nicks, tears, and pressure marks
Half-yearly	Preventive maintenance service	Technical support	Performed by manufacturer's engineer if under any contract or warranty period as per checklist or by in-house biomedical engineer as per in-house checklist specific to particular equipment
Yearly	Calibrating/ validating speed	Technical support	Performed by manufacturer as per their standard procedure or can be outsourced from a NABL-certified vendor with authoritative scope for the calibration/validation of speed with range 800–850 rpm for the centrifuge with their calibrated tachometer having a valid master traceability certificate
Yearly	Calibrating/ validating the centrifugation time	Technical support	Performed by manufacturer as per their standard procedure or can be outsourced from a NABL-certified vendor with authoritative scope for the calibration/validation of timer for the centrifuge with their calibrated stopwatch having a valid master traceability certificate

Incubator for Gel Cards

No internal part of the centrifuge is to be lubricated or oiled.

Time	Activity	Carried out by	Method
As required	Cleaning	Laboratory technician	Clean the tub, lid, outer, and housing with a lint-free cloth moistened with 70% ethyl alcohol after switching off and removing the power cord. Remove the hot plate to clean the entire tub. Allow the machine to dry
As required	Decontamination	Laboratory technician	In case of contamination, the incubator should be decontaminated immediately. *Never use cleaning agent containing chloride or ammonium*
Weekly	Checking/replacing O ring	Laboratory technician	Check the O ring for damage, e.g., nicks, tears, and pressure marks. In case it is damaged, it is to be replaced
Half-yearly	Preventive maintenance service	Technical support	Performed by manufacturer's engineer if under any contract or warranty period as per checklist or by in-house biomedical engineer as per in-house checklist specific to particular equipment
Yearly	Calibrating/validating incubation temperature	Technical support	Performed by manufacturer as per their standard procedure or can be outsourced from an NABL-certified vendor with authoritative scope for the calibration/validation of temperature with their calibrated/validated instruments such as resistance temperature devices (RTDs) and digital temperature having valid master traceability certificates

Hemo Control

Time	Activity	Carried out by	Method
As required	Cleaning	Laboratory technician	• Clean the housing and the touchscreen with a lint-free cloth lightly moistened with clear water power cord • Clean the cuvette holder with mild soap solution • Cleaning the optical unit is very delicate. It is done with a special cleaner provided by the manufacturer and no cleaning agent is used

Continued

Continued

Time	Activity	Carried out by	Method
As required	Charging and care of the battery	Laboratory technician	To maintain the full capacity, batteries should always be discharged as far as possible before being recharged
Yearly	Preventive maintenance service	Technical support	Performed by manufacturer's engineer if under any contract or warranty period as per checklist or by in-house biomedical engineer as per in-house checklist specific to particular equipment
Yearly		Technical support	Performed by manufacturer's engineer with reference quality control solution as per manufacturer procedures with all supporting documents

VDRL Shaker

Time	Activity	Carried out by	Method
As required	Cleaning	Laboratory technician	Clean the instrument with a lint-free cloth lightly moistened with mild soap water and then dry with a soft absorbent cloth
Half-yearly	Preventive maintenance service	Technical support	Performed by manufacturer's engineer if under any contract or warranty period as per checklist or by in-house biomedical engineer as per in-house checklist specific to particular equipment
Yearly	Calibrating/ validating speed	Technical support	Performed by manufacturer as per their standard procedure or can be outsourced from a NABL-certified vendor with authoritative scope for the calibration/validation of fixed 180 rpm with their calibrated tachometer having valid master traceability certificate

Microplate ELISA Reader

Time	Activity	Carried out by	Method
As required	Cleaning	Laboratory technician	• Clean the instrument with a lint-free cloth lightly moistened with mild soap water. Decontamination is done using 70% isopropanol • Clean LCD using soft cloth
Half-yearly	Preventive maintenance service	Technical support	Performed by manufacturer's engineer if under any contract or warranty period as per checklist or by in-house biomedical engineer as per in-house checklist specific to particular equipment
Yearly	Calibration/ validation	Technical support	Performed by manufacturer as per their standard procedure for the calibration/validation of ELISA reader in terms of wavelengths, filter, and detection process

Incubator

Time	Activity	Carried out by	Method
As required	Cleaning	Laboratory technician	Clean the chamber and outer surface at regular intervals with a lint-free cloth lightly moistened with mild soap water
Daily	Accuracy of thermometer	Laboratory technician	Compared against calibrated thermometer
Half-yearly	Preventive maintenance service	Technical support	Performed by manufacturer's engineer if under any contract or warranty period as per checklist or by in-house biomedical engineer as per in-house checklist specific to particular equipment
Yearly	Calibrating/ validating temperature	Technical support	Performed by manufacturer as per their standard procedure or can be outsourced from an NABL-certified vendor with authoritative scope for the calibration/ validation of temperature with their instruments such as RTDs and digital temperature loggers having valid master traceability certificates

Continued

ELISA Washer

Time	Activity	Carried out by	Method
As required	Cleaning	Laboratory technician	• Clean the instrument with a lint-free cloth lightly moistened with clear water. Decontamination is done using 70% isopropanol • Clean LCD using soft cloth
Half-yearly	Preventive maintenance service	Technical support	Performed by manufacturer's engineer, if under any contract or warranty period as per checklist, or by in-house biomedical engineer as per in-house checklist specific to particular equipment

Bench Centrifuge

Time	Activity	Carried out by	Method
As required	Cleaning	Laboratory technician	• Clean all the buckets at regular intervals • After removing the profiled rubber insert, remove any glass splinters and pore the talcum powder
Half-yearly	Preventive maintenance service	Technical support	Performed by manufacturer's engineer if under any contract or warranty period as per checklist or by in-house biomedical engineer as per in-house checklist specific to particular equipment
Yearly	Calibrating/ validating speed	Technical support	Performed by manufacturer as per their standard procedure or can be outsourced from an NABL-certified vendor with authoritative scope for the calibration/validation of rpm for the centrifuge with their calibrated tachometer having valid master traceability certificate

Blood Collection Monitor (BCM)

Time	Activity	Carried out by	Method
As required	Cleaning	Laboratory technician	Clean the blood collection monitor (BCM) using delicate detergent. Take out the tray and clean it separately. Dry the BCM before connecting it to mains
Half-yearly	Preventive maintenance service	Technical support	Performed by manufacturer's company engineer if under any contract or warranty period as per checklist or by in-house biomedical engineer as per in-house checklist specific to particular equipment
Yearly	Calibration/ validation	Technical support	Performed by manufacturer as per their standard procedure for the calibration/validation of BCM in terms of standard weight (with conversion factor in liters stored in equipment) along with its master traceability certificates

Tube Sealer

Time	Activity	Carried out by	Method
As required	Cleaning	Laboratory technician	Clean the tube sealer with soft cloth dipped in delicate detergent. In case of blood spills, disinfest the electrodes with spirit. Allow the electrodes to dry up before connecting to mains
Half-yearly	Preventive maintenance service	Technical support	Performed by manufacturer's engineer if under any contract or warranty period as per checklist or by in-house biomedical engineer as per in-house checklist specific to particular equipment
Yearly	Calibration/ validation	Technical support	Performed by manufacturer as per their standard procedure for the calibration/validation of sealer in terms of sealing time and radio frequency (RF) with standard instruments along with their master traceability certificates

Donor Station

Time	Activity	Carried out by	Method
As required	Cleaning	Laboratory technician	Before cleaning, be sure to disconnect the AC power cord. Clean the Rexine cloth of the donor station with clean cloth dipped in mild detergent solution. Blood stains are to be removed by using isopropyl alcohol. For disinfection, the surface is wiped with cloth dipped in hospital spirit or any antiseptic germicide solution
Half-yearly	Preventive maintenance service	Technical support	Performed by manufacturer's engineer if under any contract or warranty period as per checklist or by in-house biomedical engineer as per in-house checklist specific to particular equipment

Blood Storage Cabinets (Blood Center Refrigerator/Deep Freezers)

Time	Activity	Carried out by	Method
As required	Cleaning	Laboratory technician	• Clean the blood storage cabinets with clean soft cloth. *Alcohol/ spirit/ether/any other organic solvents are not to be used* • Finned condenser to be cleaned with vacuum cleaner
Daily	• Checking of temperature chart daily • Temperature to be recorded twice daily • Check uniformity of temperature in upper and lower shelves • Maintain temperature record sheet and affix on outside	Laboratory technician	Observation
Weekly	Checking of alarm system	Laboratory technician	By immersing the sensor in ice and in water at 15–20°C

Continued

Continued

Time	Activity	Carried out by	Method
Weekly	Changing of temperature chart	Laboratory technician	Chart change switch is pressed and needle moves to rest position. Pull the chart holding knob out. Replace the chart and put the knob back. Then press chart set switch to adjust the starting time of recording. When you hold the switch down, the chart rotates. Press chart change again to restart the recording
Half-yearly	Preventive maintenance service	Technical support	Performed by manufacturer's engineer if under any contract or warranty period as per checklist or by in-house biomedical engineer as per in-house checklist specific to particular equipment
Yearly	Calibration/ validation	Technical support	Performed by manufacturer as per their standard procedure or can be outsourced from an NABL-certified vendor with authoritative scope for the calibration/ validation of temperature with their instruments such as RTDs and digital temperature loggers having valid master traceability certificates

Platelet Agitator and Incubator

Time	Activity	Carried out by	Method
As required	Cleaning	Laboratory technician	• Clean the platelet agitator/ incubator using a clean dry cloth. Do not clean with wet cloth, cloth dipped in ether, or other organic solvents • Cleaning of trays is to be done with soft detergent solution after removing the trays from tray stand and rinse the trays with clean water to remove the detergent • The openings between the fins of the condenser should be cleaned with the vacuum cleaner whenever there is clogging with dust • Do not lubricate any internal parts

Continued

Continued

Time	Activity	Carried out by	Method
Half-yearly	Preventive maintenance service	Technical support	Performed by manufacturer's engineer if under any contract or warranty period as per checklist or by in-house biomedical engineer as per in-house checklist specific to particular equipment
Yearly	Calibration/validation	Technical support	Performed by manufacturer as per their standard procedure or can be outsourced from an NABL-certified vendor with authoritative scope for the calibration/validation of fixed temperature around 22°C and fixed agitating speed 60 rpm with their calibrated instruments such as RTDs, digital temperature loggers, and tachometer having valid master traceability certificates

Cryo Bath and Plasma Bath

Time	Activity	Carried out by	Method
As required	Cleaning	Laboratory technician	• Clean the external surface regularly by using clean dry cloth • Empty the water in the tank and clean with soap solution at regular intervals • Wash the coating/scaling of the inner tank surface and evaporator coil • Culture of water to be done
Half-yearly	Preventive maintenance service	Technical support	Performed by manufacturer's engineer if under any contract or warranty period as per checklist or by in-house biomedical engineer as per in-house checklist specific to particular equipment

Continued

Continued

Time	Activity	Carried out by	Method
Half-yearly	Calibration/validation	Technical support	Performed by manufacturer as per their standard procedure or can be outsourced from an NABL-certified vendor with authoritative scope for the calibration/validation of fixed temperature of 37°C for plasma thawing bath and 4°C for cryo bath with their instruments such as RTDs and digital temperature loggers having valid master traceability certificates

Refrigerated Centrifuge

Time	Activity	Carried out by	Method
Daily	Checking of temperature	Laboratory technician	Keep the thermometer in between the blood bags and check the temperature after the blood bags are centrifuged
Daily	Time	Laboratory technician	Use stopwatch to check timer accuracy
Daily	Speed	Laboratory technician	Speed check by tachometer
As required	Cleaning	Laboratory technician	Clean the external surface regularly by using clean dry cloth
Half-yearly	Preventive maintenance service	Technical support	Performed by manufacturer's company engineer if under any contract or warranty period as per checklist or by in-house biomedical engineer as per in-house checklist specific to particular equipment
Yearly	Calibration/validation	Technical support	Performed by manufacturer as per their standard procedure or can be outsourced from an NABL-certified vendor with authoritative scope for the calibration/validation of rpm, temperature, and timer with their calibrated tachometer, temperature data loggers, and stopwatch having valid master traceability certificates

Continued

Laminar Airflow

Time	Activity	Carried out by	Method
As required	Cleaning	Laboratory technician	Clean the external surface regularly by using clean dry cloth
Half-yearly	Preventive maintenance service	Technical support	Performed by a manufacturer's engineer if under any contract or warranty period as per checklist or by in-house biomedical engineer as per in-house checklist specific to particular equipment
Yearly	Calibration/validation	Technical support	Performed by manufacturer as per their standard procedure or can be outsourced from an NABL-certified vendor with authoritative scope for the calibration/validation of air velocity and particle count with their calibrated flow meter and particle count meter having valid master traceability certificates. Particle counts are measured by air particle counters as a function of concentration per unit volume (e.g., particles per cubic meter or cubic foot).

Composcale

Time	Activity	Carried out by	Method
As required	Cleaning	Laboratory technician	Clean the external surface regularly by using clean dry cloth
Half-yearly	Preventive maintenance service	Technical support	Performed by manufacturer's engineer if under any contract or warranty period as per checklist or by in-house biomedical engineer as per in-house checklist specific to particular equipment
Yearly	Calibration/validation	Technical support	Performed by manufacturer as per their standard procedure for the calibration/validation of BCM in terms of standard weight (with conversion factor in liters stored in equipment) along with its master traceability certificates

Continued

Automatic Component Extractor

Time	Activity	Carried out by	Method
As required	Cleaning	Laboratory technician	Clean the external surface regularly by using clean dry cloth
Half-yearly	Preventive maintenance service	Technical support	Performed by manufacturer's engineer as per product-specific checklist
Yearly	Calibration/ validation	Technical support	Performed by manufacturer as per their standard procedure for the calibration/validation of weights. Validation in terms of buffy coat sensors also needs to be carried out by manufacturer's engineer. Apart from these, sealing quality and time validation need to be carried out by the engineer during this procedure

Hematology Cell Counter

Time	Activity	Carried out by	Method
As required	Cleaning	Laboratory technician	Clean the housing and the touchscreen with a lint-free cloth lightly moistened with clear water power cord
As required	Cleaning and deconta-mination of instrument	Laboratory technician	To be carried out with recommended solution by LT as per product-specific standard procedure of manufacturer
Half-yearly	Preventive maintenance service	Technical support	Performed by manufacturer's engineer if under any contract or warranty period as per product-specific checklist or by in-house biomedical engineer as per in-house checklist specific to particular equipment
Yearly	Calibration/ validation	Technical support	Performed by manufacturer's engineer with reference quality control solution as per manufacturer procedures with all supporting documents

MAINTENANCE OVERVIEW

- Prepare a complete list of equipment and instruments in all sections of the blood center consisting of the following headings:
  - *Equipment name/description*
  - *Equipment ID number*
  - *Serial number*
  - *Model number*
  - *Operation*:
    - o Operating range
  - *Calibration*:
    - o Frequency
    - o Referenced documents
    - o Performed by
  - *Performance check*:
    - o Frequency
    - o Referenced documents
  - *Preventive maintenance*:
    - o Frequency
    - o Referenced documents
    - o Performed by
  - *Routine maintenance*:
    - o Frequency
    - o Referenced documents
  - *Cleaning*:
    - o Frequency
- Prepare a clear outline of the relevant procedures, routine maintenance and preventive maintenance, and cleaning of equipment. Prepare a manual of instructions for operator for each equipment. The manual must include the name of the contact person and service personnel. Maintain a documented maintenance logs for all items.
- Identify and determine the frequency of relevant procedures associated with equipment maintenance, calibration, and cleaning procedures—clearly identifying the times, e.g., daily, weekly, and monthly, etc.

Maintenance Schedule

- Draw up suitable schedules for each maintenance type and frequency or by equipment type.
- Define due dates for maintenance completion and record actual dates of performance on schedule.

Service Contracts

- All major equipment must be purchased with the maximum negotiable warranty along with fixed annual maintenance contract (AMC)/comprehensive maintenance contract (CMC) rates at the time of procurement.
- Contracts must be concluded for all externally serviced equipment agents.
- Each service contract must define exactly what/how often it will be performed and by whom it is completed.
- After completion of the service, a maintenance report signed by the contractor responsible party must be submitted. The report should contain details of the work performed by the contractor.

Repair and Breakdown

- The instruction manual for each equipment indicates the steps required to be taken in the event of a fault or breakdown and indicates the person responsible for arranging service or replacement.
- Error and corrective action logs must be maintained for all equipment. When equipment fails, it is important to clearly identify it and mark it as "out of service."

Maintenance Overdue

A quality control lab will determine the suitability for continued use of the instrument past its scheduled maintenance due date (scheduled maintenance does not include calibration). The laboratory should document the reasons for continued use of the equipment overdue for maintenance. If applicable, this must include explanation (and supportive evidence if available) that product quality has not been compromised or impacted by service delays. If possible, evidence should be obtained from the manufacturer to support this determination. In the next scheduled maintenance, steps should be taken to determine whether the delayed maintenance has caused obvious damage to the equipment.

DOCUMENTATION

- Keep all manufacturer's instructions and display them near the *equipment.*
- Maintain individual files with service reports for all equipment.
- Record details of all routine and corrective service calls made by the manufacturer's technicians in the equipment maintenance records.

- A logbook of all equipment should be maintained, detailing each failure and preventive maintenance service (PMS)/calibration verification.
- Record the name, address, and phone number of each unit's service technician who should be contacted if necessary.
- Device Do's and Don'ts should be labeled on the equipment as recommended by the manufacturer.
- Each device must be tagged with PMS and calibration verification information.

Maintenance of Automated Immunohematology Analyzer

SCOPE AND APPLICATION

This standard operating procedure (SOP) describes how to maintain ORTHO VISION Analyzer for testing of human blood using column agglutination cassettes for various serological tests to prevent erroneous test results due to potential carryover.

RESPONSIBILITY

It is the responsibility of the blood center technicians to operate and do the monthly, weekly, and daily maintenance.

EQUIPMENT AND MATERIALS REQUIRED

- *Equipment*:
  - Automated immunohematology (ORTHO VISION Analyzer)
- *Materials required*:
  - *For daily maintenance*
    - ORTHO 7% bovine serum albumin (BSA) vial
    - NaOH vials
    - Isopropyl alcohol
    - Lint cloth piece
  - *For weekly maintenance*
    - 70% isopropyl alcohol or NaOH
    - Deionized water
    - Normal saline solution
  - *For monthly maintenance*
    - 70% isopropyl alcohol or NaOH
    - Empty α-naphthaleneacetic acid (NAA) reagent rack (labeled NO1B)

PROCEDURE

The maintenance of the analyzer is done by following each step of the prompt wizard of the ORTHO VISION while performing daily/ weekly/monthly maintenance operations. In case the monthly/weekly maintenance is due, it is done followed by daily maintenance.

Daily Maintenance

1. Stop processing and enter the maintenance mode.
2. Execute daily probe maintenance.
3. Open the load station door.
4. Add 5 mL of 0.5 M NaOH to a 10 mL vial with a barcode. Place the vial into position 3 of a nonagitated reagent rack.
5. Place a new 5 mL vial of 7% BSA into position.
6. Load the reagent rack.
7. Open the maintenance door and clean probe with 70% isopropyl alcohol.
8. Close the maintenance door.
9. Open the load station door.
10. Remove the NaOH and BSA vials.

Now, daily maintenance is done and resume the processing.

Note: Ensure placing of NaOH and BSA vials in correct positions as placing of NaOH and BSA vials in the wrong position or loading only one type of solution in both positions could lead to inefficient probe decontamination and conditioning, which can potentially contribute to carryover.

Weekly Maintenance

1. Stop processing.
2. Select weekly.
3. Enter the maintenance mode.
4. Execute weekly liquid system decontamination and pump test.
5. Open the liquid access door and pull the bottle release for the liquid waste bottle.
6. Install the bottle cap and slide the liquid waste bottle into the system until it snaps into place.
7. Pull the bottle release for the liquid container and remove the liquid container from the system.
8. Remove the two bottle caps and dispose of the liquids. Fill the smaller bottle (blue) with approximately 400 mL of 70% isopropyl alcohol or NaOH and the larger bottle (white) with approximately 600 mL of 70% isopropyl alcohol or NaOH.

Note: See the reference guide for a list of other acceptable solution.

9. Slide the liquid container into the system either manually or with the bottle insertion. Tool until it snaps into place. Close the liquid access door.
10. Open the liquid access door. Pull the bottle release for the liquid container and remove the liquid container from the system.
11. Remove the bottle caps and dispose of the liquid. Fill the smaller bottle (blue) with approximately 500 mL of deionized water and larger bottle (white) with approximately 3,000 mL of deionized water.
12. Install the bottle caps and gently tilt side to side.
13. Remove the two bottle caps and fill the liquid container as labeled to reach the maximum volume of approximately 900 mL of deionized water and 4,700 mL of saline solution. Plug the openings with bottle caps.
14. Slide the liquid container into the system either manually or with the bottle insertion tool until it snaps into place. Close the liquid access door.
15. Open load station and place the tube and testing rack (S16b).
16. Open the load station door.
17. Remove and empty sample tube. Place the sample tube back into the sample rack at position 1.
18. Open the load station door.
19. Remove the sample rack and sample tube.
20. Now, weekly maintenance is done.
21. Then do the daily maintenance and resume processing.

Monthly Maintenance

1. Stop processing.
2. Select monthly.
3. Enter the maintenance mode.
4. Execute instrument cleaning.
5. Open the load station door.
6. Remove all racks and dilution trays from the agitated (inner) and nonagitated (outer) load station rotors.
7. Clean all positions of the agitated (inner) and nonagitated (outer) load station rotors. Touch help for cleaning solution.
8. Close the load station door.
9. Open the maintenance door.
10. Remove both centrifuge covers.
11. Clean all surfaces of both centrifuges. Touch help for cleaning solution.
12. Install both of the centrifuge covers.

13. Clean all surfaces of the incubator and the probe adjustment position located between the incubator and the load station.
14. Clean the probe adjustment position.
15. Close the maintenance door.
16. Starting task
17. Open the load station door.
18. Load an empty NAA reagent rack (labeled NO1B).
19. *Sample Reagent Diluent Rotor (SRDR)*: The load station will move to the reagent rack load position.
20. SRDR 1—Load an empty 10 mL reagent rack (Labeled R10b) and close the load station door.
21. Instrument will now read the barcodes of both the loaded racks and once completed successfully, dialogue "The test completed successfully" will be displayed on instrument.
22. Open load station.
23. Unload the empty NAA reagent rack.
24. SRDR 1—The load station will move to the reagent rack load position.
25. Unload the empty reagent rack and close the load station door.
26. Now, monthly maintenance is done.
27. Then do the weekly and daily maintenance and resume processing.

Note: For yearly maintenance, contact the manufacturer.

65

Maintenance of VITROS ECiQ Immunodiagnostic Assay System

SCOPE AND APPLICATION

To maintain VITROS ECiQ Immunodiagnostic Assay System for effective testing of serum/plasma for various analytes.

RESPONSIBILITY

It is the responsibility of the technical supervisor to operate VITROS ECiQ Immunodiagnostic Assay (chemiluminescence) System.

EQUIPMENT AND MATERIALS REQUIRED

- *Equipment*:
  - VITROS ECiQ Immunodiagnostic Assay System
- *Materials required*:
  - Human serum/plasma
  - VITROS ECiQ Reagent pack for various analytes, calibrators, and controls
  - VITROS ECiQ Signal Reagent
  - VITROS ECiQ Universal Wash Reagent

PROCEDURE

Daily Maintenance

1. Open the left and right front doors of the VITROS ECiQ System.
2. Remove the solid waste container and discard the solid waste, namely used tips and wells.
3. Place back the solid waste container.
4. Move the toggle switch to the "Off" position to release the pressure and vacuum.
5. Pull the liquid supply tray out.

6. Disconnect the tubes from the liquid waste container.
7. Remove the liquid waste container from the tray. Remove the cap and discard the liquid waste.
8. Clean the bottle with tap water and close the bottle with the cap.
9. Disconnect the tubes from the universal wash reagent bottle.
10. Remove the universal wash reagent bottle from the tray. Remove the cap from the bottle.
11. Replace the universal wash reagent bottle if necessary and close with the cap removed in the earlier step.
12. Clean the liquid supply tray by wiping with a soft lint-free cloth moistened with warm soapy water.
13. Wipe the liquid supply tray with a soft lint-free cloth moistened with warm water to remove any soap residue.
14. Clean the tray surface with 70% isopropyl alcohol in water solution.
15. Allow the liquid supply tray to air dry thoroughly.
16. Place back the liquid water container into position on the tray and connect tubes to the container.
17. Place back the universal wash reagent bottle into position on the tray and connect tubes to the bottle.
18. Push the tray back into the cabinet.
19. Move the toggle switch to the "On" position to apply pressure and vacuum to the system. It may take about 5 minutes to update the system with the required pressure and vacuum.
20. Close both the front doors.
21. Unload the empty reagent packs, if any, by selecting the reagent pack in the "Reagent Management" screen and then touch unload icon.
22. Unload the empty signal reagent packs and discard the same.
23. Lift the sample supply cover from the sample supply subsystem and set it aside.
24. Inspect the universal sample trays and microcollection container adapters.
25. Remove and discard any remaining samples already processed.
26. Open the top cover of the system.
27. Move the signal reagent probe assembly away from the incubator by grasping the horizontal arm of the signal reagent probe assembly and lift the arm to its topmost position and swing the arm in a counterclockwise direction until it is no longer over the incubator.
28. Inspect and clean the signal reagent probes using a soft lint-free cloth or tissue paper moistened with distilled water to wipe away any crystals formed over there in the probe tip.
29. Swing the signal reagent probe assembly clockwise until the assembly is back into position over the incubator.

30. Close the top cover of the system.
31. Touch "Return" button on the screen to return to the main menu and initialize the system.
32. Allow the system to return to READY status on the status console.
33. Verify the reagent inventory and signal reagent inventory and load the required reagents.
34. Process the quality control (QC) samples as per the requirement.

Weekly Maintenance

1. *Cleaning the sample metering proboscis*:
   - Open the sample metering safety shield in a counterclockwise direction or open the top cover of the system.
   - Wipe the outside of the sample metering proboscis with a lint-free cloth moistened with distilled water.
   - Dry the proboscis with a dry lint-free cloth.
   - If necessary, clean the proboscis with 70% isopropyl alcohol in water solution and allow to air dry thoroughly.
2. *Cleaning the tip-disposal chute/cup retainer*:
   - Remove the tip-disposal chute/cup retainer by pulling up on the three black fasteners and lifting the tip-disposal chute/cup retainer out of the system.
   - Wash the chute/cup retainer with warm soapy water.
   - Rinse the chute/cup retainer with warm water to remove any soap residue.
   - Clean the chute/cup retainer with 70% isopropyl alcohol in water solution, if necessary.
   - Allow the tip disposal chute/cup retainer to air dry thoroughly.
   - Install the tip disposal chute/cup retainer by placing it in position and pushing down on the three black fasteners.
3. *Cleaning the sample supply subsystem*:
   - Remove all the universal sample trays from the sample supply.
   - Pull up on the two black fasteners to release the retainer plate.
   - Remove the retainer plate and tray transport carriers from the sample supply subsystem and set them aside.
   - Wipe the inside surfaces of the sample supply area, sample barcode reader, retainer plate, transport carriers, universal sample trays, and sample supply cover with a soft lint-free cloth moistened with warm, soapy water and then wipe with a lint-free cloth moistened with warm water to remove any soap residue.
   - Clean the surfaces with 70% isopropyl alcohol in water solution and air dry thoroughly.
   - Assemble the sample supply subsystem by placing the tray transport carriers and retainer plate in position and pushing down on the two black fasteners. Load universal sample trays.

4. *Cleaning the touchscreen monitor and keyboard*:
   - Touch an area of the touchscreen without any buttons and continue touching.
   - Wipe the touchscreen monitor and touchscreen frame with a soft lint-free cloth moistened with warm, soapy water and then wipe with a lint-free cloth moistened with warm water to remove any soap residue.
   - Clean the surfaces with 70% isopropyl alcohol in water solution and air dry thoroughly.
   - Wipe the keyboard with a lint-free cloth moistened with warm, soapy water and then wipe with a lint-free cloth moistened with warm water to remove any soap residue.
   - Clean the surfaces with 70% isopropyl alcohol in water solution and air dry thoroughly.

5. *Cleaning the subsystem*:
   - Scan the maintenance lot card through the magnetic card scanner (only for the first time).
   - Load the maintenance pack in the autoload station and check the inventory status. The inventory should be above 20 wells to do the subsystem cleaning.
   - Touch periodic maintenance—weekly maintenance icon to display the subsystem cleaning screen.
   - Touch "Start" icon. Progress of the cleaning is displayed on the status line, counting down from step 10 to step 1 as each cleaning step is completed.
   - When the status message indicates that subsystem cleaning is complete, return to the main menu.
   - Touch "Reagent Management" icon and unload the maintenance pack. The maintenance pack should not be left in the system after the subsystem.
   - Cleaning procedure is completed.

6. *Clean the processing center*:
   - Touch "Diagnostics" icon on the main menu.
   - Touch MEDs on the Diagnostics screen.
   - Lift the sample supply cover from the sample supply subsystem and open the top cover of the system.
   - Move the signal reagent probe assembly and the well wash probe assembly away from the incubator as mentioned below:
     - Grasp the horizontal arm of the signal reagent probe assembly and lift the arm to its topmost position and swing the arm in a counterclockwise direction until it is no longer over the incubator.
     - Grasp the horizontal arm of the well wash probe assembly and lift the well wash arm to its topmost position and swing

the arm in a counterclockwise direction until it is no longer over the incubator.

- Clean the signal reagent and well wash prime/purge stations located on the top of the incubator cover by wiping any debris or moisture with a soft lint-free cloth moistened with distilled water.
- *Move the luminometer to an upright position as mentioned below*:
  - Push down on the luminometer release lever and rotate the latch clockwise.
  - Using both hands, move the luminometer up in a clockwise direction until it is in an upright position.
- Open the incubator by swinging the front edge of the cover toward the back of the system until the cover is upright.
- *Clean the incubator evaporation cover as follows*:
  - Clean all edges and openings including the retention screw openings, where fluid and debris may collect, using a swab moistened with distilled water to remove any residue.
  - Clean all areas using a dry swab.
  - Clean all areas using a swab moistened with 70% isopropyl alcohol in water solution to facilitate drying.
- Clean the bottom side of the evaporation cover including the inner and outer edges using a lint-free cloth moistened with distilled water followed by a dry lint-free cloth and then using a lint-free cloth moistened with 70% isopropyl alcohol in water solution to facilitate drying.
- *Clean the incubator rings as follows*:
  - Push the two gear wheels away from the incubator rings to release the rings.
  - Touch MEDs in the Diagnostics screen.
  - Touch Incubator in the MEDs screen.
  - Touch "Shuttle" in the Incubator screen.
  - Touch "Move" and then touch "Home" followed by "Start" icon in the Incubator screen.
  - The shuttle will be moved toward the center of the incubator.
  - Remove the incubator rings—first, lift the outer ring up and out of the system and set it in a safe place. Then, lift the inner ring up and out of the system and set it aside in a safe place.
  - Flush each ring thoroughly with warm tap water. Be sure that all openings are thoroughly rinsed.
  - If necessary, use a soft plastic bristle brush to remove any residual material.
  - Wipe off excess water from each ring with a lint-free cloth.
  - Rinse each ring thoroughly with 70% isopropyl alcohol in water solution.

- Wipe off excess isopropyl alcohol from each ring with a lint-free cloth.
- Set aside each ring to dry thoroughly.
- *Clean the well shuttle weight and recess as follows*:
  - Touch MEDs in the Diagnostics screen.
  - Touch Incubator in the MEDs screen.
  - Touch "Shuttle" in the Incubator screen.
  - Touch "Move" and then touch "Reference Read" followed by "Start" icon in the Incubator screen.
  - The shuttle will be moved from the center of the incubator to the end of travel.
  - Remove the shuttle weight using a dry swab by inserting the same into the center of the well shuttle weight and recess and lift the shuttle weight from the recess.
  - Clean the inner and outer surfaces of the shuttle weight using a swab moistened with distilled water, followed by a dry swab and by using a swab moistened with 70% isopropyl alcohol to remove any residual fibers.
  - Clean the shuttle weight recess using the same method for cleaning as the shuttle weight.
  - Clean the underside of the shuttle using the same method using a lint-free cloth moistened with distilled water followed by dry cloth and then by a lint-free cloth moistened with 70% isopropyl alcohol.
  - Allow shuttle weight, shuttle weight recess, and the underside of the shuttle to dry thoroughly before reassembly.
  - Gently place the shuttle weight back into the shuttle weight recess. Do not place the shuttle weight into the recess upside down.
  - Touch MEDs in the Diagnostics screen.
  - Touch Incubator in the MEDs screen.
  - Touch "Shuttle" in the Incubator screen.
  - Touch "Move" and then touch "Home" followed by "Start" icon in the Incubator screen.
  - The shuttle moves toward the center of the incubator.
- *Clean the lift pins as follows*:
  - Touch MEDs in the Diagnostics screen.
  - Touch Incubator in the MEDs screen.
  - Touch "Inner lift pin" in the Incubator screen.
  - Touch "Move" followed by "Read" position and then "Start" icon.
  - Touch "Outer lift pin" in the Incubator screen.
  - Touch "Up" and "Start" icons.

- Clean both the lift pins with a lint-free cloth moistened with distilled water followed by dry cloth and then by a lint-free cloth moistened with 70% isopropyl alcohol.
- Make sure that the white screw head on the inner lift pin should not be loose.
- Allow the lift pins to air dry thoroughly and then lower the lift pins.
- Touch "Inner lift pin" in the Incubator screen.
- Touch "Move" followed by "Home" position and then "Start" icon.
- Touch "Outer lift pin" in the Incubator screen.
- Touch "Down" and "Start" icons.
- *Clean the incubator heater plate as follows*:
  - Clean the incubator housing using a dry swab to remove any foreign material.
  - Clean the heater plate with a lint-free cloth moistened with distilled water followed by dry cloth and then by a lint-free cloth moistened with 70% isopropyl alcohol.
  - Allow the heater plate to air dry thoroughly.
- *Reassemble the incubator rings as follows*:
  - Place the inner ring into position in the incubator.
  - Place the outer ring into position in the incubator.
  - Push the gear wheel below the inner ring toward the front of the system and pull up on the silver knob that engages the gear wheel with the inner ring, and allow to reengage the inner ring.
  - Push the gear wheel above the outer ring toward the back of the system, pull up on the silver knob to release the gear and allow it to reengage the outer ring.
  - Close the incubator cover.
  - Clean the fiber optic bundle in the luminometer with a lint-free dry cloth.
  - Move the luminometer back into position over the incubator.
  - Push down on the luminometer release lever to secure the luminometer.
  - Clean the wash reagent probe with a lint-free cloth moistened with distilled water to remove any debris or crystals. Make sure that the sensor on the tip of the wash reagent probe should not get damaged.
  - Swing the well wash probe assembly clockwise until each probe assembly is back into position over the incubator.
- Clean the signal reagent probe with a lint-free cloth moistened with distilled water to wipe away any crystals formed over there in the probe tip. Make sure that the sensor on the tip of the wash reagent probe should not get damaged.

- Swing the well wash probe assembly clockwise until each probe assembly is back into position over the incubator.
- Clean the signal reagent probe with a lint-free cloth moistened with distilled water to wipe away any crystals formed over there in the probe tip.
- Swing the signal reagent probe assembly clockwise until the assembly is back into position over the incubator.
- Clean the reagent metering probe wash station with a lint-free cloth moistened with distilled water to wipe away any crystals formed over there.
- Clean the reagent metering probe tip by bringing down the probe by rotating the knob in the reagent metering assembly, using a lint-free cloth moistened with distilled water followed by a dry lint-free cloth and cloth moistened with 70% isopropyl alcohol.
- Allow the probe to air dry thoroughly and move the probe up by rotating the knob in the opposite direction.
- Empty the container which collects the unused wells.
- Open the door on the left side of the system.
- Look for signs of dust or dirt on the exposed surface of the filter.
- If the filter is dirty, remove and install a new dry filter and send the dirty one for cleaning.
- Close the side door of the system.
- Close the top cover of the system.
- Replace the sample supply cover.
- Touch "Return" button to return to the main menu and initialize the system.
- Allow the system to return to READY status on the status console.
- Do Incubator Reference System (IRS) calibration as follows:
  - Touch "Diagnostics" in the main menu.
  - Touch "Calibrate Subsystem" in the Diagnostics screen.
  - Touch "Luminometer" in the screen.
  - Touch "IRS Calibration."
  - Touch "Start." It will take about 5 minutes to do the IRS calibration.
  - After successful calibration, touch "Return" to return to the main menu.
  - Allow the system to return to READY status on the status console before continuing with sample processing.

The maintenance log is maintained as per **Annexure 65.1**.

ANNEXURE 65.1

Maintenance log ECiQ Immunodiagnostic System

Maintenance Log	System J Number															System Serial Number															
Month/Year	Day																														
Daily—Check (√) Box	1	2	3	4	5	6	7	8	9	10	11	12	13	14	15	16	17	18	19	20	21	22	23	24	25	26	27	28	29	30	31
Empty:																															
• Solid waste container*																															
• Liquid waste bottle*																															
Remove outdated and empty:																															
• Reagent packs and SR packs																															
• Universal wash reagents																															
Clean the reagent probe assembly																															
Inspect:																															
• Universal samples trays																															
• Micro-collection container adapters																															
Verify inventory and load:																															
• Reagent packs and SR packs																															
• Universal wash reagents																															
Verify that QC fluids have been processed																															
Operator's initials																															

Continued

Continued

Weekly—Date/Initial Boxes	WEEK 1	WEEK 2	WEEK 3	WEEK 4	WEEK 5	Monthly—Date/Initial Boxes	Date	Initials
Clean the sample metering proboscis						Back up QC, calibration and configuration files		
Clean the tip disposal chute/cup retainer						Inspect the reagent cooler filter		
Clean the sample supply subsystem						Every 2 months: Change the vapour adsorption cartridge		
Clean the touchscreen monitor						Every 3 months: Change the universal wash reservoir filter		
Clean the keyboard and keyboard cover						As required—Date/Initial Boxes	Date	Initials
Perform subsystem cleaning						Clean the system cabinetry		
Clean the processing center								
Operator's Initials								

*May require emptying more frequently depending on usage.

Reviewed By:.. Date:.................... Version:....................

66

Use and Maintenance of Laminar Airflow Workstation

SCOPE AND APPLICATION

This standard operating procedure (SOP) describes the use and maintenance of horizontal laminar airflow (LAF) workstation which provides sterile and safe working environment for the preparation of blood components by minimizing/eliminating the introduction of particulate matter, microorganisms, and other contaminants. In horizontal LAF workstations, room air is drawn into work area through a high-efficiency particulate air (HEPA) filter mounted on the back side of the cabinet. Filtered air flows horizontally to the user, creating sterile working environment.

RESPONSIBILITY

It is the responsibility of the blood center technician working in the component area to ensure that the horizontal LAF workstation is appropriately cleaned and maintained in a good working order.

MATERIALS REQUIRED

- Horizontal LAF workstation
- Lint cloth
- Disinfectant solution (70% isopropyl alcohol)

PROCEDURE

Cleaning

- Clean the outer surface and working table of LAF workstation with a lint-free cloth moistened with 70% isopropyl alcohol.

- Clean the working table of LAF workstation before and after every operation.
- Clean the outer surface of LAF workstation.

Operation

- Make sure the area is clean and free of previous products and other materials associated with previous products.
- Make sure the instrument is set up clean and dusted so that dust in the air does not affect the positive pressure when the airlock door is open. Turn the power "ON."
- Make sure that the manometer reads zero reading before starting.
- There is a side panel for three switches of instruments and a pressure barometer.
  - Switch (1) AIR-FLOW
  - Switch (2) LIGHTS
  - Switch (3) ultraviolet (UV) light
- Press "switch (1)" to start AIR-FLOW through the HEPA filter and press "switch (2)" to turn the fluorescent lamp "ON."
- The AIR-FLOW should be left "ON" for approximately 5 minutes before using LAF workstation.
- When AIR-FLOW is "ON," check the manometer/pressure gauge pressure and it should be >0.5 inches of water/15 mm Wc (millimeter water column).
- Always "turn (3)" to "ON" 15–20 minutes before and after using the LAF workstation.
- A UV lamp sterilizes the work area before use.
- Perform the activities.
- *Please note that the fluorescent and UV lights are not ON at the same time.*
- Turn "OFF" the instrument when not in use.

PRECAUTIONS

- Check the manometer calibration status.
- Do not turn ON the UV light during the processing time.
- Turn on the "AIR-FLOW" on the LAF workstation for approximately 15 minutes before working under laminar flow.
- If the manometer reading is less than or more than 0.5 inches of water, contact the manufacturer or engineering department immediately.
- In the event of spill, stop work if possible and switch off the blower motor. Follow the standard spill management guidelines to clean and disinfect the workstation surface.

MAINTENANCE

- Check the condition of the instrument and power cord/plug for safe operation.
- Keep the instrument clean. *Do not use alcohol* or *organic solvents on PLEXIGLAS.*
- UV lamp replacement frequency is after 700 burn hours and UV lamp usage records are maintained in accordance with **Annexure 66.1**.
- If the exit velocity cannot be maintained at 90 ± 20 feet per minute (FPM), the HEPA filter should be replaced. Below this exit velocity, the airflow is no longer unidirectional and the area within the hood cannot be safely kept sterile.
- Vendor annual plan certification and regular maintenance should be adhered to. (As the actual time of hood use is low, the manufacturer's annual filter check should cover all recommended service intervals.)
- Certification is documented by labeling the equipment with the certification date and certification expiration date.
- Additional maintenance/service must be performed by the authorized personnel and the unit must be recertified in writing.

Laminar airflow efficiency can be checked periodically after installation using one of the following methods:

- HEPA filter integrity test
- Particle count test
- Air velocity measurement test
- Smoke profile test (video shooting/photography to be arranged by customer)

Smoke test: Smoke tests are performed to demonstrate proper and effective unidirectional airflow. Smoke is produced using a portable glycol-based smoke generator (nebulizer). During the airflow smoke test, the airflow flows inward along the entire perimeter of the work access area. Smoke flows down the housing without dead spots or backflow. No airflow escapes the cabinet and does not swell or invade the work surface.

The calculated average intake air velocity should be between 100 and 130 FPM or 30 and 40 ft/min.

ANNEXURE 66.1

Date	Manometer reading/ Magnetic gauge mm (7.0–15.0)	UV light usage hours	Start time	Off time	Remarks	Used by	Checked by

CHAPTER 67

Documentation and Record Keeping in Blood Centers

DOCUMENT

All written procedures, instructions, records, quality control procedures, and recorded test results related to the manufacture of products or the provision of services are referred to as documentation. The documentation contains explanations or instructions about what should happen. They are active and can only be changed by authorized personnel.

Documents are approved and can be in written or electronic form. They define a quality system for external inspectors and internal staff. Examples include written policies, process descriptions, standard operating procedures (SOPs), forms, computer software, manufacturer inserts, instruction manuals, process descriptions, flowcharts, and copies of regulations and standards.

RECORD

A record indicates that an activity was performed or a result was achieved. Records are evidence of work been done in the past and are dead, fixed, and cannot be changed. Examples include worksheets, instrument printouts, tags, labels, or other written or electronic media that record the results or results of activities and tests.

Unfilled blood requisition form is a document but the filled blood requisition form is a record.

Documentation is the process of preparing documents which provide proof or evidence of something or are a record of something.

AIMS OF DOCUMENTATION

- To provide evidence that specified standards have been followed in donor selection, blood collection, serological testing, transfusion transmissible infection (TTI) testing, blood component preparation, and issue of blood/blood components

- Availability of donor traceability records for any evidence of error and the staff involved
- Ensuring consistency and reliability at every stage of blood transfusion service
- To provide evidence for the investigation in event of adverse reactions or complaints

DOCUMENT CONTROL

Document control refers to documents and records that can only be used at a specific facility and cannot be reproduced elsewhere. This is integral to the quality management system and proper document control processes should be implemented to define the controls required to approve, review, update, identify changes, identify revision status, and grant access. The document management process should clearly define the scope, purpose, methods, and responsibilities required to implement these parameters.

Each document should have a unique numbering system that combines the section/organization code, document control, and document serial number according to the sample format shown in **Table 1**.

The procedure for document control shall ensure the following:

- Documents are approved by authorized personnel before issue.
- Documents include a unique identifier, a review date, revision version, total page count, and authorized signatories.
- Invalid or expired documents will be revoked.
- Documentation should be readable, easily identifiable, and searchable.
- Documentation is reviewed regularly and updated as necessary.
- Handwritten changes to existing documents are clearly defined.
- Where applicable, only the latest version of the documentation is available.
- All records and registers must be maintained for 5 years.

Table 1: Unique numbering system.		
Document level	**Document type**	**Numbering plan**
1	Quality manual	BC/QM
2	Standard operating procedure	BC/SOP/WW/xx
3	Forms and formats	BC/FM/WW/xx

- No unauthorized person should have access to the confidential information that is contained in the records.
- Records should ideally be destroyed after 5 years or according to SOP by shredding according to procedures/SOPs approved by the facility's document disposal committee.

Records Required to be Maintained as per Schedule F of the Drugs and Cosmetics Rules 1945

- *Blood donor record*: It shall indicate serial number, date of bleeding, name, address and signature of donor with other particulars of age, weight, hemoglobin, blood grouping, blood pressure, medical examination, bag number, and patient's detail for whom donated in case of replacement donation, category of donation (voluntary/replacement) and deferral records and signature of medical officer in charge. Specimen format is given in **Annexure 67.1**.
- *Master records for blood and its components*: It shall indicate bag serial number, date of collection, date of expiry, quantity in milliliter, ABO/Rh group, results for testing of human immunodeficiency virus I (HIV I) and HIV II antibodies, malaria, venereal disease research laboratory (VDRL), hepatitis B surface antigen and hepatitis C virus antibody and irregular antibodies (if any), name and address of the donor with particulars, utilization issue number, components prepared or discarded, and signature of the medical officer in charge. A specimen format is given in **Annexure 67.2**.
- *Issue register*: It shall indicate serial number, date and time of issue, bag serial number, ABO/Rh group, total quantity in milliliter, name and address of the recipient, group of recipients, unit/institution, details of crossmatching report, and indication for transfusion. A specimen format is given in **Annexure 67.3**.
- *Records of components supplied*: Quantity supplied; compatibility report, details of recipient, and signature of the issuing person

  Note: The record of components supplied has been merged in **Annexure 67.3** for convenience.

- Records of acid-citrate-dextrose (ACD)/citrate-phosphate-dextrose (CPD)/citrate-phosphate-dextrose-adenine (CPDA)/saline-adenine-glucose-mannitol (SAGM)/any other approved anticoagulant and preservative bags giving details of manufacturer, batch number, date of supply, and results of testing, mfg./exp. dates. The format is given in **Annexure 67.4**.
- *Register for diagnostic kits and reagents used*: Name of the kits/reagents, details of batch number, and manufacturer's name, date of expiry, and date of use. A sample format is given in **Annexure 67.5**.

- *Crossmatching/compatibility report*: The blood center should issue the crossmatching report of the blood/components to the patient together with the blood/component unit.
- Blood transfusion record/adverse transfusion reaction record: Specimen format is given in **Annexure 47.2**.
- Records of purchase, use and stock in hand of disposable needles, syringes, blood bags, and diagnostics reagents shall be maintained.

Other Records

- Component preparation records (if applicable). A sample format is given in **Annexure 67.6**.
- Crossmatch Register **Annexure 67.7**.
- Blood/blood components discard record register and autoclaving log sheet. Sample formats are given in **Annexure 67.8** and **Annexure 73.1**, respectively.
- Daily stock register/record (group-wise) showing collection, processing, issue, and balance of whole blood/PRBC/FFP/RDP units. Sample formats are given in **Annexures 67.9 to 67.11**.
- Quality control record. Sample formats are given in **Annexures 67.12 to 67.17**.
- Record of external quality control
- Stock register of consumable articles
- Stock register of nonconsumable articles
- Record of equipment maintenance
- Record of document control
- Records of communication with the State Blood Transfusion Council
- Records of communication with State Licensing Authority/CLAA, etc.
- Hemovigilance reporting records
- Staff attendance register or any other recording system
- Documentation of staff qualifications and training
- Documentation of staff competency and proficiency tests
- Grievance redressal reporting register
- Personnel health records

ANNEXURE 67.1

Blood Donor Register

Logo

Name of Blood Centre:

S. No.	Date of Bleeding	Name and Address of Donor	Sign. of Donor	Age	Weight	Hb g/dL	Blood Grouping	BP	Med. Exam.	Blood Unit No.	Blood Bag Segment No.	Patient Detail for Whom Donated (in case of Replacement)	Category of Donation (V/R)	Deferral Records	Sign. of Medical Officer In-Charge

ANNEXURE 67.2

Blood/Blood Components Master Record Register

Name of Blood Centre:

License No.:

S. No.	Unit No.	Volume	Segment No.	Date of Collection	Name and Address of Donor	Age/Sex	Type of Donor	ABO/Rh	HIV I and II	HBsAg	HCV	VDRL	MP	Irregular Antibodies
0001														
0002														

Continued

Continued

Logo

S. No	Blood/Blood Components	Date of Expiry	Qty in mL	Utilization No.	Date of Issue	Name of Recipient	MR No./ IP No.	ABO/Rh	X-Match Detail	Ward/ Bed No	Diagnosis	Reason for Discard	Signature of Technologist	Signature of Medical Officer	Remarks
0001	Whole Blood														
	PRBCs														
	FFP														
	Random platelet														
	SDP														
	CRYO Poor Plasma														
	Cryoprecipitate														
0002	Whole Blood														
	PRBCs														
	FFP														
	Random platelet														
	SDP														
	CRYO Poor Plasma														
	Cryoprecipitate														

Continued

Continued

0003		0004	

Continued

Continued

	Whole Blood	PRBCs	FFP	Random platelet	SDP	CRYO Poor Plasma	Cryoprecipitate
0003							

	Whole Blood	PRBCs	FFP	Random platelet	SDP	CRYO Poor Plasma	Cryoprecipitate
0004							

ANNEXURE 67.3

Issue Register

(Blood and Blood Components)

Logo

Name of Blood Center:

License No.: PAGE NO.: ....

S. No.	Date of Issue	Time of Issue	Unit No.	ABO/ Rh	Segment No.	Blood Component	Total Qty. (Vol.)	Patient's Name	MR No/ IPD No.	Blood Group	Name of Hospital Ward/Bed No.	Consultant In-Charge	Indication for Transfusion	Crossmatch Report	Sign of Issuing Person	Received by

ANNEXURE 67.4

Crossmatching Register

Logo

Name of Blood Center:

License No.:

PAGE NO: ....

Req. No.	Patient's Name	MR No./ IPD No.	ABO/ Rh	Patient ABS III Cells Panel Screening	Blood Component	Unit No.	Blood Group	Segment No.	DOE	Crossmatch Technique	Crossmatch Report	Signature of Technician and ID No.	Remarks

ANNEXURE 67.5

Record for CPDA Bags

Logo

Name and Address of Blood Center:

License No:

PAGE NO: ....

S. No.	Date of Receipt	Name of Supplier/ Manufacturer	Invoice No. and Date	Batch No.	Date of Expiry	Quantity Receipt	COA of Manufacturer No. and Date	Date of Issue	Quantity Issue	Balance	Signature of MO I/C

ANNEXURE 67.6

Register for Diagnostic Kits and Reagents

Logo

Name of Blood Center:

License No:

PAGE NO: ....

S. No.	Date of Receipt	Name of Supplier/ Manufacturer	Invoice No. and Date	Batch No.	Date of Expiry	Quantity Received	Date of Issue	Quantity Issued	Balance	Sign of MO (I/C)

ANNEXURE 67.7

Blood Component Preparation Record

Name of Blood Center:

License No:

Logo

PAGE NO: ....

S. No.	Date of Collection	Unit No.	Type of Blood Bag Used	Whole Blood Volume	Blood Group	Leukoreduced PRBCS		PRBCs			FFP			RDP			CRYO-PPT			CPP			TOC	TOP	TOS	Prepared by	Remarks
						VOL. (mL)	Expiry	VOL. (mL)	Expiry		VOL. (mL)	Expiry		VOL. (mL)	Expiry		VOL. (mL)	Expiry		VOL. (mL)	Expiry						

*TOC: Time of Collection, ***TOP:** Time of Preparation, ***TOS:** Time of Storage

*WB: Whole Blood, ***PRBCs:** Packed Red Blood Cells, ***FFP:** Fresh Frozen Plasma,

*RDP: Random Donor Platelet, ***CRYO-PPT:** Cryoprecipitate, ***CPP:** Cryo Poor Plasma

Signature of Technical Supervisor: _____

Signature of Medical Officer: _____

ANNEXURE 67.8

Blood/Blood Components Discard Record Register

Name of Blood Center:

License No:

Logo

S. No.	Date	Unit No.	DOC	DOE	Segment No.	Blood Group	Blood/Blood Component	Reason for Discard	Signature of Technician	Signature of Technical Supervisor	Signature of Medical Officer

ANNEXURE 67.9

Daily Stock of PRBC/Whole Blood

Name of Blood Center:

License No:

Logo

Date.............

S. No.	"A" Positive				"B" Positive				"O" Positive				"AB" Positive			
	Whole Blood		PRBC		Whole Blood		PRBC		Whole Blood		PRBC		Whole Blood		PRBC	
	Unit No.	DOE	Unit No.	DOE	Unit No.	DOE	Unit No.	DOE	Unit No.	DOE	Unit No.	DOE	Unit No.	DOE	Unit No.	DOE
1																
2																
3																
4																
5																
6																
7																
8																
9																
10																
11																
12																

Continued

Continued

13																				
14																				
15																				
16																				
17																				
18																				
19																				
20																				
21																				
22																				
23																				
24																				
25																				
26																				
27																				
28																				
29																				
30																				
Total																				

S. No.	"A" Positive Whole Blood Unit No.	"A" Positive Whole Blood DOE	"A" Positive PRBC Unit No.	"A" Positive PRBC DOE	"B" Positive Whole Blood Unit No.	"B" Positive Whole Blood DOE	"B" Positive PRBC Unit No.	"B" Positive PRBC DOE	"O" Positive Whole Blood Unit No.	"O" Positive Whole Blood DOE	"O" Positive PRBC Unit No.	"O" Positive PRBC DOE	"AB" Positive Whole Blood Unit No.	"AB" Positive Whole Blood DOE	"AB" Positive PRBC Unit No.	"AB" Positive PRBC DOE
1																
2																
3																
4																
5																
6																
7																
8																
9																
10																
Total																

Daily Blood Stock Inventory of Whole Blood/PRBC

a	b	c	d	e	f	g	h
BALANCE	Whole Blood	Whole Blood	PRBCs	Total Stock	PRBC/whole	PRBC/whole	PRBC/whole

ANNEXURE 67.10

Daily Stock of Fresh Frozen Plasma (FFP)

Name of Blood Center: **Logo**

License No:

	"A" Positive		"B" Positive		"O" Positive		"AB" Positive	
	FFP		FFP		FFP		FFP	
S. No.	Unit No.	DOE	Unit No.	DOE	Unit No.	DOE	Unit No.	DOE
1								
2								
3								
4								
5								
6								
7								
8								
9								
10								
11								
12								
13								
14								
15								
16								
17								
18								
19								
20								
21								
22								
23								
24								
25								
26								

Continued

Continued

27									
28									
29									
30									
Total									

	"A" Positive		"B" Positive		"O" Positive		"AB" Positive	
	FFP		FFP		FFP		FFP	
S. No.	**Unit No.**	**DOE**	**Unit No.**	**DOE**	**Unit No.**	**DOE**	**Unit No.**	**DOE**
1								
2								
3								
4								
5								
6								
7								
8								
9								
10								
Total								

Daily Blood Stock Inventory of Fresh Frozen Plasma

a	b	c	g	
Balance (FFP)	FFP Prepared	FFP Discard	FFP Issued	Total

ANNEXURE 67.11

Daily Stock of Random Donor Platelet (RDP)

Name of Blood Center: **Logo**

License No:

S. No.	"A" Positive RDP Unit No.	DOE	"B" Positive RDP Unit No.	DOE	"O" Positive RDP Unit No.	DOE	"AB" Positive RDP Unit No.	DOE
1								
2								
3								
4								
5								
6								
7								
8								
9								
10								
11								
12								
13								
14								
15								
16								
17								
18								
19								
20								
21								
22								
23								
24								
25								
26								

Continued

Continued

27								
28								
29								
30								
Total								

	"A" Positive		"B" Positive		"O" Positive		"AB" Positive	
	FFP		FFP		FFP		FFP	
S. No.	**Unit No.**	**DOE**	**Unit No.**	**DOE**	**Unit No.**	**DOE**	**Unit No.**	**DOE**
1								
2								
3								
4								
5								
6								
7								
8								
9								
10								
Total								

Daily Blood Stock Inventory of Random Donor Platelet

a	b	c	g	
Balance (FFP)	FFP Prepared	RDP Discard	RDP Issued	Total

ANNEXURE 67.12

Logo

Quality Control for PRBC

Name of Blood Center:

License No:

S. No.	Unit No.	DOC	DOE	DO Test	Volume	HCT	WBC Observed value	Total Leukocytes/ Bag Accepted criteria	Viral Markers — All Nonreactive/Negative HBsAg	HCV	HIV	VDRL	HBc	MP	Sterility Testing Sterile	Remarks
					250 ± 10% mL + 100 mL SAGM (for 450 mL bag) 150 ± 10% mL + 100 mL SAGM (for 350 mL bag)	50–60%		<5x10⁶/Bag							Blood Culture	

ANNEXURE 67.13

Logo

Quality Control for Platelet (RDP)

Name of Blood Center:

License No:

S. No.	Unit No.	DOC	DOE	DO Test	PLT Count $\times 10^3$	HCT %	WBC Count $\times 10^3$	Volume	pH	PLT Yield	RBC Yield	WBC Yield
										Accepted criteria		
								60–80 mL	≥6.0 at the end of 5 days storage	>5.5 × 10¹⁰/ Bag	TRACES- 0.5 mL/ Bag	<0.12 × 10⁹/ Bag
1												
2												
3												
4												
5												
6												
7												
8												
9												
10												
11												
12												

Continued

Continued

13	14	15	16	17	18	19	20	21	22	23	24	25	26	27	28	29	30	31	32	33	34

Continued

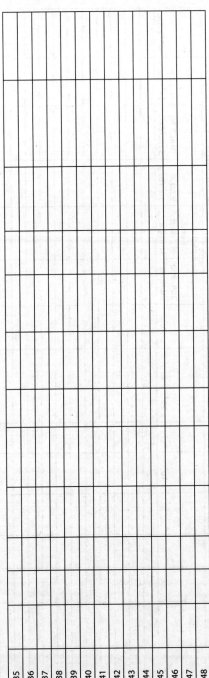

Continued

35
36
37
38
39
40
41
42
43
44
45
46
47
48

ANNEXURE 67.14

Quality Control for SDP

Logo

Name of Blood Center:

License No:

S. No.	Unit No.	DOC	DOE	DO Test	Platelet Post-Count	HCT	WBC Count	Donor Pre Count	Target PLT Yield	Unit Vol.	pH	PLT Yield	RBC Yield	WBC Yield	Cell Separator Make
					$\times 10^3$	%	$\times 10^3$	$\times 10^3$	$\times 10^{11}$	200–300 mL/BAG	≥ 6.0 at the end of 5 days storage	$\geq 3.0 \times 10^{11}$/Bag	TRACE TO 5 mL/BAG	$<0.12 \times 10^9$/Bag	MACHINE

Accepted criteria

ANNEXURE 67.15

Quality Control for Fresh Frozen Plasma (FFP)

Name of Blood Center: Logo

License No:

								Stable Coagulation Factor		
S. No.	Unit No.	Date of Collection	Date of Expiry	Date of Test	Vol of FFP (mL)	PT (in sec)	aPTT (in sec)	Fibrinogen 200–400 mg/dL	Factor VIII 60–150%	
								Accepted criteria		
					180–300 mL			Atleast 150 mg/ Bag	Atleast 70 iu/ Bag	Remarks
								Observed Value mg/dL	Observed value iu/Bag	
1										
2										
3										
4										
5										
6										
7										
8										
9										
10										
11										
12										
13										
14										
15										
16										
17										
18										
19										
20										
21										
22										

Continued

Continued

23									
24									
25									
26									
27									
28									
29									
30									
31									
32									
33									
34									
35									
36									
37									
38									
39									
40									
41									
42									
43									
44									
45									

ANNEXURE 67.16

Quality Control for Cryoprecipitate

Name of Blood Center: **Logo**

License No:

S. No.	Unit No.	Date of Collection	Date of Expiry	Date of Test	Vol. of Cryo (mL)	FACTOR VIII	
						Accepted criteria	
						Atleast 80 iu/Bag	
					15–20 mL	Observed Value%	.....iu/Bag
1							
2							
3							
4							
5							
6							
7							
8							
9							

ANNEXURE 67.17

Daily Quality Control of Reagents

Name of Blood Center:

License No:

Logo

I. Lot No. and Expiry of Antisera:

	Anti-A (IgM)	Anti-B (IgM)	Anti-AB (IgM)	Anti-D (IgM)	Anti-H (IgM)
Manufacturer					
Lot No.					
Date of Expiry					

II. Physical Appearance:

a. Reagent Antisera (any precipitate/gel formation/turbidity)_____

_____

b. Reagent cells/pooled saline washed 5% cells suspension any hemolysis/clot/contamination_____

III. Specificity:

Donor unit not used for Pooling Reagents Cells			Reagent Cells 5%	Anti-A (IgM)	Anti-B (IgM)	Anti-AB (IgM)	Anti-D (IgM)
			A1 Cells				
			B Cells				
			O Cells				

IV. Avidity and Reaction Strength:

Titre	Anti-A (IgM) 1:256	Anti-B (IgM) 1:256	Anti-AB (IgM) 1:256	Anti-D (IgM + IgG) 1:32–1:64	Anti-H 1:16
Avidity	3–6 sec	3–4 sec	3–4 sec	10–20 sec	15–20 sec
Reaction strength	+++	+++	+++	+++	++
Observed avidity					
Observed Reaction strength					

Signature of Technician/Technical Supervisor: .... **Date:** ....

Daily Quality Control of Reagents		
Quality Control of Normal Saline		
Normal Saline 0.9% w/v Lot No.: Manufacturer: Expiry:		
Parameters:		
a) Appearance	Turbidity/Particles	Yes/No
b) pH	6.0–7.4	Observed Value:
c) Hemolysis	(Centrifuge 10 Drops of 5% RBC suspension with 10 drops of Normal Saline 0.9% at 3,500 rpm) for 10 minutes. Look for Hemolysis	Present/Absent
Quality Control of Distilled Water		
Lot No.: Manufacturer: Expiry:		
Parameters:		
a) Appearance	Turbidity/Particles	Yes/No
b) pH	6.0–8.0	Observed Value:
Quality Control of DILUENT BLISS/LISS		
Lot No.: Manufacturer: Expiry:		
Parameters:		
a) Appearance	Turbidity/Particles	Yes/No
b) pH	6.0–8.0	Observed Value:

Signature of Technician/Technical Supervisor: .... **Date:** ....

Quality Control of Column Cards ABO and Reverse Grouping

Lot No.:

Manufacturer:

Expiry:

Parameters:

1. Appearance				
• Clear liquid layer should appear on top of the opaque gel in each microtube	No/Yes			
• Discoloration	No/Yes			
• Bubbles, crystals, or other artifacts	No/Yes			
2. Intact Foil Seals	No/Yes			
3. Testing with Known cells along with Control	A cells	B Cells	Rh +ve cells	Control

Signature of Technician/Technical Supervisor: ....   **Date:** ....

CHAPTER 68

Audit of Blood Center

INTRODUCTION

Audit is a system of evaluation, investigation, and measurement as well as a means of continuous assessment and, therefore, improvement in any kind of system with the sole purpose of improvising and assuring the quality as well as the services. Auditing, which can be prospective, concurrent, or retrospective, is based on set guidelines, but in practice, it is about determining the difference between the instructions and what has actually been done.

In prospective audit, individual transfusion requests are reviewed in real time, i.e., before the issue of blood/blood components, and the treating physician can be contacted if the request is inappropriate. Though this method is helpful in immediate intervention and prevention of unnecessary transfusion, it may cause friction with the treating physician.

In concurrent audit, a review of each transfusion is done after 12 or 24 hours. Here, immediate intervention is not possible, but future transfusion practice can be modified.

Retrospective audits are usually performed by a team from the hospital and the results are reviewed in the Hospital Transfusion Committee meetings. The frequency of audit may vary from 6 monthly to yearly. These audits help to examine aggregate transfusion data and trends in transfusion utilization and also to understand the practice among various clinical specialties.

Audits in blood center services are valuable which must be written with the intent to review thoroughly all the crucial systems within the blood center. All audits are conducted in accordance with specified methods designed by the management. It formally represents a review of all factors involved in assuring the quality of blood, blood components, blood products, and blood transfusion services.

TYPES OF AUDITS

There are two types of audits:
1. Quality audit
2. Medical audit

Quality Audit

A well-planned comprehensive quality audit covers all activities of transfusion service and assesses how the various elements of the service relate to each other. But it can also be selective and specific, focusing on specific areas. The procedures for the audit may be internal or external.

Internal Audit

Internal audit may be carried out by:
- Periodic departmental or departmental self-assessment procedures in activity area, using the mechanism of peer review circles wherever possible
- Regular inspections by directors, managers, or supervisors in accordance with established standard operating procedures (SOPs)
- All blood transfusion services must maintain an adequate and cost-effective internal audit system. Regular audits should be conducted by senior staff members, and regular spot-checks should be conducted by the director.

Fields of Activity of Internal Audit

An internal audit may include a review of multiple factors, which may be addressed individually or collectively, in one or more areas of activity. Selected aspects considered suitable for internal audit in the different areas of activity are:
- Donor aspects such as planning, deferrals, SOPs, interviews, screening, and adverse donor reactions
- Blood component production, e.g., process, control, documentation, and efficiency of blood component manufacturing, e.g., systems for tracking the blood or blood products from the donor to the patient
- Shortage of blood or blood component
- Inventory control
- Issue and shipping of blood and/or components
- Labeling
- Quality control testing, documentation, quarantine, and blood component issue mechanisms
- Equipment installation and preventive mechanisms
- Personnel training
- Documentation

External Audit

Document trails and product audits are often used for external audits.

The *document trail* addresses SOPs, documentation systems, batch records, complaint files, transfusion board and ad hoc committee reports and actions, and corrective action files.

A product audit consists of selecting and tracking specific blood units or blood components approved for transfusion and identifying unsuitable units or components for transfusion. This path is traced from the donor to the recipient (or from the recipient back to the donor).

External audits are conducted by qualified and trained individuals with the necessary skills and resourcefulness for the task. Professional standards and guidelines are used to compare established standards, other systems, or within the same system over time and are used to assess improvements and deficiencies. Appropriate indicators are used that can be quantitatively assessed using a checklist.

Data from external audits facilitates operational decisions. External assessments can correct any preconceived notions about the status of the quality assurance systems, procedures, methods, communications, and training requirements. There is often a discrepancy between what is actually happening and what management thinks, e.g., by determining whether established guidelines are being implemented and are adhered to.

External audits provide an objective and unbiased assessment of system health (efficiency and safety) and are particularly useful in identifying the need for appropriate corrective procedures, including training and retraining. The results of external audits help obtain the resources necessary to meet the requirements of an institution's quality assurance policy or guidelines. External audits also help to facilitate communication and dialogue within and between various departments and services. If the audit is to be a rewarding educational experience, respect and mutual trust between the auditor and the auditee are highly desirable for audits.

MEDICAL AUDIT

National AIDS Control Organization (NACO)/National Blood Transfusion Council (NBTC) standards apply only to safe donors and safe blood, not the third component of blood safety. According to national blood policy guidelines, state and union governments must ensure that hospital transfusion committees (HTCs) are established in all hospitals to guide, monitor, and control the clinical use of blood/blood components.

Recently, the Hospital Transfusion Committee has been named as Patient Blood Management Committee (PBMC). Whether the committee is called a PBMC or remains as HTC, expectations are the same; the committee plays a critical role in ensuring that blood/blood components are used appropriately, safely, efficiently, and effectively in accordance with national guidelines and standards. It is also a key driver of change as PBMC principles and strategies are adopted.

Blood transfusion practices are reviewed by the transfusion committee of both hospitals. The purpose of a transfusion audit is to determine the adequacy of transfusion practices and to provide guidance for improving transfusion practices. Medical audits in blood centers help improve the processes of ordering, distributing, handling and managing blood/blood components, and monitoring transfusion reactions. The rational use of blood requires a study of existing blood transfusion practices and the collection of background information on the types of existing blood transfusion practices, i.e., requests for individual unit transfusion of blood, fresh blood transfusion, use of blood component therapy, use of autologous blood transfusion, and change these policies for proper use of blood in every hospital setting after regular analysis.

MEMBERS OF HOSPITAL TRANSFUSION COMMITTEE

According to NACO guidelines on appropriate use of blood [adapted from the World Health Organization (WHO) document on Global Blood Safety Initiative], an HTC should consist of the following members:

- Major blood consumers, e.g., obstetricians, pediatricians, surgeons, anesthesiologists, internal medicine specialists, intensivists, and hematologists
- Member from nursing staff
- Representative of medical management
- *The service provider group*:
  - The medical director/transfusion service officer (or representative), who is the member secretary
  - The quality assurance manager or equivalent

The committee is chaired by a senior physician, preferably a doctor, and the frequency of meetings is determined by local guidelines.

Functions of Hospital Transfusion Committee
Policies, Procedures, and Compliance

- Development and implementation of standardized blood transfusion guidelines and procedures across institutions—developing Maximum surgical blood ordering schedule (MSBOS) for surgical procedures, developing guidelines for the use of blood components, and issuing blood units without appropriate testing in emergencies

- Facilitate collaboration between clinical disciplines to ensure that transfusion therapy policies and procedures comply with applicable regulations.
- Evaluate and implement blood storage techniques and transfusion alternatives as appropriate.

Staff Training and Education
- Providing orientation and educational seminars
- Annual validation of transfusion skills
- Schedule regular self-assessments of blood administration practices.
- Conduct an unannounced independent evaluation of blood administration practices.
- Exchange of root cause analysis (RCA) results and recommendations
- Organization of process improvement events
- Displaying educational posters

Blood Utilization Review and Peer Review Program
- Develop a unified approach to monitoring the use of blood/blood components and overseeing blood consumption peer review programs.
- Establish systems to generate physician-specific and peer review-specific reports of blood/blood components for the approval or renewal of hospital privileges for medical staff.

Performance Improvement (Root Cause Analysis)
- *Reactive*: Participate in RCA of transfusion-related adverse events. RCAs should be done to ensure that RCA recommendations are disseminated, implemented, and evaluated for efficacy.
- *Proactive*: Improving patient safety through ongoing proactive assessment and performance improvement in blood ordering, collection, pretransfusion bedside testing, and transfusion reaction reporting practices

Blood Center Reports
- Review and analysis of blood center reports, e.g., regarding usage of blood/blood components, discard and wastage of blood/blood components, adverse transfusion reactions, and transfusion errors/accidents.

Communication
- Provide meaningful and relevant feedback to clinical departments.
- Provide executive leadership with comprehensive blood/blood component usage reports and recommend corrective actions as needed.

- Submission of blood/blood component usage reports to the accrediting and regulatory agencies and, where appropriate, governing bodies

INDICATORS FOR MONITORING OF BLOOD TRANSFUSION SERVICE

The blood transfusion services must have the following information available to continuously control the basic quality of operations:

- Total number of blood units or components transfused over a specified time period
- The number of patients who received blood transfusions during this period compared to the total number of hospitalized patients (it is *recommended* to treat each component separately)
- Number of each blood component transfused per transfused patient
- Ratio of whole blood used to packed red blood cells (PRBCs)
- *Transfusion probability (TP)*: This represents the probability of blood transfusion for a particular patient group/surgery/procedure. A TP of >30% represents a significant blood utilization for a particular procedure/surgery.

  Transfusion probability monitoring can help the blood center to implement the type and screen policy which can be safely implemented in procedures/surgeries where TP is <10%; in cases where it is >30%, maximum surgical blood ordering schedule is advised and type and crossmatch policy are implemented.
- *Crossmatch to transfusion ratio (C:T ratio)*: Monitoring of C:T ratio is a very good way to minimize wastage of blood components. A C:T ratio of 2–2.5 is generally accepted as the standard. An AQ ratio >2.5 is associated with higher units of blood getting reserved for particular population. This leads to unnecessary exhaustion of blood stock of excessive reservations.
- *Transfusion index (TI)*: Number of units transfused/number of patients crossmatched × 100.
- *Maximum surgical blood ordering schedule*: TI is used to set MSBOS for a particular patient group/surgery and is calculated by multiplying TI by 1.5. MSBOS gives an average/safe requirement of blood for specific surgery/patient group and is calculated by considering an average of at least 6 months. MSBOS can also vary depending upon the Surgeon and therefore, an annual revision of the same is recommended.
- *Issuable stock index (ISI)*: It is an average stock available in the blood center and is the number of unreserved red cell units in all groups/ number of red cell units issued in a month/number of day in that

month. An ISI of 6 would mean that the blood center has a stock which would be sufficient to fulfill blood requirement for 6 days. As the packed cells have an expiry of an average 42 days, it is advisable to keep ISI in the range of 6–10 days. In case of platelets which have an expiry of 5 days, it is advisable to keep an ISI of 2.

- Mean number of units transfused per procedure/surgery
- *Wastage rates of blood/blood components*: Wastage rates of blood/ blood components may help a blood center to evaluate its internal process control and find the critical weak points after a thorough root cause analysis. It could be due to expiry, poor storage, leakage (mainly plasma), or reactive for transfusion transmitted diseases. The wastage is calculated as a percentage of issue (WAPI) = Number of units wasted/number of units issued × 100.
- Number of inappropriate transfusions for each component (Red Cells, Platelets, FFP)
- Number and type of transfusion reactions
- The workload and output of the various sections within the blood transfusion service
- Number of urgent and uncrossmatched units issued
- The number of urgent requests compared to the number of routine requests
- Number of unused units returned
- Number of surgeries canceled due to lack of blood
- Number of late preoperative requests, indicating ward or clinic, and surgeon who raised the requests
- Number of units issued to other hospitals
- Number of replacement versus volunteer donors

After monitoring the basic operational quality of blood transfusion services in hospitals, HTC can improve blood transfusion practices in the following ways:

- *Resolve blood transfusion issues with one-on-one discussions with physicians*:
  - When it comes to crossmatching and blood transfusion, clinical practice varies greatly between obstetricians. Many obstetric patients are "grouped and held" or crossmatched unnecessarily, leaving a significant portion of their requested blood unused. This practice increases the workload of blood centers and impacts efficiency and quality.
  - *Holding conferences and seminars*: This approach has been shown to improve obstetric and gynecological transfusion practices by reducing blood transfusions by 60%.
- *Regular monitoring of transfused patients and determination of daily requirements*.

- *Review each request prior to issuance (concurrent review), and refer any disputes to HTC.*
  - With this methodology, a reduction in fresh frozen plasma (FFP) requirements has been achieved.
- *Implement transfusion algorithms and policies in all clinical settings.*

The use of single-unit blood transfusions can be reduced through a regular review of blood requirements, proper documentation, and application of approaches outlined above. Reducing inappropriate blood transfusions reduces the risk of transfusion infections, side effects, and transfusion sensitization. Blood transfusions should be used only when the clinical benefits outweigh the risks, especially when one transfusion only increased his/her hemoglobin by 1 g/dL and is therapeutically insignificant.

Hospital transfusion committee aims to promote rational transfusion practices and enable blood centers to maximize the use of blood units available at each blood center. It helps blood center managers plan needs and avoid unnecessary waste, reducing effort, costs, errors, and risks associated with blood transfusions. All these efforts, therefore, improve the rational use of limited resources.

CHAPTER 69

Hemovigilance

INTRODUCTION

Hemovigilance is defined as a set of surveillance procedures covering the entire transfusion chain, from blood collection to the recipient follow-up, designed to collect information about unanticipated or adverse effects, to prevent their occurrence and recurrence. A hemovigilance program helps to collect information about transfusion-related adverse events related to blood donations and transfusions. Therefore, the ultimate goal of the hemovigilance system is to improve transfusion safety. The primary objective of the intensive hemovigilance program is to improve transfusion safety and quality by collecting, compiling, analyzing, and distributing information on the many common serious side effects associated with blood/blood component transfusions.

INTERNATIONAL HEMOVIGILANCE

Hemovigilance started in France in 1994 with the establishment of a nationwide surveillance and warning system. Then, in 1995, the European Council issued a resolution regulating the law enforcement for the hemovigilance system. Today, the International Haemovigilance Network (IHN) operates on a global level. The purpose of the IHN is to develop and maintain a common structure for blood and blood component safety worldwide.

NATIONAL HEMOVIGILANCE PROGRAM

On December 10, 2012, a national hemovigilance program was launched in India as an integral part of the pharmacovigilance program to monitor adverse reactions associated with blood and blood product transfusions. Further, National Donor Vigilance Program, i.e., reporting of adverse reactions associated with blood donation, was launched on June 14, 2015. In these programs, predonation, postdonation, and adverse reactions occurring during or after transfusion are reported to the National Coordinating Center, i.e., National Institute of Biologicals.

DONOR HEMOVIGILANCE

Systematic monitoring of the adverse reactions or complications in blood donors associated with blood donation is called donor hemovigilance. Monitoring of such reactions is important as they may directly harm the blood donor or indirectly harm the recipient by influencing the quality of the product.

RECIPIENT HEMOVIGILANCE

Recipient hemovigilance includes monitoring, evaluation, reporting, and analysis of transfusion reactions that occur in patients during or after blood transfusion.

Early recognition, prompt cessation of transfusion, and proper evaluation are the keys to a successful outcome of any transfusion reactions. Many common signs and symptoms are associated with these transfusion reactions.

WORKUP OF A TRANSFUSION REACTION

Evaluation of a transfusion reaction involves a combination of bedside clinical examination of the patient along with laboratory investigations to determine the nature of reaction. Signs and symptoms suggestive of a transfusion reaction should be attended to immediately at the patient's bedside. The doctor should stop the transfusion and contact the blood center immediately. If a transfusion reaction is suspected, the following steps should be taken:

1. *Patient-centric steps*:
   - Immediately stop the transfusion and use a new infusion set to keep the intravenous (IV) line patency with normal saline.
   - Perform bedside clerical recheck and check all labels on the blood component and patient's medical records (name and unique identification number) for patient identification errors or mix-ups with another patient.
   - Inform the doctor on duty about patient management and appropriate laboratory tests.
2. *Component-centric steps*:
   - Send the implicated blood bag with attached blood transfusion set and posttransfusion patient sample taken from another

vein in ethylenediaminetetraacetic acid (EDTA) and plain vacutainers to the blood center for evaluation.

- Further transfusions to the patient should be given only after consultation with the transfusion medicine team.

3. *Standard laboratory protocol*:

- Perform a clerical recheck of all the records in the laboratory and at the issue counter. Cross-check patient identity from the pretransfusion sample, requisition form, and crossmatch and issue registers. Check all the donor unit labels and match with the donor record register. If any discrepancy is found, immediately retrieve back all nontransfused and partially transfused units. It is important to note that another patient may also be involved due to a similar name or identification number. Such errors are known as "companion errors," and timely recognition can prevent transfusion reaction in another patient.

- A visual inspection of the patient's posttransfusion sample can be the first indication of hemolysis. Centrifuge the posttransfusion sample and observe the color of the supernatant and compare with pretransfusion sample. A pink to reddish-colored supernatant may be an indicator of hemolysis. This method detects free plasma hemoglobin when it is >20–50 mg/dL. A yellow discoloration of supernatant plasma may indicate increased bilirubin. Check the color of the blood unit for any discoloration or clots which may indicate bacterial contamination or hemolysis. Compare the color of blood in the bag with the attached segment.

- Perform a repeat blood grouping on the patient's pre- and posttransfusion samples and implicated blood unit. In case of platelet or plasma components, check blood group from the records.

- Perform a direct antiglobulin test (DAT) on the EDTA sample. DAT may be positive in an immune-mediated hemolytic transfusion reaction. It is important to note that DAT may be negative if all transfused cells have been cleared or if few antibody-coated cells are present. If postreaction DAT is positive, then perform DAT on the pretransfusion sample for confirmation or exclusion.

- *Compatibility testing*: Repeat the compatibility testing on both pre- and posttransfusion samples of the patient.

- Perform an indirect antiglobulin test which may be positive if the patient has an underlying antibody due to exposure from previous transfusion or pregnancy. If it is positive, then antibody screening and identification should be done to identify antibodies to other blood group systems. All tests should also be performed on the pretransfusion sample.

- Donor units can also be tested for irregular antibodies and DATs.
- Send a blood culture of the implicated unit and the patient. If the culture is positive and the same organism is detected in both samples, the reaction could be due to bacterial contamination of the blood component.

4. *Other laboratory investigations indicating hemolysis*:
   - First voided urine should be sent for analysis of free hemoglobin. Urine hemoglobin may be present if free hemoglobin exceeds the haptoglobin-binding capacity. Presence of cola-colored urine after initiation of transfusion can indicate hemoglobinuria.
   - Plasma hemoglobin levels may be increased in intravascular hemolysis due to an acute immune-mediated transfusion reaction.
   - Plasma haptoglobin levels are reduced in acute intravascular hemolysis as free hemoglobin initially binds with haptoglobin.
   - Serum lactate dehydrogenase levels may be elevated due to red cell hemolysis.
   - Serum bilirubin levels can be increased at a later stage, 5–7 hours after transfusion.

5. *Ancillary investigations*:
   - Complete blood count, reticulocyte count, and peripheral blood film should be performed. Spherocytes may be seen in delayed hemolytic transfusion reaction.
   - Coagulation profile in the form of prothrombin time, activated partial thromboplastin time, fibrinogen, and D-dimer tests can identify the development of disseminated intravascular coagulation (DIC) in patients with acute hemolytic transfusion reaction.
   - Renal function tests such as blood urea and serum creatinine should be closely monitored in suspected hemolytic transfusion reaction to detect early renal damage.
   - If the reaction manifests with pulmonary symptoms, a chest X-ray should be ordered.

Note:
- It is important to take a complete history of the patient with respect to age, diagnosis, pregnancy, previous transfusion, historic blood group, date and time of issue and start of transfusion, storage and transportation details of blood component, and drug history as all these could give an important clue to the probable cause of the reaction.

Table 1: Immutability* levels.	
Immutability levels	**Assessment scale**
Definite (certain)	When there is conclusive evidence beyond reasonable doubt that the adverse event can be attributed to the transfusion
Probable (likely)	When the evidence is clearly in favor of attributing the adverse event to the transfusion
Possible	When the evidence is indeterminate for attributing the adverse event to the transfusion or an alternate cause
Unlikely (doubtful)	When the evidence is clearly in favor of attributing the adverse event to causes other than the transfusion
Excluded	When there is conclusive evidence beyond reasonable doubt that the adverse event can be attributed to causes other than the transfusion

*Immutability means the likelihood that an adverse reaction in a recipient can be attributed to the blood or blood component transfused.

- If hemolysis is associated with the transfusion and immune and nonimmune causes have been ruled out, it is possible that the patient has an intrinsic red cell defect, and further investigations may be done accordingly.

6. *Documentation and reporting*:
   - All reactions should be documented in detail after the completion of workup. Each reaction should be classified and assigned immutability **(Table 1)** according to hemovigilance guidelines. The final report of workup of transfusion reaction should be shared with the clinician. Further transfusions should be based upon the results of reaction workup, and due care should be taken to prevent future reactions.
   - After complete documentation, reactions should be reported to the national hemovigilance program.

7. *Conclusion*:
   - Early recognition and thorough evaluation of every transfusion reaction are key to safe transfusion practice.
   - Appropriate management of donor adverse reaction instills satisfaction in blood donors and improves donor safety. Such blood donors may continue as repeat donors leading to a positive impact on national blood supply.

- All donor and recipient adverse reactions should be classified following standard definitions and reported to the national hemovigilance program.
- Each transfusion reaction should be classified and reported to National Haemovigilance Propgramme and State Blood Transfusion Council.

ROLE OF BLOOD CENTER

- Blood centers must participate in the Haemovigilance Programme of India (HvPI) and be registered with the Haemo-Vigil software (www.nib.gov.in) for reporting of adverse transfusion reactions.
- The blood centers should develop a process to obtain complete details of adverse transfusion reactions to be able to report to HvPI.
- The blood centers should ensure that clinical and emergency medical staff are trained to properly report adverse transfusion reactions to transfusion services.
- The blood center should delegate responsibility for reporting adverse reactions to his/her HvPI transfusion on a regular basis after proper training. Regular monitoring and analysis of all reported adverse transfusion (both donor and recipient) reactions is done by blood center and reports as per format given at **Annexures 69.1 and 69.2** are uploaded monthly on the website of Haemovigilance Programme of India.
- Physicians and nurses caring for patients with suspected transfusion complications must perform the following documentation and reporting functions:
  - Attending nursing staff should immediately report any suspected transfusion reaction to the attending physician.
  - Document patient data as well as the implicated units/products and retain them in the patient's file.
  - Submit details of the transfusion reaction to the Department of Transfusion Medicine/Blood Center in appropriate documents accompanied by the patient samples and unit transfused, required for tests.
  - Work with the transfusion department/blood center to assess the consistency of side effects.
  - Maintain a record of complications in the patient's medical record, including transfusion department/blood center laboratory reports.
- The transfusion service is responsible for documenting and reporting them to national hemovigilance program.
- A detailed clinical and laboratory report should be submitted to the appropriate clinical department and hospital blood transfusion committee.

- Investigations should be done according to the workup form and record the results.
- Enter the required details according to the documentation required for the transfusion reaction-traceability document (TR-TD).
- Determine the immutability levels of the adverse transfusion reaction.
- Ensuring the integrity of the TR-TD.
- Report the details to the Pharmacovigilance Program of India (PvPI) technical officer according to the transfusion reaction reporting form through the website.
- To assure the completeness of the TR-TD.
- TR-TD is kept on record.
- Hospital transfusion committees regularly review reported adverse events and provide guidance and support for improvement.

ANNEXURE 69.1

National Institute of Biologicals
Ministry of Health & Family Welfare, Govt. of India
(National Coordinating Center)
HAEMOVIGILANCE PROGRAMME OF INDIA

Transfusion Reaction Reporting Form (TRRF) For Blood & Blood Components & Plasma Products (Version-2)

*Mandatory Field

(A) Patient Information

Hospital Code No.:

Patient Initials*:   Gender*:   Blood Group*:

Hospital Admission No.*:   Age/Date of Birth*:   ....Yrs ....Month ....Days ....Hrs ....Mins

Primary Diagnosis*:

Medical History:

(B) Transfusion Reaction Details*

Was the patient under anaesthesia during transfusion: Yes/No if Yes type: GA/Spinal/LA

Pre-transfusion Vitals:	Temp:	Pulse:	BP:	RR:	SpO₂:
Vitals at the time of reaction:	Temp:	Pulse:	BP:	RR:	SpO₂:

Please tick mark the relevant signs and symptoms listed below

Generalised	Pain	Respiratory	Renal	Circulatory
☐ Fever	☐ Anxiety	☐ Chest Pain	☐ Dyspnoea	☐ Haematuria	☐ Tachycardia
☐ Chills	☐ Itching (Pruritus)	☐ Abdominal	☐ Wheeze	☐ Haemoglobinuria	☐ Hypertension
☐ Rigors	☐ Edema (Site)____	☐ Back/Flank Pain	☐ Cough	☐ Oliguria	☐ Hypotension
☐ Nausea	☐ Jaundice	☐ Infusion Site Pain	☐ Hypoxemia	☐ Other____	☐ Raised JVP

Continued

Continued

☐ Urticaria	☐ Other_____	☐ Other_____		☐ Arrhythmias
☐ Flushing			☐ Bilateral Infiltrates on Chest X-ray	☐ Other_____
☐ Restlessness				
☐ Vomiting			☐ Other_____	

Any Other (Specify):..............

(C) Transfusion Product(s) Details*

Select*	Select Component	Date & Time of Issue of Blood Component	Date & Time of onset Transfusion	Unit Id (Transfused)	Blood Group	Volume Transfused (ml)	Expiry date of Blood Component	Manufacturer of Blood Bag	Batch/Lot No. of the Blood Bag	1st time/repeat Transfusion
☐	Whole blood									☐ 1st Time
☐	Packed Red blood cells (PRBC)									
☐	Buffy coat depleted PRBC									☐ Repeat 1 to 10
☐	Leucofiltered PRBC									
☐	Random Donor platelets/pooled									☐ Repeat > 10
☐	Apheresis Platelets									
☐	Fresh Frozen Plasma									
☐	Cryoprecipitate									
☐	Any Other									

Add New Plasma Product

Select	Plasma Product	Indication	Date of Administration	Manufacturer	Expiry Date of the Plasma Product	Batch No./Lot No.	1st Time/Repeat
							☐ 1st Time
							☐ Repeat 1 to 10
							☐ Repeat >10

Continued

Continued

(D) Investigations

☐ Clerical Checks — Specify Error Found if any: _____

Investigation	Pre-transfusion sample			Post-transfusion sample		
☐ Visual Check						
* ☐ Repeat Blood Grouping	O+/A+/B+/AB+/O-/A-/B-/AB-			O+/A+/B+/AB+/O-/A-/B-/AB-		
* ☐ Repeat Crossmatch	☐ Compatible	☐ InCompatible	☐ Not Done	☐ Compatible	☐ InCompatible	☐ Not Done
* ☐ Repeat Antibody screen	☐ Negative	☐ Positive	☐ Not Done	☐ Negative	☐ Positive	☐ Not Done
☐ Antibody Identification						
* ☐ Direct antiglobulin test	☐ Negative	☐ Positive	☐ Not Done	☐ Negative	☐ Positive	☐ Not Done
☐ Hemoglobin						
☐ Plasma Hemoglobin						
☐ Urine hemoglobin						
☐ Bilirubin (Total/conjugated)						
☐ Platelet count						
☐ PT/INR						

Continued

Continued

		Negative	Positive	Not Done	Specify Organism if positive _____	
*	Blood culture of Blood Bag	☐	☐	☐		
*	Blood culture of Patient	☐ Negative	☐ Positive	☐ Not Done	☐ Negative ☐ Positive ☐ Not Done	
		Specify Organism if positive _____			Specify Organism if positive _____	
☐	Chest X-ray of the patient in case of suspected TRALI					
In case of Non-immune hemolysis (which of the following was the case?)						
☐	Hemolysis due to freezing of PRBC Units					
☐	Hemolysis due to inappropriate warming of PRBC Units					
☐	Hemolysis due to infusion of any other fluid through same BT set.		Specify Fluid: _____			
☐	Mechanical damage					
In Case of ABO Mismatch (which of the following was the case?)						
☐	Wrong Blood in tube					
☐	Grouping error					
☐	Labelling error					
☐	Wrong unit transfused					

Continued

Continued

(E) Nature of Adverse Reaction(s)*

Select	Reaction	Date & Time of Onset of Reaction	Date & Time of Recovery	Outcome
☐	Febrile Non Haemolytic Reactions (FNHTR) 1°C rise in temperature ☐ ☐ ☐ 2°C rise in temperature ☐ ☐ Only Chills and Rigors			☐ 1. Death following the Adverse Reaction(s)
☐	Allergic reaction			
☐	Anaphylaxis			
☐	Immunological Haemolysis due to ABO Incompatibility			
☐	Immunological Haemolysis due to other Allo-Antibodies			
☐	Non Immunological Haemolysis			
☐	Hypotensive Transfusion Reaction			☐ 2. Recovered
☐	Transfusion Related Acute Lung Injury (TRALI) Definite ☐ ☐ Possible ☐			
☐	Transfusion Associated Dyspnoea (TAD)			
☐	Transfusion Associated Circulatory Overload (TACO)			
☐	Transfusion Transmitted Bacterial Infection			
☐	Transfusion Transmitted Parasitic Infection (Malaria)			☐ 3. Recovered with Sequelae
☐	Post-transfusion Purpura			
☐	Transfusion-associated Graft-versus-host Disease (TA-GvHD)			
☐	Other Reaction (s) ☐ ☐ Add New			☐ 4. Unknown

Continued

IMPUTABILITY ASSESSMENT

(F) Imputability Assessment*

S. No.	Reaction Term	Transfusion Product/Component	*Imputability Assessment (Please mention from the below list)

*Imputability: 1. Definite (Certain), 2. Probable (Likely), 3. Possible, 4. Unlikely (Doubtful), 5. Excluded, 6. Not Assessed

Monthly Denominator Reporting Form*

Hospital Code: _____ Month/Year: _____

Blood Component	No. of Units Issued
1) Fresh Frozen Plasma	
2) Whole Blood	
3) Packed Red Blood Cells (PRBCs)	
4) Buffy Coat Depleted PRBC	
5) Leucofiltered PRBC	
6) Random Donor Platelets/ Pooled	
7) Apheresis Platelets	
8) Cryoprecipitate	
9) Any Other_____	

ANNEXURE 69.2

I) Donor Information	

Donor Id:_____	Type of Donation:
	(a) Whole Blood
	(b) Apheresis
	    1. RBC
	    2. Platelets
	    3. Plasma
	    4. Plasma + Platelets

Sex:_____	Donor Type:
	(a) Voluntary
	(b) Replacement
	(c) Family Donor
	    1. first-time
	    2. repeat

Weight of Donor (KG):_____	Venipuncture: **(a)** 1 **(b)** 2 **(c)** >2
	Data Captured: **(a)** Onsite **(b)** Call back by donor **(c)** Call back by Blood Centre
Age/Date of Birth:_____	Site of Donation: **(a)** Camp **(b)** Blood Centre
II) Details of Blood Collected	
Lot No. of Blood Bag _____	Volume of Blood Collected (mL) _____ Expiry date of Blood Bag _____ Date & Time of Reaction _____

Continued

Continued

III) Type of Complications (Refer Annexure I)

A1-Complications mainly characterized by the occurrence of blood outside the vessels
- (a) Haematoma (bruise)
- (b) Arterial puncture
- (c) Delayed (bleeding/Re-bleeding)

A2-Complications mainly characterized by pain
- (a) Nerve injury/irritation
- (b) Other Painful arm

A3-Localised infection/inflammation along the course of a vein
- (a) Thrombophlebitis
- (b) Cellulitis

A4-Other major blood vessel injury—Serious conditions needing specialist medical diagnosis and attention
- (a) Deep venous thrombosis (DVT)
- (b) Arteriovenous fistula
- (c) Compartment syndrome
- (d) Brachial artery pseudoaneurysm

B-Complications mainly with generalized symptoms: Vasovagal reactions
- (a) LOC (Loss of Consciousness) <60 sec
- (b) LOC (Loss of Consciousness) >60 sec
- (c) Without loss of consciousness (LOC)
- (d) With injury
- (e) Without injury
- (f) Within Blood collection facility
- (g) Outside blood collection facility

C-Complications related to apheresis
- (a) Citrate reaction
- (b) Haemolysis
- (c) Air embolism
- (d) Infiltration of IV fluids

D-Allergic reactions
- (a) Allergy (local)
- (b) Generalised allergic reaction (anaphylactic reaction)

E-Other serious complications related to blood donation
- (a) Acute cardiac symptoms
- (b) Myocardial infarction (MI)
- (c) Cardiac arrest
- (d) Transient ischemic attack (TIA)
- (e) Cerebrovascular accident
- (f) Death

F-Other Reactions_____

Continued

Continued

IV) Outcomes	V) Imputability (Refer Annexure II)
☐ Resolved	☐ Definite (Certain)
☐ On Follow Up	☐ Probable (Likely)
☐ Recovered with Sequelae	☐ Possible
☐ Permanently Disabled	☐ Unlikely (Doubtful)
☐ Death following the Adverse Reactions	☐ Excluded
☐ Unknown	
VI) Reporter_____	**Date of Report**_____

CHAPTER 70

Accreditation of Blood Centers

INTRODUCTION

Blood transfusion services (BTS) are regulated under the Drugs and Cosmetics Act 1940 and Rules 1945. Therefore, each blood center must obtain a license from the State Licensing Authority/Drugs Controller General of India before starting blood center operations. However, there is a growing need to focus on quality rather than on quantitative benchmarks.

Accreditation is a nongovernmental, voluntary process of evaluating institutions, agencies, and educational programs. It is defined as the process by which a government agency or association publicly recognizes a laboratory or blood center as meeting certain established standards determined by initial and periodic evaluations. Expert teams include evaluations by independent panels or committees. To be accredited, facilities and/or laboratories must establish and maintain a quality system that includes all activities that determine the purpose and responsibilities of a quality policy, taking into account the principles of good manufacturing practice.

GOALS OF ACCREDITATION

- Achieve highest quality self-sufficiency.
- Appropriate and rational use of blood
- Ensure safe and economical processing of blood.
- Continue regulatory impact to improve blood/blood component quality.

ACCREDITATION DYNAMICS

- The Consumer Protection Act 2019
- The Clinical Establishments (Registration and Regulations) 2010

- Regulations of insurance companies
- Empanelment by Central Government Health Scheme (CGHS), Ex-Servicemen Contributory Health Scheme (ECHS), corporate, etc.
- Community awareness and response
- Medical tourism

BENEFITS FOR USERS/PATIENTS/DONORS

- Accreditation leads to improved quality and safety in the collection, processing, testing, transfusion, and distribution of blood and blood components.
- Accreditation guarantees that services are provided by qualified health professionals and that their rights are respected and protected.
- User's/patient's/donor's satisfaction is assessed regularly.
- Increase public confidence that the organization cares about patient safety and quality care.
- Encourage nonstop improvement.
- Actively prevent problems from occurring.
- Customer satisfaction is maximized.
- Enable blood centers to demonstrate their commitment to quality.
- Increase community confidence in blood center services.
- Give blood centers an opportunity to compete with the best.

BENEFITS FOR THE STAFF

- Staff is provided with continuous learning, a good work environment, and leadership.
- Define critical interfaces between processes, departments, and employees.
- Provide a safe and efficient environment that contributes to job satisfaction.
- Improve the overall professional development of all employees.

SYSTEMS FOR ACCREDITATION

Various systems for accreditation are enumerated below:
- International Organization for Standardization 9000 (ISO 9000)
- ISO 17025 accreditation
- Joint Commission on the Accreditation of Healthcare Organizations and Specialty Accreditations
- College of American Pathologists
- American Association of Blood Banks (AABB)
- South African National Accreditation System

- Central Board of Accreditation for Healthcare Institutions
- National Accreditation Board for Hospitals and Healthcare Providers, India (NABH)

International Organization for Standardization 9000

It guarantees that the process of developing products is documented and carried out in a high-quality manner, but it does not guarantee the quality of products.

International Organization for Standardization 17025 Accreditation

It is recognized as the global standard for laboratory accreditation. It is required by many private and public institutions as a requirement of business contracts, and such accredited status significantly enhances the image of the laboratory and its employees.

Joint Commission on Accreditation of Healthcare Organizations and Specialty Accreditations

It is one of the highest standards in healthcare and is a voluntary accreditation for participants to assess an organization's compliance with set standards of the Joint Commission. During the onsite visit, surveyors will review more than 700 criteria for quality of care, safety, and service performance. This survey is conducted every 3 years, and the results determine whether a hospital is accredited.

College of American Pathologists

Its goal is to improve the quality of clinical laboratory services through voluntary participation, expert peer review, education, and adherence to established performance standards. When the inspection process is completed successfully, the American Society of Pathologists grants accreditation to the laboratory which becomes part of an exclusive group of over 6,000 laboratories worldwide that meet the highest standards of excellence.

American Association of Blood Banks

Its goal is to improve the quality and safety of blood/blood component collection, processing, testing, distribution, and administration and to improve the quality in tissues and BTS.

South African National Accreditation System

It is based on a combination of the ISO 9000 and ISO 17025 systems and is internationally recognized as a nationally accredited program in Saudi Arabia.

Central Board of Accreditation for Healthcare Institutions

This is Saudi Arabia's national accreditation program for healthcare facilities across the country to improve service quality and patient safety. Blood center standards have been adapted from AABB, College of American Pathologists, and Joint Commission International.

NATIONAL ACCREDITATION BOARD FOR HOSPITALS AND HEALTHCARE PROVIDERS, INDIA

A constituent board of the Quality Council of India was established to set up and administer accreditation programs for healthcare organizations. NABH was established to improve health system and promote continuous quality improvement and patient safety. The board is supported by all stakeholders, including industry, consumers, and government, but has full functional autonomy in its operations. The accreditation program assesses quality and operational systems within the facility and/or blood centers/blood centers and transfusion services. The accreditation includes compliance with NABH standards and applicable laws and regulations.

Accredited standards for blood center/transfusion services improve the quality and safety of blood during (1) collection/donation, (2) processing, (3) testing, and (4) issuing/distribution/transfusion. Accreditation results in quality patient care by ensuring that safe blood and blood components are provided to the right patients at the right time and in the right amount.

An overview of the NABH standard:
- Organization and management
- Accommodation and environment
- Staff
- Equipment
- External services and supplies
- Process control
- Identification of deviations and adverse events
- Improved performance
- Document control
- Record
- Internal audits and management reviews

ADVANTAGES OF BLOOD CENTER ACCREDITATION

- Unique program. Few countries have blood center accreditation programs in place.
- Ensures protocol standardization leading to adherence to quality and safety in blood centers.
- Improves the skills and competencies of the blood center staff.
- Increased community confidence as meeting accreditation standards ensures safe delivery of blood and blood components for transfusion.
- Contributes to promotion of medical tourism

CRITERIA FOR ACCREDITATION OF BLOOD CENTERS

- Licensed operational blood center
- Blood center has a responsibility to improve the quality of its care and services.
- Blood centers provide services according to NABH standards.
  Apply for accreditation online. Fee structure can be checked on the NABH website.

QUALITY INDICATORS FOR BLOOD CENTER

The following 10 quality indicators have been defined by NABH. All blood centers are encouraged to capture the data for these indicators. Further, out of these 10, the first 5 indicators have been mandated for accredited blood centers to monitor and report to NABH every 6 months.

Quality indicators	Calculation of values
TTI %	$\dfrac{\text{Combined TTI cases (HIV + HBV + HCV + Syphilis + MP)}}{\text{Total no. of donors}} \times 100$
Adverse transfusion reaction rate %	$\dfrac{\text{No. of adverse transfusion reactions}}{\text{Total no. of blood and components issued}} \times 100$
Wastage rates	$\dfrac{\text{No. of blood/blood components discarded}}{\text{Total no. of blood and components issued}} \times 100$
Turnaround time (TAT) of blood issues*	$\dfrac{\text{Sum of time taken}}{\text{Total no. of blood and blood components crossmatched}}$
Component failures in QC (for each component)	$\dfrac{\text{No. of component failures in QC}}{\text{Total no. of components tested}} \times 100$

Continued

Continued

Quality indicators	Calculation of values
Adverse donor reaction rate %	$\dfrac{\text{No. of donors experiencing adverse reaction}}{\text{Total no. of donors}} \times 100$
Donor deferral rate %	$\dfrac{\text{No. of donor deferrals}}{\text{Total no. of donations + Total no. of deferrals}} \times 100$
Percentage of components	$\dfrac{\text{Total components issued}}{\text{Total whole blood + components issued}} \times 100$
TTI outliers %	$\dfrac{\text{No. of deviations beyond} - 2}{\text{Total no. of batch assays}} \times 100$
Delays in transfusion beyond 30 minutes after issue	Sample audit by blood center every month

*Turnaround time is the time to be calculated from the time the request/sample is received in the blood center till the blood is crossmatched/reserved and available for transfusion. Blood centers have separate limits for routine and emergency cases.

(HBV: hepatitis B virus; HCV: hepatitis C virus; HIV: human immunodeficiency virus; MP: malaria parasite; QC: quality control; TTI: transfusion transmitted infection)

CHAPTER 71

Sterility Testing of Blood/Blood Component Units

SCOPE AND APPLICATION

Whole human blood IP must comply with the quality standards as provided under Second Schedule of the Drugs and Cosmetics Act, 1940 which further stipulates it to be as per "Indian Pharmacopoeia" (IP) standards. IP 2022 (which is the current edition and book of standards in Indian context) mandates its compliance to "sterility" in addition to various other quality tests to be complied with for ensuring its quality. A detailed method for performing this test of sterility including use of various types of growth media for detection of anaerobic, aerobic bacteria and fungi followed by incubation at appropriate temperatures to observe microbial growth have been given under Chapter 2.2.11 of Indian Pharmacopoeia 2022.

Aseptic collection and processing of blood and blood components is of paramount importance as each and every blood/component unit cannot be subjected to "test for sterility," it being a destructive test. According to guidelines issued by the National AIDS Control Organisation (NACO) and the provisions under Schedule F of the Drugs and Cosmetics Rules, 1945, 1% of collected whole human blood units must be tested for sterility. Up to 1% of packed red blood cells (PRBC) and 1% of total platelets prepared must be tested for sterility according to Schedule F of the Drugs and Cosmetics Rules, 1945. Keeping in view the importance of whole human blood and the fact that it can only be obtained from human volunteers, it is advised to use expired blood/blood components to perform "sterility test."

RESPONSIBILITY

Testing of blood/blood components for "sterility" is the responsibility of the blood center technician under direct supervision of a medical officer. This test can also be outsourced to any approved [by SLA/CLAA] commercial drug testing laboratory; however, efforts must be made to have in-house testing facilities by the blood centers to ensure safe blood. Most of the hospital-based blood centers have in-house pathological laboratories where blood and blood components can be subjected to "sterility test" by culture method simulating statutory method. There are numerous commercially available testing systems in the market such as BD BACTEC (Becton Dickinson and Company), BacT/ALERT (bioMérieux), and VersaTREK (Thermo Scientific) which can be put to use to perform "sterility test" precisely, accurately, speedily, and conveniently. The authors would like to discuss alternate methods of sterility testing of blood/blood components using the BD BACTEC system, guarantying equivalent accuracy and precision as well as easy availability and convenience to perform. To further add, IP 2022 has also provided provisions for the "alternative methods" to use for analysis in its Chapter 1 of Indian Pharmacopoeia 2022 under heading "General Notices," which is reproduced below.

Alternative methods: *"The tests and methods described are the official methods upon which the standards of the Pharmacopoeia are based. Alternative methods of analysis may be used for control purposes, provided that the methods used are shown to give results of equivalence accuracy and enable an unequivocal decision to be made as to whether compliance with the standards of the monographs would be achieved if the official methods were used. Automated procedures utilizing the same basic chemistry as the test procedures given in the monograph may also be used to determine compliance. Such alternative or automated procedures must be validated and are subjected to approval by the authority competent to authorized manufacturer of the substance or product.*

In the event of doubt or dispute, the method of analysis of the Pharmacopoeia are alone authoritative and only the result obtained by the procedure given in the Pharmacopoeia is conclusive."

Note: *As mentioned in the IP 2022, the blood center or any other organization intending to perform sterility testing on blood/blood components can follow IP 2022 method or any other method of equivalent accuracy subject to approval from the regulatory authorities.*

MATERIALS REQUIRED

- *Equipment*:
  - Laminar air flow bench
  - BACTEC blood culture bottles
  - BACTEC continuous blood culture monitoring system (alternative method)

- 37°C incubator
- Blood agar, MacConkey agar, Sabouraud's dextrose agar culture media
- Biosafety cabinet

BD BACTEC FX40 Instrument (US FDA Approved)

BD BACTEC FX40 instrument is an automated system designed for the rapid detection of presence of bacteria and fungi in blood specimens. Samples are drawn from blood units (to be tested) and injected directly into BACTEC culture vials, which are placed into the instrument vial stations for incubation and testing.

Cultures found positive are immediately pointed out by an indicator light on the front of the BACTEC FX40 instrument and an audible alarm is displayed. The positive vials are taken out of the instrument after they are identified for further confirmation of results, isolation, and identification of the organism.

Media used in BACTEC

Various kinds of growth media are available which can be put to use with the BD BACTEC FX40 system.

Different types of media can be used for culture purposes for detection of bacteria as well as fungus. Some of the media available for use are described in **Table 1**. Each medium type has default test protocol duration (modifiable in the lab configuration display). The default protocol can be overridden on each media vial entered in the BACTEC instrument.

Table 1: Types of media for sterility testing.

Type of media	Indications
BD BACTEC Plus Aerobic/F	• Contains resins for antibiotic neutralization • Indicated for 3.0–10.0 mL (8.0–10.0 mL optimal) blood volume
BD BACTEC Plus Anaerobic/F	• Contains resins for antibiotic neutralization • Indicated for 3.0–10.0 mL (8.0–10.0 mL optimal) blood volume
BD BACTEC Mycosis IC/F	• Selective culture medium specifically designed for the recovery of fungi from blood culture specimens • Accepted specimen volume range is 3.0–10.0 mL

Incubation Subsystem of BACTEC

This incubation subsystem is designed to maintain the temperature of the contents of any culture vial in any station at 35.0 ± 1.5°C. The temperature is achieved by forced air convection over the media vials. Incubation hardware includes blowers, heaters, and temperature sensors. The incubation system heats air according to the temperature set point and actual temperature measurements.

Vial Agitation in BACTEC

Vial stations are agitated so that their fluid contents achieve a homogeneous distribution of nutrients and microbial by-products. Vials are arranged in separate row modules that are coupled by a gang linkage to a motor. The motor causes each row module to agitate over a range of 0–20° relative to the horizontal.

Specimens

• Blood units to be tested

Reagents/Glassware/Miscellaneous

• Disposable syringe
• Bunsen burner
• Glass slide
• Gram stain reagents
• Microscope

PROCEDURE

Sample Collection at Blood Center Facility

Blood samples are typically completely drawn from a satellite tube attached to a blood bag, thoroughly mixed, and washed with a disinfectant such as povidone-iodine solution or methanol. A typical sample volume is 8–10 mL. We recommend inoculating this blood sample into a BACTEC vial and bringing it to the test laboratory as soon as possible.

Remove the flip-off cap from the top of the BACTEC vial and inspect the vial for cracks, contamination, excessive cloudiness, and bulging or chipped stoppers. Do not use if defects are found. Wipe the septum with alcohol prior to inoculation and aseptically inject or directly withdraw 8–10 mL of sample per vial. This medium is designed for use with blood samples ranging from 3 to 10 mL. If the sample is <3 mL, the recovery is not as good as for larger volumes.

Sterility Testing in Microbiology Section

The vials inoculated with the blood specimens are placed in the BACTEC instrument at the earliest possible for incubation and evaluation. If shifting of inoculated vials in BACTEC instrument is delayed leading to visible growth, it should not be tested in the *BACTEC* fluorescent series instrument, and rather it should be subcultured, appropriately stained, and treated as a presumptively positive bottle.

Vials which are placed and entered into the instrument will be automatically tested every 10 minutes for the duration of the testing protocol period which can be extended to 14 days as provided under the IP 2022 [Drugs and Cosmetic Rules, 1945 (Schedule F, Part XII-B), Government of India].

Positive vials are determined by the *BACTEC* fluorescent series instrument and identified as such. The sensors in the bottles do not appear visually different between positive and negative vials, but the *BACTEC* fluorescent series instruments can detect the difference in fluorescence. At the end of the test period, if a negative *BACTEC* Mycosis-IC/F vial is visually positive (i.e., Septal bulge and/or turbid), it must be subcultured, appropriately stained, and treated as a presumptive positive. Positive vials should be subcultured and stained appropriately. In most cases, microorganisms are found and can be notified to the in-charge of the blood center in advance.

Subculturing: Prior to subculturing, hold the vial in an upright position, and place an alcohol swab over the septum. To depressurize the vial, insert a sterile needle fitted with an appropriate filter or pledget through the alcohol wipe and septum. The needle should be removed after the pressure is released and before the sample is taken from the vial for subculture. Needle insertion and withdrawal should be done in a straight line, avoiding twisting movements.

All positive vials/bottles are smeared and subcultured on blood agar and MacConkey agar. If Gram-stained smear shows budding yeast cells, Sabouraud's dextrose agar plates are also used for subculture.

INTERPRETATION

Positive or negative culture vial/bottles are determined by decision-making software contained in the BACTEC microbial detection system, which signals a culture vial/bottle either positive or negative.

QUALITY CONTROL

Quality control requirements must be performed in accordance with applicable state and national regulatory or accreditation requirements and in-house laboratory standard quality control procedures/protocols.

The user should comply with the quality standards set out in the Drugs and Cosmetics Rules, 1945, IP 2022, in conjunction with the Manual of Blood Transfusion Medical Technology, Director General of Health Services (DGHS), Ministry of Health and Family Welfare, Government of India 3rd Edition, 2022 and National Standards for Blood Centers by NACO.

Culture tubes should be used within the expiration date and should be free of cracks or defects. Anything deemed unusable should be properly disposed of. A quality control certificate is typically provided by the manufacturer with each carton of media showing test organisms containing American Type Culture Collection (ATCC™) cultures specified in the Clinical and Laboratory Standards Institute (CLSI) Standard, Quality Control for Commercially Produced Microbial Culture Media. Each shipment of media should be performance tested using positive and negative control vial tests. Positive vials should be inoculated with 0.1 mL of 0.5 McFarland standard of *Candida albicans* (ATCC 10231) or *Candida (Torulopsis) glabrata*. This vial must be logged into the BACTEC instrument and tested together with the noninoculated vial. Inoculated vials should be recognized as positive by the device within 72 hours. Negative control vials must remain negative to pass the proficiency test. This also ensures that media have not been exposed to improper storage or shipping conditions prior to arrival at the laboratory. If any of these vials do not give the expected results, do not use the medium.

SAFETY

- All specimens used in testing should be considered potentially infectious.
- General precautions should be followed for the handling and disposal of blood/blood components during and after adminis-tration.
- Use soap for regular hand washing.
- Use biohazard disposal techniques.

Note: There are various "sterility testing systems" available commercially with their respective claims and counterclaims over the others. The user is free to opt and use any such available systems after proper validation of the test method in compliance to the IP 2022 and seeking approval from the respective regulatory authorities [FDA/CDSCO (Central Drugs Standard Control Organisation), etc.]. Authors have discussed one of such sterility testing systems available in the market (by BACTEC) as an alternative method to the one prescribed in IP 2022, without any recommendations for its use by the institutions performing such tests. Blood centers and other similar institutions are advised to adopt the most suitable system after complying with the statutory provisions.

CHAPTER 72

Biomedical Waste Management

SCOPE AND APPLICATION

This standard operating procedure (SOP) defines the guidelines for segregation, handling, storage, transportation, and disposal of various kinds of biomedical waste (BMW) as per Biomedical Waste Management Rules, 2016 and Biomedical Waste Management (Amendment) Rules, 2018.

This SOP applies to all employees who generate, collect, receive, store, transport, treat, dispose of, or handle any form of biomedical waste. These regulations do not apply to radioactive waste, Municipal Solid Wastes (MSW), lead-acid batteries, hazardous waste, electronic waste, and hazardous microorganisms.

RESPONSIBILITY

It is the responsibility of laboratory technicians and laboratory attendants working in the blood center to dispose of the waste generated to ensure proper and safe management of BMW. The technical supervisor in a blood center needs to cross-check the method of disposal and documentation.

MATERIALS REQUIRED

- 1% sodium hypochlorite (NaOCl) solution
- Color-coded plastic buckets
- White (translucent) puncture-, leak-, and tamper-proof containers
- Red, yellow, blue, and black plastic bags

TYPES OF WASTE GENERATED, ON-SITE SEGREGATION, AND STORAGE

Segregation at source is the most important step toward a well-functioning waste management system. Mixing infectious and noninfectious waste makes it impossible to separate, increasing risk for all involved. When mixed, noninfectious also becomes infectious. The Biomedical Waste Management Rules 2016 color-coded waste segregation is shown in **Table 1**.

Blood Center Section-wise Waste Segregation, Disinfection, and Disposal Procedures

The different types of waste materials generated in various areas of the blood center and their segregation in various color-coded plastic bags are given in **Tables 2 to 6**.
1. *Blood donation centers and blood donation camps*
2. *Component preparation laboratory*
3. *Transfusion transmissible infections (TTI) testing*
4. *Pretransfusion testing lab*
5. *Apheresis section*

CLEANING OF GLASSWARE

Glassware include slides, tubes, and pipettes. The cleaning steps are as follows:
1. Immerse in water immediately after use to avoid desiccation of serum proteins.
2. Then soak in a mild detergent solution (e.g., Labolene) or chromic acid mixture for 1 hour or overnight.
3. Rinse thoroughly under running water.
4. Rinse with distilled water.
5. Keep upside down in a wire basket.
6. Dry in a hot air oven at 150°C.

DUTIES OF OCCUPIER (HOSPITAL/HEALTHCARE FACILITY)

- Pretreatment of laboratory waste, microbiological waste, blood samples, and blood bags by on-site disinfection and sterilization is to be carried out as directed by the World Health Organization (WHO) or National AIDS Control Organisation (NACO).
- Major incidents such as needlestick injuries, broken mercury thermometers, fire-related mishaps, and explosions while handling BMW must be reported, along with any corrective actions

performed, and the details must be documented in Form I accident reporting form—*see rule 4(o), 5(i), and 15(2) of BMW Rules, 2016.*

- According to the regulations, hospitals or healthcare facilities (residents) are not allowed to set up on-site treatment and disposal facilities if there is a "common biomedical waste treatment facility" (CBMWTF) available within 75 km.
- Under the Biomedical Waste Management (Amendment) Rules 2018, it is the responsibility of the occupant to provide a safe and ventilated place to store the segregated BMW on the premises.
- The use of chlorinated plastic bags (except blood bags) and gloves should be phased out.
- All medical personnel and everyone involved in the handling of BMW must also be trained in accordance with these regulations.
- Establish a barcode system for sending BMW bags or containers containing BMW off-site and provide immunization against hepatitis B and tetanus for workers who handle BMW.
- All healthcare workers must use personal protection equipment (PPE) in the form of gloves and masks while handling BMW.
- At the time of filing an annual report to Central Pollution Control Board (CPCB), accidents such as needlestick injuries and spills need to be reported.
- Mercury is a dangerous element having serious adverse effects on healthcare workers and environment, and its use has been banned in hospitals on the orders of the Government of India.
- Waste management is the responsibility of everyone who is directly or indirectly involved in its handling in any form as its mismanagement has wider medical, ethical, legal, ecological, and social implications.

Table 1: Color coding for waste segregation of biomedical waste. (*For color version of Bins, see Plates 12*)

Category	Type of bag or container to be used	Type of waste
Yellow	Yellow-colored nonchlorinated plastic bags	• Human anatomical waste • Animal anatomical waste • Soiled waste • Expired or discarded medicines • Chemical waste • Chemical liquid waste • Discarded linen, mattresses, beddings contaminated with blood or body fluid

Continued

Continued

Category	Type of bag or container to be used	Type of waste
		• Microbiology, biotechnology, and other clinical laboratory waste: Blood bags, laboratory cultures, stocks or specimens of microorganisms, live or attenuated vaccines, human and animal cell cultures used in research, industrial laboratories, production of biological, residual toxins, dishes and devices used for cultures
Red	Red-colored nonchlorinated plastic bags or containers	• Contaminated waste (recyclable) • Wastes generated from disposable items such as tubing, bottles, intravenous tubes and sets, catheters, urine bags, syringes (without needles and fixed-needle syringes and vacutainers with their needles cut), and gloves
White	Puncture-proof, leak-proof, tamper-proof containers	Waste sharps including metals
Blue	Cardboard boxes with blue-colored marking	• Broken or discarded and contaminated glass, including medicine vials and ampoules, except those contaminated with cytotoxic wastes • Metallic body implants

Table 2: Blood donation centers and blood donation camps.

Type of waste	Treatment at source and segregation
Copper sulfate solution	Disinfected by 1% sodium hypochlorite (30 minutes hold time) and discharged after treatment in effluent treatment plant
Lancets, needles, and Luer lock adapter needles in the diversion pouch system	White puncture-proof, leak-proof, tamper-proof containers
Cotton swabs used to clean phlebotomy site and cotton swabs applied to phlebotomy area postdonation	Yellow biomedical waste (BMW) disposal bags
Empty phlebotomy bags without needle	Yellow BMW disposal bags
Expired medicine	Yellow BMW disposal bags
Gloves	Red BMW disposal bags

Table 3: Component preparation laboratory.

Type of waste	Treatment at source and segregation
Buffy coat bags (if available) and diversion pouches and blood unit unfit for transfusion	Autoclave in autoclave bags and discard in yellow BMW disposal bags
Blood bag tubings	Discard in red BMW disposal bags
Leaked blood bags, waste bags generated at the time of preparation of washed red cell, IUT procedure	Autoclave in autoclave bags and discard in yellow BMW disposal bags
Tube segments, lab-side leukofilters	Autoclave in autoclavable disposable bags and discard in red BMW disposal bags
Evacuated blood collection tubes (nonreactive only)	Discard in red BMW disposal bags
(BMW: biomedical waste; IUT: intrauterine transfusion)	

DUTIES OF A COMMON BIOMEDICAL WASTE TREATMENT FACILITY OPERATOR

- Inform the State Pollution Control Board (SPCB) of any significant incidents, such as fire-related mishaps or explosions that occurred when managing BMW, as well as the corrective measures that were implemented by recording in Form I.
- BMW to be collected from healthcare facilities.

Table 4: Transfusion transmissible infections (TTI) testing.

Type of waste	Treatment at source and segregation
Blood bags (reactive) with all satellite bags of components and the sample evacuated tubes (reactive)	Autoclave in autoclavable disposable bags and segregated in yellow BMW bags (at 121°C at 15 psi pressure for minimum 30 minutes hold over time—autoclaved in separate runs in autoclave bag and segregated in yellow BMW bags)
RPR cards	Treated with sodium hypochlorite solution and discarded in red BMW disposal bag
Rapid diagnostic test (card/cassette/strips)	Treated with sodium hypochlorite solution and discarded in red BMW disposal bag
Used plastic bottles with positive controls for ELISA and CLIA and cardiolipin antigens used in RPR test	Treated with sodium hypochlorite solution and discarded in red BMW disposal bag
ELISA microplates and microtips	Treated with sodium hypochlorite solution (immerse in 1% sodium hypochlorite for 30 minutes) and discarded in red BMW disposal bag
Used plastic bottles of chemiluminescence (CLIA) reagent bottles	Treated with sodium hypochlorite solution and discarded in red BMW disposal bag
Hitachi cups	Treated with sodium hypochlorite solution and discarded in red BMW disposal bags
Waste solutions generated using ELISA and CLIA	Disinfected with 1% sodium hypochlorite solution (30 minutes hold over time) and to be discharged in sewerage drain
Peripheral blood films	Treated with sodium hypochlorite solution and segregated in puncture-proof, leak-proof, tamper-proof containers with blue lining Or Cardboard boxes with blue lining
Evacuated blood collection tubes (nonreactive only)	Discard in red BMW disposal bags
(BMW: biomedical waste; CLIA: chemiluminescence immunoassay; ELISA: enzyme-linked immunosorbent assay; RPR: rapid plasma reagin)	

Table 5: Pretransfusion testing lab.

Type of waste	Treatment at source and segregation
Tissue paper contaminated with blood, cotton swabs, gauzes contaminated with blood	Segregated in yellow biomedical waste (BMW) bags
Syringes (without needle), gel cards, microtiter plates, microtips, empty reagent plastic bottles, gloves	Segregated in red BMW bags
Scalpels and blades	White puncture-proof, leak-proof, tamper-proof containers
Slides, antisera vials, beakers, test tubes, and glass pipettes if not *reusable*	White puncture-proof, leak-proof, tamper-proof containers with blue lining Or Cardboard boxes with blue lining
Gloves	Red BMW disposal bag
Blood/plasma/serum in glass containers, e.g., sample vials/ test tubes/slides/glass pipettes to be reused	• Discard in plastic bins containing 1% sodium hypochlorite solution for 30 minutes minimum (10,000 ppm chlorine) to liquid effluent treatment plant • Glassware treated in chromic acid, washed thoroughly, and dried in hot air oven (at temperature 100°C, holding period of 60 minutes)

Table 6: Apheresis section.

Type of waste	Treatment at source and segregation
Used apheresis and therapeutic plasma exchange kits, bags for saline, ACD, waste	Autoclave in autoclavable disposable bags and discard in red BMW disposal bags
Plastic tray of apheresis and TPE kits	Red BMW disposal bags
IV fluid bottles, IV set, BT set, three-way cannula, fistula tubings (without needles)	Red BMW disposal bags

Continued

Continued

Type of waste	Treatment at source and segregation
Used injections, vials, and empty albumin bottles	White puncture-proof, leak-proof, tamper-proof containers with blue lining Or Cardboard boxes with blue lining
Empty phlebotomy bags	Yellow BMW disposal bags
Plasma collection bag (waste) generated during TPE	Autoclave in autoclavable disposable bag and discard in yellow BMW disposal bags
Needles	Destroyed in needle destroyer and discarded in white puncture-proof, leak-proof, and tamper-proof containers
Gloves	Red BMW disposal bag

(ACD: acid-citrate-dextrose; BMW: biomedical waste; BT: blood transfusion; IV: intravenous; TPE: therapeutic plasma exchange)

- Introduction of barcodes and global positioning systems to address regulations on disposal of Biomedical Waste.
- To aid healthcare facilities in staff training.
- Upgrading of present incinerators and meeting of standards for secondary chamber.

ANNUAL REPORT FROM OCCUPIER AND COMMON BIOMEDICAL WASTE TREATMENT FACILITY

- Every CBMWTF operator or occupier must submit an annual report to the designated authorities by June 30 of each year.
- The prescribed authority is responsible for compiling, reviewing, and analyzing the report, and finally submitting to the Central Pollution Control Board (CPCB) annually (on or before July 31).
- The CPCB must submit a report to the Ministry of Environment, Forest, and Climate Change by the end of every year.
- The websites of the occupier, SPCB, and CPCB must all have access to the annual reports.

ACCIDENT REPORTING BY HEALTHCARE FACILITIES OR COMMON BIOMEDICAL WASTE TREATMENT FACILITY

The designated person is required to notify others immediately in the event of a serious accident and provide a report outlining the corrective measures taken within 24 hours.

OPERATIONAL GUIDELINES FOR WASTE MANAGEMENT IN BLOOD CENTER

- The specified segregation point should be as close as possible to the generation point.
- Appropriate consumables are used for segregation, e.g., good quality and appropriately sized containers, chlorine-free plastic bags, needle cutters, and safety boxes.
- The specifications and color coding specified in the biomedical rules are strictly adhered to.
- Do not fill the waste collection container more than three-fourth. Empty at least once a day.
- The containers are kept closed all the time.
- Always dispose of sharps yourself.
- Do not pass used sharps directly from person to person.
- Procedures involving risk of exposure should minimize the risk of injury by ensuring that the operator has the best possible visibility. Position the donor, adjust the light source, and control bleeding.
- Do not reseal, bend, or break single-use needles.
- Place needles and syringes in the designated containers immediately after use.
- Do not dispose of used sharps in other waste containers.
- Make sure that there is no secondary handling, pilferage of recyclables, or inadvertent scattering or spillage by animals, and the BMW from such place or premises is directly transported into the CBMWTF.
- Pursuant to the Biomedical Waste Management (Amendment) Rules, 2018:
  - Laboratory waste, blood samples, and blood bags should be pretreated on-site by disinfection or sterilization in accordance with the WHO guidelines for the safe management of medical waste and the WHO Blue Book (2014) and then sent to the CBMWTF for final disposal.
  - A barcode system must be established for off-site shipping of bags or containers containing BMW or for further treatment and disposal in accordance with guidelines issued by the CPCB.
  - The use of chlorinated plastic bags (except blood bags) and gloves has been phased out.

HANDLING SYRINGES AND NEEDLES (TABLE 7)

The do's and don'ts for handling syringes and needles are shown in **Table 7.**

Table 7: Do's and Don'ts for handling syringes and needles.	
Do's	**Don'ts**
Pass syringes and needles in a tray, preferably cut with needle cutter	Never pass syringes and needles directly to the next person
Put needles and syringes in 1% sodium hypochlorite solution if needle cutter is not available	Do not bend or break used needle with hand
Remove cap of needle near the site of use	Never test the fineness of the needle's tip before use with bare or gloved hand
Pick up open needle from tray/drum with forceps	<ul><li>Never pick up open needles by hands</li><li>Suck air in and out of syringe and needle after removing from packing and before taking blood sample</li><li>Never recap used needles</li></ul>

DOCUMENTATION

Enter the time, type of material, quantity, and reason for disposal in the waste management/disposal register with initials of designated technician.

According to the guidelines, records of generation, collection, reception, storage, transit, treatment, and disposal of BMW must be kept at least for 5 years.

CHAPTER 73

Autoclaving of Blood Bags after Use

SCOPE AND APPLICATION

As blood bags are a class of hazardous materials that require pretreatment under the Biomedical Waste Management (Amendment) Regulations, 2018, this standard operating procedure (SOP) covers the safe disposal of blood bags [transfusion transmitted infection (TTI) reactive and others]. This SOP describes the method of autoclaving to disinfect or sterilize blood bags on site according to the World Health Organization (WHO) guidelines and WHO Blue Book (2014) for the safe management of medical waste before sending to a common biomedical waste disposal facility for final disposal.

RESPONSIBILITY

It is the responsibility of the blood center technician to get the used blood bags autoclaved under the supervision of technical supervisor/nursing staff.

MATERIALS REQUIRED

- *Autoclave*: Autoclaves should be dedicated to BMW disinfection and processing.
- *Blood bags*:
  - Expired
  - Under-/overcollected
  - Reactive after screening for mandatory testing
  - Blood unsuitable for transfusion due to any other reason (hemolyzed, used for quality control purpose, clotted, leaked, etc.)
  - Blood bag received back for the follow-up of adverse transfusion reaction
  - Unused blood returned from wards
  - Other potentially infected materials

PROCEDURE

1. Enter the particulars of the blood bag in the register, e.g., donor ID, collection date, expiry date, screening report, reason for disposal.
2. Keep the bag in vertical position (standing) in polybags.
3. Follow universal precautions while handling the blood bags.
4. Autoclave the container with bags at 121°C and 15 lbs of pressure for 60 minutes.
5. After autoclaving, hand over the container with the bag to the authorized person of the BMW management and take his signature as per hospital policies for disposal in accordance with the BMW rules.
6. Maintain the entries in the register.
7. Type 4 chemical indicators are used with every cycle, and record of this is maintained in the BMW record register. The chemical indicator indicates that a temperature of 121°C has been achieved within the autoclave. The chemical indicators change color when exposed to a temperature of 121°C.
8. Biological indicators are used once a month. Biological indicator vials contain spores of *Bacillus stearothermophilus*, a microorganism that is inactivated by exposure to saturated steam at 121°C for at least 20 minutes. Autoclaves used to process biological waste are evaluated monthly with biological indicators, and vials are sent to the microbiology department for processing. A report from the department of microbiology is documented.

Note: Medical waste is not considered properly processed unless time, temperature, and pressure indicators show that the required time, temperature, and pressure have been achieved during autoclaving. If, for any reason, the temperature or pressure gauges indicate that the required temperature, pressure, or time has not been achieved, remove all medical waste until the correct temperature, pressure, and time has been achieved. The load should be reautoclaved.

DOCUMENTATION

1. Enter the date, time, and status of blood bags into waste management/disposal register with initials of the designated technician/nursing staff countersigned by the technical supervisor/authorized official.
2. Paste the steam type 5 chemical indicator after use in the record register.
3. Enter the screening status of blood/blood components.
4. Maintain the autoclave log sheet as per **Annexure 73.1**.
5. Take the signature of person of the Common Biomedical Waste facility to whom autoclaved biomedical waste material is handed over on proper receipt.

ANNEXURE 73.1

NAME OF BLOOD CENTER: ....

LICENSE NO.: ....

AUTOCLAVE MAKE/MODEL ....

AUTOCLAVE SERIAL NO ....

AUTOCLAVE LOG SHEET

LOGO

Date	Cycle start time	Cycle end time	Waste (type)	Weight (kg)	Temperature	Pressure	Chemical indicator (class IV)	Affix chemical indicator used	Biological indicator used?	Operator signature	Comments
							☐ Pass ☐ Fail		☐ Yes ☐ No		
							☐ Pass ☐ Fail		☐ Yes ☐ No		
							☐ Pass ☐ Fail		☐ Yes ☐ No		
							☐ Pass ☐ Fail		☐ Yes ☐ No		
							☐ Pass ☐ Fail		☐ Yes ☐ No		

CHAPTER 74

Management of Blood Spill

SCOPE AND APPLICATION

This standard operating procedure (SOP) describes the method to disinfect the blood spillage area to avoid the spread of infection and to prevent the personnel from exposure to infection which has a potential of transmitting through blood.

RESPONSIBILITY

In case of spilling of blood or blood components by a person, he/she should take the responsibility to adhere to the standard recommendations as per Centers for Disease Control and Prevention (CDC)/World Health Organization (WHO) guidelines for containment, thereby preventing any inadvertent accident to the healthcare staff or visitors/patients. If spilled material is unscreened and/or positive for transfusion transmitted infection (TTI), extra precaution should be taken. Laboratory attendant/housekeeping staff is to clean the surface under the guidance of blood center staff.

MATERIALS REQUIRED

A spillage kit should be kept in donor section, immunohematological laboratory, TTI laboratory, and component area so that all the equipment for dealing with spillage is available at one place. This kit contains:
- Written spill cleanup procedures
- A "Do Not Enter" door sign with universal "biohazard" symbol
- Protective equipment, including latex gloves, protective clothing, disposable plastic apron, safety glasses, boots, and respiratory protection
- Tape or marking device to mark off the spill area
- Absorbent material (cotton balls, incontinent pads, or paper towels)

- Suitable disinfectant supplies (check expiry date and dilution) which deliver available chlorine at 10,000 ppm (1%)
- Scoop and scraper
- Sharps collector and forceps for picking up broken glass or sharps (dustpan and broom)
- Appropriate containers or autoclave bags (disposal bags—leakproof, autoclavable, and labeled with a biohazard symbol)

PROCEDURE

Small Spills of Blood or Other Potentially Infectious Materials (OPIM) (Up to 30 cm or 30 mL)

1. Put on appropriate protective clothing such as gloves and gowns.
2. Remove any sharp objects with forceps and discard as contaminated sharps in puncture-proof container.
3. Spills on the floor, of infected or potentially infected material, should be covered with paper towel/blotting paper/newspaper.
4. Pour an adequate amount of 1% sodium hypochlorite solution and cover the area of spillage with paper towel/blotting paper/ newspaper on the area.
5. Keep it covered for at least 20–30 minutes.
6. Remove the soaked paper towel/blotting paper/newspaper with gloved hands and discard in a yellow bag.
7. Use the same 1% sodium hypochlorite disinfectant solution to wipe over the area likely to have been contaminated.
8. Carefully mop up the spill and disinfection solution, and transfer all contaminated materials for disposal.
9. Remove protective clothing and wash hands.

Major Spills (>30 cm or 30 mL)

1. Evacuate immediately.
2. Remove the laboratory gown, any other garment or shoes which are suspected of being contaminated, and place in a biohazard bag.
3. If spilled material has soaked through the laboratory clothing, take a complete body shower.
4. Close the door and place a "Do Not Enter" sign on the door.
5. Stay out of the spill area for at least 30 minutes.
6. Notify the area supervisor of the spill.

Procedure

1. *Assemble a cleanup team consisting of three people*: One to observe and direct the cleanup procedure and the other two to carry out the procedure.

2. Wear protective clothing, respiratory protection, goggles, and boots.
3. Place absorbent material such as paper towels, cotton balls, or incontinent pads.
4. Put 1% sodium hypochlorite over the spill.
5. Leave it for at least 20 minutes to effect disinfection. Discard in a yellow bag.
6. Carefully remove any sharp objects with forceps and dispose of as contaminated sharps.
7. Take a disposable scrapper (e.g., cardboard) or scoop, and starting from outside, wipe toward the center of the spill.
8. Dispose of into a yellow biohazard bag.
9. Using the same 1% sodium hypochlorite disinfectant solution, wash the affected area.
10. Also, by using the same 1% sodium hypochlorite disinfectant solution, wipe the surrounding area.
11. Each member of the cleanup team has to decontaminate boots, discard respirator, gloves, and gowns, and decontaminate clothing.
12. Replenish spillage kit.
13. Ventilate and make area safe.
14. Complete the hazard incident report in accordance with biomedical waste management committee regulations.

DOCUMENTATION

- Enter the time and nature of material spilled in the waste management/disposal register with the initials of the designated staff/technician.
- Enter the screening status of spilled blood/blood components.

Management of Sharps/Needlestick Incidents and Other Exposure Cases

SCOPE AND APPLICATION

Needlestick injuries are common in medical settings and can lead to serious complications. The introduction of universal precautions and safety-focused needle designs has reduced needlestick injuries, but they still occur. Awareness of needlestick injuries began to grow shortly after human immunodeficiency virus (HIV) was identified in the early 1980s. However, today, the main concern after a needlestick injury is not HIV, but hepatitis B or C. Guidelines have been established to help healthcare facilities treat needlestick injuries and when to initiate postexposure HIV prevention and prophylaxis. These guidelines apply to all healthcare professionals to adopt a responsible attitude in preventing and reporting such incidents of coming into contact with patients' blood or body substances. Accurate documentation is essential to the success of this policy. Therefore, the objectives of this standard operating procedure (SOP) are as follows:

- Identify the epidemiology of needlestick injuries.
- Identify risk factors for needlestick injuries.
- Describe the risk of acquiring bloodborne pathogens as a result of a needlestick injury.
- To discuss the importance of improving care coordination among multidisciplinary team members to improve outcomes for patients with needlestick injuries.

RESPONSIBILITY

The Hospital Infection Control Committee (HICC) is responsible for safely treating needlestick injuries that occur during caregiving. Personnel are responsible for reporting all incidents of contaminated needle-related exposures and taking appropriate action to prevent them from occurring in the first place and are responsible for adherence to safe practices, including provision of resources to identify appropriate use of personal protective equipment (PPE), immunization programs in place, and incidents reviewed, and follow-up actions, where necessary, are taken. Training should be provided on all aspects of managing needlestick injuries. The infection control team is responsible for ensuring that training is available, and staff are required to attend such training.

- *Infection control officer (ICO):*
  - Must conduct audit every month.
  - Keep records (incidents and actions taken).
  - Make postexposure prophylaxis (PEP) drugs available in hospitals.
  - Make sure that PPE are provided at all concerned locations.
  - All needlestick injuries, including the exposure code and the HIV status code, must be reported to the state AIDS (acquired immunodeficiency syndrome) control societies.
  - Ensure compliance with hospital infection control practices.
- *Infection control nurse (ICN):*
  - Conduct daily rounds in all departments.
  - Ensure that puncture-proof containers (PPCs) are available at all locations. Make sure that all needles are disposed of in puncture-resistant containers.
  - Ensure disposal of PPC as per biomedical waste (BMW) policy.
  - All needlestick injuries should be reported to the infection control team/committee.
  - Notify all nonconformities to ICO/chairperson.
  - Keep track of all hospital incident reports.

PROCEDURE AND GUIDELINES

The following steps must be taken to manage needlestick and exposure incidents:
1. Reporting
2. First aid administration
3. Risk assessment and exposure assessment
4. Source assessment
5. Management of the exposed person
6. Follow-up with the injured person and healthcare worker (HCW)

Reporting

The exposure should be reported to the appropriate authorities [ICO/ medical officer (MO)], and the situation should be treated as an emergency. Prompt reporting is essential as HIV PEP (post-exposure prophylaxis) is recommended in some cases and should be started as soon as possible, preferably within hours.

First Aid Administration

- *Needlestick, sharps injury, or cut:*
  - Wash needlesticks and cuts with soap and water.
  - Cover with a waterproof bandage if necessary.
  - Do not reflexively put your pricked finger in your mouth.
  - Carefully dispose of sharps in an approved sharps container.
- *Splash to mucous membrane, conjunctiva, or nonintact skin:*
  - Immediately wash exposed areas with water.
  - If possible, identify the source of the information.

No topical antiseptic creams or disinfectants are required.

Risk Assessment and Evaluation of Exposure

A risk assessment requires knowledge of the following:
- Infectious status and/or risk factors for infection in the baseline patient, if identified. Identification of potential risk factors in baseline patients includes:
  - Transfusion/injection with blood products.
  - Birth in areas where HIV, hepatitis B or hepatitis C are endemic.
  - Close contacts infected with HIV, hepatitis B or hepatitis C.
- Individuals with identified risk factors for HIV, hepatitis B, or hepatitis C, e.g., intravenous drug users, susceptibility of the HCW to blood-borne viruses, e.g., previous immunization history and immune status
- Type of exposure and bodily fluid. The risk of transmission of postexposure blood-borne viral infections is increased with percutaneous exposures, including:
  - Serious injuries to medical personnel
  - Visible blood on equipment that caused injury
  - Devices previously inserted in the veins or arteries of the source patient (e.g., phlebotomy needles rather than suture needles)
  - Devices previously used in a patient with a high viral load (e.g., advanced disease)
  - Volume of blood injected or exposed to mucous membrane or skin involving:
    - o Prolonged contact with blood
    - o Large areas of skin where skin integrity is compromised

The HCW should be assessed for its potential to acquire HIV based on the type of biological material involved, route of injury, and severity of exposure as indicated in **Flowchart 1**.

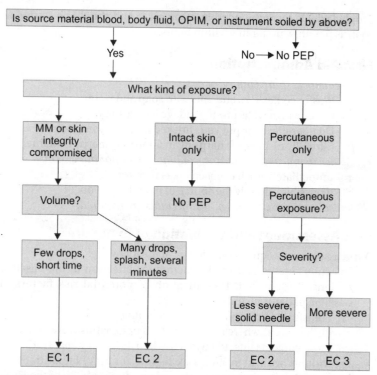

FLOWCHART 1: Algorithm for determination of exposure code (EC) of an injury. (MM: mucous membrane; OPIM: other potentially infectious material; PEP: postexposure prophylaxis)

Susceptibility to hepatitis B is determined by hepatitis B virus (HBV) vaccination status and antibody response.

Baseline HCW for hepatitis B surface antigen (HBsAg), antihepatitis C virus (HCV), and anti-HIV should be performed within 72 hours of injury.

Cost (Staff)

The hospital bears all costs, including all laboratory tests and treatments recommended by HICC.

Recommendation of the same will be provided by the HICC.

Evaluation of the Source

The clinical team will be notified as soon as the original patient is known. A clotted blood sample will be taken after written consent and pretest

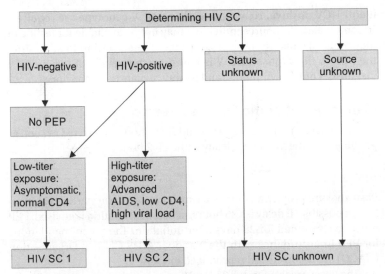

FLOWCHART 2: Determining human immunodeficiency virus (HIV) source status code (SC).

(AIDS: acquired immunodeficiency syndrome; PEP: postexposure prophylaxis)

consultation. Urgent testing for HBsAg, hepatitis C antibody, and HIV antibody is done. Confidentiality is maintained in HIV testing.

The HIV testing is routinely performed in many circumstances such as antenatal patients and patients who are referred for surgery. Patients being tested will not be discriminated against, and their information will be kept confidential. *An HIV test will not affect the current and future life and other insurance policies as long as the person is HIV-negative.* HIV source status code is determined by the algorithm shown in **Flowchart 2**.

If HIV antibody is positive, assess absolute lymphocyte count/ CD4 count, viral load, history of antiretroviral (ARV) therapy (ART), and clinical stage of the disease. Drug resistance should be pursued whenever possible in patients with poor treatment outcomes.

Confidentiality

Patients being tested will not be discriminated against and their information will be kept confidential and confidentiality will be maintained in testing. If the HIV test is positive, refer the case to a specialist for further treatment. The HIV status of source patients and injured persons must be kept strictly confidential. If the source is HBsAg-positive, hepatitis B e-antigen (HBeAg) testing is required, and if anti-HCV positive, HCV viral load and HCV genotype are required. In some cases, the source individual may not be available for testing or may refuse testing. In these circumstances, the decision to administer the PEP to the exposed HCW is based on the details of her medical diagnosis, clinical symptoms, and history of high-risk behavior.

Management of the Exposed Person

For optimal effect, the PEP for HIV and HBV should be started as soon as possible after the incident, ideally within 1–2 hours.

HIV

Postexposure prophylaxis for HIV exposure should be started within an hour if possible. If delay is >36 hours, expert consultation is advised. PEP must be continued for 28 days after initiation. The recommendations for PEP in accordance with the National AIDS Control Organisation (NACO) are followed and reproduced in **Table 1**.

The latest recommended ARV regimens by the Government of India (GOI) are shown in **Table 2**.

The first dose of PEP should be administered immediately (preferably within 2 hours) and at most within 72 hours after exposure. The duration of a PEP is 28 days, regardless of regimen.

HBV

Following the guidelines in **Table 3**, PEP for HBV should be started immediately, preferably within 24 hours, but in any case, within 7 days.

	Table 1: Postexposure prophylaxis (PEP).	
Exposure code (EC)	**Human immunodeficiency virus status code**	**PEP recommendation**
1	1	PEP may not be warranted
1	2	Consider basic regimen (negligible risk)
2	1	Recommend basic regimen (most exposures are in this category)
2	2	Recommended expanded regimen
3	1 or 2	Recommended expanded regimen
2 or 3	Unknown	If setting suggests a possible risk (epidemiological risk factors) and EC is 2 or 3, consider basic regimen

Table 2: Latest recommended antiretroviral (ARV) regimens.

Exposed person	Preferred regimen for postexposure prophylaxis	Alternate regimen (if the preferred regimen is not available or contraindicated)
Adolescents and adults (>10 years of age and >30 kg of weight)	Tenofovir (300 mg) + lamivudine (300 mg) + dolutegravir (300 mg) (FDC: One tablet OD)	Tenofovir (300 mg) + lamivudine (300 mg) (FDC: One tablet OD) + lopinavir (200 mg) + ritonavir (50 mg) (two tablets BD) Or tenofovir (300 mg) + lamivudine (300 mg) (FDC: One tablet OD) + efavirenz (600 mg) (FDC: One tablet OD)
Children (≥6 years old or ≥20 kg weight)	Zidovudine + lamivudine (dosage as per weight band) + dolutegravir (50 mg) (one tablet OD)	If Hb <9 g/dL: Abacavir + lamivudine (dosage as per weight band) + dolutegravir (50 mg) (one tablet OD)
Children (<6 years old or <20 kg weight)	Zidovudine + lamivudine + lopinavir/ ritonavir (dosage as per weight band)	If Hb <9 g/dL: Abacavir + lamivudine + lopinavir/ ritonavir (dosage as per weight band)

(FDC: fixed-dose combination; Hb: hemoglobin)

Table 3: Postexposure prophylaxis in hepatitis B virus (HBV).

Hepatitis B prophylaxis for reported sharps, injuries, and mucocutaneous exposure to blood or other body fluids

Hepatitis B status of the healthcare worker (HCW)	Hepatitis B status of source		
	Negative	Unknown/ untested	Positive
One dose or less of hepatitis B vaccine prior to exposure	Initiate/ continue course of hepatitis B vaccine	Accelerated course of hepatitis B vaccine	Accelerated course of hepatitis B vaccine and one dose of hepatitis B immunoglobulin*

Continued

Continued

Hepatitis B status of the healthcare worker (HCW)	Hepatitis B status of source		
	Negative	Unknown/ untested	Positive
Two or more doses of hepatitis B vaccine prior to exposure but antibody titer not known	• Check HbsAb titer • Complete course of hepatitis B vaccine if indicated	• Check HbsAb titer • Complete course of hepatitis B vaccine if indicated	Check HbsAb titer. One dose of hepatitis B vaccine immediately and complete the course as indicated
Responder to hepatitis B vaccine (anti-HBs >10 IU/L)	No action required	Booster dose of hepatitis B vaccine may be required depending on risk assessment	A booster dose of hepatitis B vaccine is required
Known nonresponder to hepatitis B vaccine (titer <10 IU/L, 2 months after course or booster)	Consider reimmunization if not previously attempted	Following risk assessment, consider two doses of HBIG 1 month apart and consider reimmunization if not previously attempted[†]	Two doses of HBIG 1 month apart and consider reimmunization if not previously attempted[†]

*An accelerated vaccination course consists of vaccinations at 0, 1, and 2 months intervals. An HCW receiving accelerated vaccination may need the fourth dose in 12 months. 1.0 mL of hepatitis vaccine contains 20 µg of hepatitis B surface antigen (HBsAg) protein and is administered intramuscularly into the deltoid region of adults and children 10 years and older.

[†]HBIG should be provided as soon as possible and within 48 hours after exposure if deemed appropriate by risk assessment. The dose of HBIG is 1,000–2,000 IU intramuscularly for adults. There are 0.5 mL ampoules containing 1,000 IU and 1 mL vials containing 2,000 IU.

(HBIG: hepatitis B immunoglobulin; HbsAb: hepatitis B surface antibody)

The dose of hepatitis B immunoglobulin (HBIG) is 32–48 IU/kg body weight intramuscularly for children.

People who lack HBsAg or who have not previously developed an adequate immune response to the virus may be susceptible to infection. Hepatitis B immunoglobulin may be offered for immediate protection from serious HBV exposure. A risk-assessed, individualized approach is recommended for the management of HCWs with unknown susceptibility to hepatitis B vaccination, persons of unknown source, and patients with unknown source of hepatitis. In such circumstances, the HBV status of the source and/or exposed should be determined when appropriate and available. It can be treated in the same way as a personal injury.

A comprehensive strategy to eliminate transmission of HBsAg is the universal vaccination of HCW.

HCV

There are currently no PEP recommendations for HCV immunoglobulins and oral anti-HCV direct-acting antiviral (DAA) agents. One of the reasons DAAs were not used in his PEP setting is that in most cases, these agents can provide complete cures even when long-standing chronic HCV infection is detected. Conversely, in the case of occupational exposure to HIV, PEP can prevent subsequent infections that cannot be cured by direct-acting therapies. PEP use would treat about 100% of HCV-exposed persons where as only 2% become infected after occupational exposure, so a "wait-and-wait" strategy may actually make the most sense as the DAA is expensive and the "wait-and-wait" strategy is cost-effective. A basic anti-HCV antibody test is guaranteed to the source. Perform anti-HCV and alanine aminotransferase (ALT) baselines of exposed HCW. For management, efforts should be made to determine the original HCV genotype.

Management of the Source Person

The clinical team will be notified as soon as the original patient is known. Clotted blood samples are taken after written consent. Urgent testing for HBsAg, hepatitis C antibody, and HIV antibody is done.

If the source is HBsAg positive, one needs hepatitis B core antigen (HBcAg). If anti-HCV positive, HCV viral load and HCV genotype are required. If HIV antibody positive, assess absolute lymphocyte count/CD4 count, viral load, history of ART, and clinical stage of disease. Drug resistance should be pursued whenever possible in patients with poor treatment outcomes. In some cases, the source individual may not be available for testing or may refuse testing. In these circumstances, the decision to administer the PEP to the exposed HCW is based on the details of her medical diagnosis, clinical symptoms, and history of high-risk behavior.

Consent and Cost (Source Person)

In order to give informed consent to receive PEP, the exposed person (the client) must be provided with sufficient information about what PEP is and the risks and benefits of PEP. Clearly, a PEP is not required.

If viral markers have not been performed on any patient, the attending consultant/physician must obtain consent to do the same. Consent is signed by the patient, and if the patient is unable to give consent for any reason, the patient's relatives give consent. Patients bear the cost of laboratory tests. Many people feel anxiety after exposure. Exposed persons must be informed of the risks and measures to be taken. This helps alleviate some of the anxiety. Some clients may require additional professional psychological support.

Follow-up of the Healthcare Worker or Injured Person

HBV

Healthcare workers exposed to hepatitis should be tested for HBsAg at 6 weeks, 1 month, and 3 months. If vaccinated, she will be tested for anti-HBs antibodies 2 months after her last vaccination. However, anti-HBs cannot be done if HBIG has been administered within the last 6–8 weeks. Healthcare professionals are advised to use barrier measures (condoms) and refrain from donating blood/plasma/organs/tissues or semen during the follow-up period.

HCV

Healthcare workers exposed to HCV should be tested for anti-HCV and ALT 4–6 weeks and at least 4–6 months after exposure. Confirm repeat positive anti-HCV enzyme-linked immunosorbent assay (ELISA) results with additional tests [recombinant immunoblot assay (RIBA) or HCV ribonucleic acid (RNA)]. HCV RNA test, if available, can be done in 4 weeks for early diagnosis. HCV seroconversion occurs silently. Therefore, tests should be performed on a regular basis. If seroconversion has occurred, genotyping can aid in treatment planning. Genotypes 2 and 3 are more responsive to pegylated interferon therapy in combination with ribavirin than genotype 1.

Currently, a combination of 400 mg sofosbuvir and 100 mg velpatasvir in one tablet orally once daily with or without food is given. It is used as a pan-genotypic drug to treat all the HCV genotypes. The duration of treatment is 12 weeks in both naive and experienced patients and in patients with compensated cirrhosis. Previously, multiple RNA polymerase chain reaction (PCR) tests were required. However, current guidelines only require two tests before treatment (6 months) and 12 weeks after treatment to confirm a sustained virologic response (SVR). The patients with mild degree of liver fibrosis (0–2) fibrosis do not require specific additional follow-up after SVR, whereas those with advanced degree of liver fibrosis (3–4) are monitored by a hepatologist/gastroenterologist and screening for hepatocellular carcinoma is recommended.

HIV

Exposed individuals should be followed for at least 6 months and asked to report signs/symptoms of acute HIV seroconversion. Blood sampling should be done immediately after injury, 6 and 12 weeks after exposure, and when there is evidence of seroconversion. If you test positive for HIV at any time within 12 weeks, your healthcare provider should refer you to a doctor for treatment. Long-term follow-up of 12 months is recommended for HCWs exposed to coinfectious sources of HIV–HCV. The liver function test (LFT), including complete blood count, serum creatinine, and enzymes, should be repeated every other week. Blood glucose levels should be monitored in patients receiving protease inhibitors. Urinalysis should be included if the patient is receiving indinavir (IDV) or tenofovir disoproxil fumarate (TDF). Blood donation, semen and organ/tissue donation, and sexual intercourse should be discouraged. Additionally, HCW women should not breastfeed the infant during the follow-up period. Individuals starting chemoprevention should also be monitored for drug toxicity and tolerability.

The needlestick/sharps/body fluid exposure protocol is summarized as follows:

1. Do not compress the area; let it bleed freely. Wash the injured area with soap and water (antiseptics can be used).
2. Check patient's HIV, HBsAg, and HCV status. If not known, it should be ascertained.
3. Promptly go to the *casualty/triage* or other designated location within the healthcare facility.
4. Must complete and sign a needlestick injury protocol with the help of the MO/ICO and provide pretest consultations to employees.
5. Inform Infection control nurse during working hours and on next day after working hours.
6. Give blood samples for HIV, HBsAg, and HCV in the laboratory (needlestick injury protocol form should be shown).
7. Follow-up treatment regimen within 2 hours of the injury.
   a. If source patient is HIV (+), start ARV treatment as soon as possible as per the hospital protocol.
   b. If the patient is HBsAg (+), initiate treatment as per protocol.
8. If source patient is HIV (–), then test for HCW is repeated after 6 and 12 weeks. If source patient is HBsAg (–), the HCW should be observed, and anti-HBs levels should be monitored.
9. If the source is unknown, then follow the protocol as per 7a and b.

TRAINING AND PREVENTION

Patients and most HCWs who work with biological samples, are at risk of incidental exposure to blood and bloodborne pathogens, prolonged exposure to blood or other infectious liquids, even on intact skin/mucous membranes, cuts with contaminated blood collection equipment and wounds with blood-filled hollow needles.

Workplace exposure controls must be instilled in all healthcare providers from the time of hiring through regular HICC training of all employees on safe work practices and sharps use.

An important component of any needlestick injury prevention program is the education and training of HCWs in sharps and sharps injury prevention as part of continuing medical education. Healthcare professionals need to know how to properly use, assemble, disassemble, and dispose of needles. An effective program should address all aspects of needlestick injuries, including injury risks, potential hazards, and recommended precautions.

All HCWs should be vaccinated against hepatitis B (three doses) and have antibody levels checked 1 month after completing the three doses (anti-HBs). The protective antibody level is 10 IU/L or more.

DOCUMENTATION

Documentation of exposure is essential. ICN will be responsible for maintaining record of the following:
- All needlestick injuries
- Reason of injury
- Treatment in emergency department
- Follow-up treatment of staff member
- All other documentations

SAFE WORK PRACTICES

Infection control and occupational hygiene measures to prevent transmission of blood-borne viruses:
- Wash your hands regularly and practice basic hygiene.
- Cover existing wounds and skin lesions with a waterproof dressing.
- Appropriate disposable gloves should be worn at all times where contact with blood, saliva, or other bodily fluids is known or expected.
- Avoid invasive procedures if you have chronic skin lesions on your hands.
- Avoid contamination by wearing suitable personal protective clothing.

- Protect the mucous membranes of the eyes, mouth, and nose from blood splashes.
- Care should be taken when opening the ampoule to avoid small cuts.
- Nondisposable clothing contaminated with blood should be placed separately for washing.
- Establish safe procedures for handling and disposal of needles and other sharp objects.
- Do not sheath the needle by hand.
- All needles, syringes, and sharps should be disposed of in puncture-resistant sharps disposal bins.
- Bins for sharps objects should not be filled above the specified level. They must be carefully sealed before disposal.
- Be aware that you are responsible for its immediate disposal, while using sharps objects.
- Establish sterilization and disinfection procedures for instruments and instruments.
- Apply 1% of sodium hypochlorite before wiping. If the spill is in the ground, granules of sodium hypochlorite should be used.
- Establish safe disposal procedures for contaminated waste.
- Ensure vaccination of all clinical and laboratory workers for hepatitis B. There is no vaccine against bad habits.

MANAGEMENT OF SHARPS INSTRUMENTS

Remember the following seven points:

1. Special care must be taken in the use and disposal of sharps instruments.
2. People who use sharp objects should dispose them safely.
3. Always dispose of used sharps directly into an approved sharps disposal container.
4. Do not sheath the needle by hand.
5. Do not overfill sharps container—replace when three-fourths is full.
6. If possible, bring a sharps disposal box to the point of use.
7. Report all sharps injuries to the ICO/MO immediately.

Know the rules: Become a sharps safety stickler

Regulatory Guidelines

CHAPTER 76

Scenario of Regulations for Blood Centers

INTRODUCTION

Blood transfusion services (BTS) are an important part of the National Health Service, and there is no substitute for human blood and its components. Advances in transfusion technology have necessitated tighter control of the quality of blood and its components. Most developed countries have evolved blood banking systems in all aspects of donor management, blood storage, grouping and crossmatching, contagious disease testing, rational use of blood, and distribution. Although governments have full responsibility for their blood programs, some countries delegate all or part of the administration of BTS to appropriate nongovernmental organizations (NGOs) operating on a nonprofit basis, e.g., Red Cross Society. When NGOs are given this responsibility, governments should formally recognize them and give them clear mandates to formulate the country's blood policy. It is important to consider policy decisions to implement appropriate regulations or necessary health service functions to ensure quality transfusion services and safe blood.

Blood transfusion services in India are one of the most important elements of the healthcare system. As this is a life-saving procedure, blood and blood components must be of safe and consistent quality to be clinically effective. The Government of India has taken necessary steps from time to time to improve the standards of whole human blood and its constituents by making necessary changes to legislation and creating additional regulatory functionaries. The Central Government, through the Drug Controller General of India, has developed comprehensive legislation to ensure better quality control systems for the collection, storage, testing, and distribution of blood and its components. The Government of India has made many changes to the Drugs and Cosmetics Act, 1940 and the underlying Drugs and Cosmetics Rules, 1945 to meet the latest standards.

To ensure adequate availability of blood and transfusion facilities in the first referral unit, the Drugs and Cosmetics Rules, 1945, was amended to provide blood storage facilities for First Referral Unit (FRU)/ Community Health Center (CHC)/Primary Health Center (PHC). The primary purpose of this amendment was to make human blood and components available to these hospitals without taking license under the Drugs and Cosmetics Rules, 1945.

Furthermore, in order to check growth and mushrooming of stand-alone blood centers in the country, the Government of India further amended the Drugs and Cosmetics Rules, 1945, by prohibiting such stand-alone blood centers to apply for grant/renewal of blood center.

NATIONAL BLOOD POLICY

National blood policies and frameworks aim to ensure the implementation of blood and blood component quality and safety standards. The Government of India notified the National Blood Policy on blood safety in 2002. The objective of this policy was to provide safe and sufficient blood and its components to the masses in distress. The primary purpose of this policy was to obtain blood from unpaid regular blood donors by the blood centers. The policy also addresses various issues related to technical, personal, research and development, and elimination of profiteering by blood centers. The directive also stipulates that no new licenses will be issued to private sector stand-alone blood centers and that renewals of such blood centers require thorough scrutiny.

The National Standards for Indian Blood Centers and BTS was first published in 2007 and has become the primary technical guidance for Indian Blood Centers and BTS. Due to numerous developments and advancements in the field of blood banking, National Blood Transfusion Council (NBTC) and National AIDS Control Organisation (NACO) initiated their review and revision, and second editions of the NBTC standards have been released recently in 2022 to improve and standardize blood transfusion practices in the country with the approval of Ministry of Health and Family Welfare, Government of India.

SCENARIO OF LEGAL FRAMEWORK

Whole human blood is included in the definition of "drug" under Section 3(b) of the Drugs and Cosmetics Act, 1940. Accordingly, medical institutions/organizations involved in the collection, storage, processing, distribution, etc., of whole human blood, blood drawn from donors, and/or the preparation, storage, and distribution of blood components are subject to provisions of the Drugs and Cosmetics Act, 1940, and Drugs and Cosmetics Rules, 1945.

With the onset of prevalence of acquired immunodeficiency syndrome (AIDS) virus spread in the country, human immuno-deficiency virus (HIV) testing of all blood units, before they were issued for transfusion, was mandated by the Government of India's Ministry of Health and Family Welfare through a notification no. GSR-600(E) dated 27.08.2002 issued under Drugs and Cosmetics Act, 1940, and Rules, 1945.

The Government of India further notified the Department of Microbiology, National Institute of Infectious Diseases, Delhi; National Institute of Virology, Pune; and Center for Advanced Research in Virology, Christian Medical College, Vellore, to test for HIV antibodies with respect to human blood and its components, under Rule 3-A(6) of the Drugs and Cosmetics Rules, 1945.

Following report by a Management Consultancy Firm (M/s A.F Ferguson & Co.) in 1990 highlighting various deficiencies in the quality control of blood and blood components, etc., and the concerns expressed in various forums and Parliament, the Drugs and Cosmetics Rules, 1945, were again amended (Rule 68A, Part XB and Part XII-B of Schedule F) in 1992–1993. These amendments provided for Central License Approving Authority (CLAA) to obtain uniformity in blood centers licensing throughout the country, and some other amendments were made. The Government of India notified the Drugs Controller General of India as the CLAA to approve licenses for blood, blood components and blood products, intravenous (IV) fluids, vaccines, sera, etc., to achieve uniformity nationwide.

The Government of India further amended existing provisions for proper and safe functioning and operation of blood centers and/or the preparation of blood components by inserting Part XII-B under Schedule F of the Drugs and Cosmetics Rules, 1945 vide notification G.S.R. 28(E) dated January 22, 1993. Various requirements such as accommodations, technical staff, equipment, and instruments for operation of blood center as well as for blood components were included in this part. Licensing authorities under the provisions of the Drugs and Cosmetics Rules, 1945 are authorized to issue licenses to operate blood centers in the country. For the first time, it included legal restrictions for organizing blood donation camps outdoors. Only licensed designated Regional Blood Transfusion Centers, licensed Government blood centers, and the Indian Red Cross were permitted to organize offsite blood collection camps as provided in Part XII-B of Schedule F of the Drugs and Cosmetics Rules, 1945. Standards for "whole human blood," "packaged red blood cells," and "platelet concentrate" were prescribed in the Indian Pharmacopoeia.

The Government of India, further in the year 2002, put regulatory control on "in vitro diagnostic devices" which were being used for testing of human blood and its components for HIV, hepatitis B surface antigen (HBsAg), and hepatitis C virus (HCV) by notifying these devices as "drug" under Section 3(b) of the Drugs and Cosmetics Act, 1940. The National Institute of Biologicals, Noida, was notified central drug testing laboratory to carry out testing of these notified drugs including blood grouping sera under Rule 3-A(8) of Drugs and Cosmetics Rules, 1945. The procedure of making applications by a blood center, fees to be paid for grant/renewal of license, and conditions of license to be followed after grant/renewal of licenses were inserted under the added Rules. Good manufacturing practices, standard operating procedures, validation of equipment, etc., were also made mandatory for the blood centers.

The Government of India further amended Rule 122-G of Drugs and Cosmetics Rules, 1945, by inserting Rule 122-G(2) vide notification G.S.R. 733(E) dated December 21, 2005, in order to check the growth and mushrooming of stand-alone blood centers in the country. Further amendments to allow transfer of whole human blood and components from one blood center to another and holding of outside blood donation camps by private hospital-based blood centers (not by stand-alone blood centers) were made in the year 2020 by the Government of India keeping in view the larger public interest. The number of personnel required for such outside blood donation camps has also been expressly provided in Drugs and Cosmetics Rules, 1945. The requirement of a blood center counselor was also made mandatory for those blood centers holding outside blood donation camps and provisions for counseling area in the blood center. Provisions for identified area for quality control of components have also been made in the component area. Even the condition of captive consumption limit of 2,000 units of blood/blood components in the FRU, CHC, PHC, and/or any hospital for blood storage center was also scrapped to promote such centers in the country. "Blood Center" was also renamed as "Blood Center" as per the notification number G.S.R. 166(E) dated March 11, 2020. Simultaneously, various types of apheresis procedures and categories of blood components were defined under the blood components part discussed in details in the preceding chapters. Scope of the requirement for blood donation was also widened by amending "Criteria for Blood Donors" under heading "H" of the Schedule F attached to the Drugs and Cosmetics Rules, 1945. The Government of India has recently issued guidelines to allow transfer of surplus plasma by the blood centers to the indigenous fractionators for use in manufacturing of blood products so as to make proper use of such human tissue.

Guidelines for recovery of 'Processing Charges' for the blood centers were issued on February 12, 2014 for the blood and blood components by the Government of India, which has recently been revised on 14.6.2022 to achieve uniformity and transparency throughout the country.

CHAPTER 77

Drugs and Cosmetics Rules, 1945 (Part X-B)

REQUIREMENTS FOR THE COLLECTION, STORAGE, PROCESSING AND DISTRIBUTION OF WHOLE HUMAN BLOOD, HUMAN BLOOD COMPONENTS BY BLOOD CENTERS; MANUFACTURE OF BLOOD PRODUCTS AND COLLECTION, PROCESSING, TESTING, STORAGE, BANKING AND RELEASE OF UMBILICAL CORD BLOOD STEM CELLS

RULE 122-EA OF THE DRUGS AND COSMETICS RULES, 1945

Definitions

1. In this Part and in the Forms contained in Schedule A and in Part XII-B, Part XII-C and Part XII-D of Schedule F, unless there is anything repugnant in the subject of context—
   a. "apheresis" means the process by which blood drawn from a donor, after separating plasma or platelets or leukocytes, is re-transfused simultaneously into the said donor;
   b. "autologous blood" means the blood drawn from the patient for re-transfusion into himself later on;
   c. "blood" means and includes whole human blood, drawn from a donor and mixed with an anticoagulant;
   d. Blood Center is an authorized premises in an organization or institution as the case may be, for carrying out all or any of the operations including collection, apheresis, processing, storage and distribution of blood drawn from donors or received from another licensed Blood Center and for preparation, storage and distribution of blood components;

e. "blood component" means a drug prepared, obtained, derived or separated from a unit of blood drawn from a donor;

f. "blood product" means a drug manufactured or obtained from pooled plasma of blood by fractionation, drawn from donors;

f(a). "cord blood bank" means a place or organization or unit for carrying out and responsible for operation of collection, processing, testing, banking, selection and release of cord blood units;

g. "donor" means a person who voluntarily donates blood after he has been declared fit after a medical examination, for donating blood, on fulfilling the criteria given hereinafter, without accepting against donated blood in return any consideration in cash or kind from any source, but does not include a professional or a paid donor;

Explanation: For the purpose of this clause, benefits or incentives like pins, plaques, badges, medals, commendation certificates, time-off from work, membership of blood assurance program, gifts of little or intrinsic monetary value shall be construed as consideration.

h. "leukapheresis" means the process by which the blood drawn from a donor, after leukocyte concentrates have been separated is re-transfused simultaneously into the said donor;

i. "plasmapheresis" means the process by which the blood drawn from a donor, after plasma has been separated, is re-transfused during the same sitting into the said donors;

j. "plateletpheresis" means the process by which the blood drawn from a donor, after platelet concentrates have been separated, is re-transfused simultaneously into the said donor;

k. "professional donor" means a person who donates blood for a valuable consideration, in cash or kind, from any source, on behalf of the recipient-patient and includes a paid donor or a commercial donor.

l. "replacement donor" means a donor who is a family friend or a relative of the patient-recipient.

m. "umbilical cord blood" is the whole blood including Hematopoietic Progenitor Cells collected from placental and or Umbilical cord blood vessels after the umbilical cord have been clamped.

n. "erythrocytapheresis" means selective collection of one or two units of red cells from a donor or patient using a cell separator and re-transfusing the remaining blood into the donor or patient.

122-F. Form of application for licence for operation of Blood Center/processing of whole human blood for components/manufacture of blood products for sale or distribution

(1) Application for grant and/or renewal of licence for the operation of a blood center/processing of human blood for components/ manufacture of blood products (collection, processing, testing, storage, banking and release of umbilical cord blood stem cells) shall be made to the Licensing Authority appointed under Part VII in Form 27-C, or Form 27-E, or Form 27-F as the case may be, and shall be accompanied by licence fee of ₹ 6,000 and an inspection fee of ₹ 1,500 for every inspection thereof or for the purposes of renewal of licence.

Provided further that a licensee holding a license in Form 28-C, Form 28-E, or 28-F as the case may be, for operation of Blood Center/ processing of whole human blood for components/manufacture of blood products/collection, processing, testing, storage, banking and release of umbilical cord blood stem cells shall apply for renewal of license under sub-rule (1) before the expiry of the said license in Form 27-C, Form 27-E, or Form 27-F as the case may be, and he shall continue to operate the same till the orders on his application are communicated to him.

(2) A fee of ₹ 1,000 shall be paid for a duplicate copy of a license issued under this rule, if the original is defaced, damaged or lost.

(3) Application by a licensee to manufacture additional drugs listed in the application shall be accompanied by a fee of ₹ 300 for each drug listed in the application.

(4) On receipt of the application for the grant or renewal of such license, the Licensing Authority shall—

  (i) verify the statements made in the application form;

  (ii) cause the manufacturing and testing establishment to be inspected in accordance with the provision of Rule 122-I; and

  (iii) in the case the application is for renewal of license, call for informations of past performance of the licensee.

(5) If the Licensing Authority is satisfied that the applicant is in a position to fulfill the requirements laid down in the rules, he shall prepare a report to that effect and forward it along with the application and the license (in triplicate) to be granted or renewed, duly completed to the Central License Approving Authority:

Provided that if the Licensing Authority is of the opinion that the applicant is not in a position to fulfill the requirements laid down in these rules, he may, by order, for reasons to be recorded in writing, refuse to grant or renew the license, as the case may be.

(6) If, on receipt of the application and the report of the licensing authority referred to in sub-rule (5) and after taking such measures including inspection of the premises, by the Inspector, appointed by the Central Government under Section 21 of the Act, and/or along with the expert in the field concerned if deemed necessary, the Central License Approving Authority is satisfied that the applicant is in a position to fulfill the requirements laid down in these rules, he may grant or renew the license, as the case may be:

Provided that if the Central License Approving Authority is of the opinion that the applicant is not in a position to fulfill the requirements laid down in these rules he may, notwithstanding the report of the Licensing Authority, by order, for reasons to be recorded in writing, reject the application for grant or renewal of license, as the case may be, and shall supply the applicant with a copy of the inspection report.

122-G. Form of license for the operation of a Blood Center/processing of whole human blood for components and manufacture of blood products/collection, processing, testing, storage, banking and release of umbilical cord blood stem cells and the conditions for the grant or renewal of such license

(1) A license for the operation of a Blood Center or for processing whole human blood for components and manufacture of blood products/ collection processing, testing, storage, banking and release of umbilical cord blood stem cells shall be issued in Form 28-C or Form 28-E or Form 28-F or Form 26-G or Form 26-I, or Form 26-J, as the case may be. Before a license in Form 28-C or Form 28-E Form or 28-F or Form 26-G or Form 26-I or Form 26-J, as the case may be is granted or renewed, the following conditions shall be complied with by the applicant:

    (i)   The operation of Blood Center and/or processing of whole human blood for components shall be conducted under the active direction and personal supervision of competent technical staff consisting of at least one person who is whole time employee and who is Medical Officer, and possessing:

       (a) Degree in Medicine MBBS having experience of working in Blood Center, not <1 year during regular service and also has adequate knowledge and experience in blood group serology, blood group methodology and medical principles involved in the procurement of blood or preparation of its components or both; or

   (b) Degree in Medicine MBBS with Diploma in Clinical Pathology or Diploma in Pathology and Bacteriology with 6 months experience in a licensed Blood Center; or

   (c) Degree in Medicine MBBS with Diploma in Transfusion Medicine or Diploma in Immunohematology or Blood Transfusion with 3 months experience in a licensed Blood Center; or

   (d) Doctor of Medicine Pathology or Diplomate of National Board Pathology with 3 months experience in a licensed Blood Center; or

   (e) Postgraduate degree in Transfusion Medicine—Doctor of Medicine Transfusion Medicine or Diplomate of National Board Transfusion Medicine, Doctor of Medicine Immunohematology and Blood Transfusion, the degree or diploma being from a University recognized by the Central Government or State Government.

Explanation: For the purposes of this condition, the experience in Blood Center shall not apply in the case of persons who are approved by the Licensing Authority or Central Licence Approving Authority or both prior to the commencement of the Drugs and Cosmetics (Second Amendment) Rules, 1999.

  (ii) The applicant shall provide adequate space, plant and equipment for any or all the operations of blood collection or blood processing. The space, plant and equipment required for various operations is given in Schedule 'F', Part XII-B and/or XII-C or XII-D.

 (iii) The applicant shall provide and maintain adequate technical staff as specified in Schedule 'F', Part XII-B and/or XII-C or XII-D.

 (iv) The applicant shall provide adequate arrangements for storage of whole human blood, human blood components and blood products.

  (v) The applicant shall furnish to the Licensing Authority, if required to do so, data on the stability of whole human blood, its components or blood products which are likely to deteriorate, for fixing the date of expiry which shall be printed on the labels of such products on the basis of the data so furnished.

(2) Applications for grant or renewal of license for operation of Blood Center or processing of Human Blood components shall be made by the Blood Center run by the Government, Indian Red Cross Society, Hospital, Charitable Trust or Voluntary Organization and Blood Center run by Charitable Trust or Voluntary Organization

need to be approved by a State or Union Territory Blood Transfusion Council as per procedure laid down in this regard by the National Blood Transfusion Council.

Explanation: For the purpose of this sub-rule, "renewal" shall include renewal of any license issued after the commencement of the Drugs and Cosmetics (Sixth Amendment) Rules, 2005.

122-H. Duration of license

An original license in Form 28-C or Form 28-E or 28-F or a renewed license in Form 26-G or Form 26-I or Form-26-J unless sooner suspended or cancelled shall be valid for a period of 5 years on and from the date on which it is granted or renewed.

122-I. Inspection before grant or renewal of license for operation of Blood Center, processing of whole human blood for components and manufacture of blood products

Before a license in Form 28-C or Form 28-E or Form 28-F is granted or a renewal of license in Form 26-G or Form 26-I or Form 26-J is made, as the case may be, the Licensing Authority or the Central License Approving Authority, as the case may be, shall cause the establishment in which Blood Center is proposed to be operated/whole human blood for components is processed/blood products are manufactured to be inspected by one or more Inspectors, appointed under the Act and/or along with the Expert in the field concerned. The Inspector or Inspectors shall examine all portions of the premises and appliances/equipments and inspect the process of manufacture intended to be employed or being employed along with the means to be employed or being employed for operation of blood center/processing of whole human blood for components/manufacture of blood products together with their testing facilities and also enquire into the professional qualification of the expert staff and other technical staff to be employed.

122-J. Report by Inspector

The Inspector or Inspectors shall forward a detailed descriptive report giving his findings on each aspect of inspection along with his recommendation in accordance with the provisions of Rule 122-I to the Licensing Authority or to the Central License Approving Authority.

122-K. Further application after rejection

If within a period of 6 months from the rejection of application for a license the applicant informs the Licensing Authority that the conditions laid down have been satisfied and deposits an inspection fee of ₹ 250, the Licensing Authority may after causing further inspection to be made, is satisfied that the conditions for the grant or renewal of a license have been complied with, shall grant or renew the license in Form 28-C or Form 28-E or Form-F:

Provided that in the case of a drug notified by the Central Government under Rule 68-A, the application, together with the inspection report and the Form of license (in triplicate to be granted or renewed), duly completed shall be sent, to the Central License Approving Authority, who may approve the same and return it to the Licensing Authority for issue of the license.

122-L. Delegation of powers by the Central License Approving Authority

The Central License Authority may, with the approval of the Central Government, by notification delegate his powers of signing licenses and any other power under rules to persons under his control having same qualifications as prescribed for Controlling Authority under Rule 50-A, for such areas and for such period as may be specified.

122-M. Provision for appeal to the State Government by a party whose license has not been granted or renewed

Any person who is aggrieved by the order passed by the Licensing Authority or Central License Approving Authority, as the case may be, may within 30 days from the date of receipt of such order, appeal to the State Government or Central Government, as the case may be and the State Government or Central Government may after such enquiry into the matter as it considers necessary and after giving the said person an opportunity for representing his view in the matter may pass such order in relation thereto as it thinks fit.

122-N. Additional information to be furnished by an applicant for license or by a licensee to the Licensing Authority

The applicant for the grant of license or any person granted a license under the Part shall, on demand, furnish to the Licensing Authority, before the grant of the license or during the period the license is in force, as the case may be, documentary evidence in respect of the ownership or occupation, rental or other basis of the premises, specified in the application for license or in the license granted, constitution of the firm or any other relevant matter, which may be required for the purpose of verifying the correctness of the statement made by the applicant or the licensee, while applying for or after obtaining the license, as the case may be.

122-O. Cancellation and suspension of licenses

(1) The Licensing Authority or Central License Approving Authority may for such licenses granted or renewed by him after giving the licensee an opportunity to show cause why such an order should not be passed by an order in writing stating the reason thereof, cancel a license issued under this part or suspend it for such period as he thinks fit, either wholly or in respect of some of the substances to which it relates or direct the licensee to stop collection, storage, processing, manufacture and distribution of the said substances and thereupon order the destruction of substances and stocks thereof in the presence of an Inspector, if in his opinion, the licensee has failed to comply with any of the conditions of the license or with any provision of the Act or Rules thereunder.

(2) A licensee whose license has been suspended or cancelled may, within 3 months of the date of the order under sub-rule (1) prefer an appeal against that order to the State Government or Central Government, which shall decide the same.

122-P. Conditions of license

A license in Form 28-C, Form 28-E, Form 28-F, Form 26-G, Form 26-I or Form 26-J shall be subject to the special conditions set out in Schedule F, Part XII-B and Part XII-C, XII-D, as the case may be, which relate to the substance in respect of which the license is granted or renewed and to the following general conditions, namely:

    (i)   (a)   The licensee shall provide and maintain adequate staff, plant and premises for the proper operation of a Blood Center for processing whole human blood, its components and/or manufacture of blood products.

           (b)   The licensee shall maintain staff, premises and equipment as specified in Rule 122-G. The licensee shall maintain necessary records and registers as specified in Schedule F, Parts XII-B and XII-C.

           (c)   The licensee shall test in his own laboratory whole human blood, its components and blood products and maintain records and registers in respect of such tests as specified in

Schedule F, Part XII-B and XII-C or XII-D. The records and register shall be maintained for a period of 5 years from the date of manufacture.

(d) The licensee shall maintain/preserve reference sample and supply to the Inspector the reference sample of the whole human blood collected by him in an adequate quantity to conduct all the prescribed tests. The licensee shall supply to the Inspector the reference sample for purpose of testing.

(ii) The licensee shall allow an Inspector appointed under the Act to enter, with or without prior notice, any premises where the activities of the Blood Center are being carried out for the processing of Whole Human Blood and/or Blood Products, to inspect the premises and plant and the process of manufacture and the means employed for standardizing and testing the substance.

(iii) The licensee shall allow an Inspector appointed under the Act to inspect all registers and records maintained under these rules and to take samples of the manufactured product and shall supply to the Inspector such information as he may require for the purpose of ascertaining whether the provisions of the Act and rules thereunder have been observed.

(iv) The licensee shall from time to time report to the Licensing Authority any changes in the expert staff responsible for the operation of a Blood Center/processing of whole human blood for components and/or manufacture of blood products and any material alterations in the premises or plant used for that purpose which have been made since the date of last inspection made on behalf of the Licensing Authority after the grant of the license.

(v) The licensee shall on request furnish to the Licensing Authority, or Central License Approving Authority or to such Authority as the Licensing Authority, or the Central License Approving Authority may direct, from any batch unit of drugs as the Licensing Authority or Central License Approving Authority may from time to time specify, sample of such quantity as may be considered adequate by such Authority for any examination and, if so required, also furnish full protocols of the test which have been applied.

(vi) If the Licensing Authority or the Central License Approving Authority so directs, the licensee shall not sell or offer for sale any batch/unit in respect of which a sample is, or protocols are furnished under the last preceding sub-paragraph until a certificate authorizing the sales of batch/unit has been issued to him by or on behalf of the Licensing Authority or the Central License Approving Authority.

(vii) The Licensee shall on being informed by the Licensing Authority or the Controlling Authority that any part of any batch/unit of the substance has been found by the Licensing Authority or the Central License Approving Authority not to conform with the standards of strength, quality or purity specified in these rules and on being directed so to do, withdraw, from sales and so far as may in the particular circumstances of the case be practicable recall all issues already made from that batch/unit.

(viii) No drug manufactured under the license shall be sold unless the precautions necessary for preserving its properties have been observed throughout the period after manufacture. Further no batch/unit manufactured under this license shall be supplied/distributed to any person without prescription of a Registered Medical Practitioner.

(ix) The licensee shall comply with the provisions of the Act and of these Rules and with such further requirements, if any, as may be specified in any Rules subsequently made under Chapter IV of the Act, provided that where such further requirements are specified in the Rules, these would come in force 4 months after publication in the Official Gazette.

(x) The licensee shall maintain an Inspector Book in Form 35 to enable an Inspector to record his impression and defects noticed.

(xi) The licensee shall destroy the stocks of batch/unit, which does not comply with standard tests in such a way that it would not spread any disease/infection by way of proper disinfection method.

(xii) All biomedical waste shall be treated, disposed of or destroyed as per the provisions of the Biomedical Wastes (Management and Handling) Rules, 1996.

(xiii) The licensee shall neither collect blood from any professional donor or paid donor nor shall he prepare blood components and/or manufacture blood products from the blood drawn from such a donor.

(xiv) The whole human blood and blood components may be transferred, under prescribed storage conditions, to another blood center which have facilities to store and monitor blood distribution.

(xv) The recipient blood center shall not further transfer units obtained from another blood center except to another blood storage center or a patient.

CHAPTER 78

Extract of Schedule K under the Drugs and Cosmetics Rules, 1945

Class of drugs	Extent and conditions of exemption
5B. Whole Human Blood I.P. and/or its components stored for transfusion by a First Referral Unit, Community Health Centre, Primary Health Centre and a Hospital	The provisions of Chapter IV of the Act and the Rules thereunder which require obtaining of a license for operation of a Blood Center or processing Whole Human Blood and/or its components, subject to the following conditions, namely: 1. The First Referral Unit, Community Health Centre, Primary Health Centre and/or any Hospital shall be approved by the State/Union Territory Licensing Authority after satisfying the conditions and facilities through inspection. 2. **Omitted** 3. The Whole Human Blood and/or its components shall be procured only from Government Blood Centre and/or Indian Red Cross Society Blood Centre and/or Regional Blood Transfusion Centre duly licensed. 4. The approval shall be valid for a period of two years from the date of issue unless sooner suspended or cancelled and First Referral Unit, Community Health Centre, Primary Health Centre or the Hospital shall apply for renewal to the State Licensing Authority three months prior to the date of expiry of the approval.

Continued

Continued

Class of Drugs	Extent and Conditions of Exemption
	5. The First Referral Unit, Community Health Centre, Primary Health Centre and/or any Hospital shall have the following technical staff for storage of blood or its components.
	a. A trained Medical Officer for proper procurement, storage and crossmatching of blood and/or its components. He/she shall also be responsible for identifying haemolysed blood and ensure non-supply of date expired blood or its components.
	b. A blood centre technician with the qualification and experience as specified in Part XII B of Schedule F or an experience laboratory technician trained in blood grouping and crossmatching.
	6. The First Referral Unit, Community Health Center Primary Health Center and Hospital shall have an area of 10 sq. metres. It shall be well lighted, clean and preferably air-conditioned. Blood centre refrigerator of appropriate capacity fitted with alarm device and temperature indicator with regular temperature monitoring shall be provided to store blood units between 2°C to 8°C and if the components are proposed to be stored, specialized equipments as specified in Part XII B of Schedule F shall also be provided.
	7. The First Referral Unit, Community Health Center, Primary Health Center and Hospital shall maintain records and registers including details of procurements of Whole Human Blood IP and/or blood components, as required under Part XII B of Schedule F.
	8. The First Referral Unit, Community Health Center, Primary Health Center and Hospital shall store samples of donor's blood as well as patient's sera for a period of seven days after transfusion.

Continued

Continued

Class of Drugs	Extent and Conditions of Exemption
30. Whole Human Blood collected and transfused by Centers run by Armed Forces Medical Services in border areas, small mid-zonal hospitals including peripheral hospitals, field ambulances, mobile medical units and other field medical units including blood supply units in border, sensitive and field areas.	All the provisions of Chapter IV of the Act and rules made thereunder which require them to be covered by a licence to operate a Blood Centre for collection, storage and processing of whole human blood for sale or distribution subject to the following conditions: i. These Centers shall collect, process and transfuse blood in emergent situations, which require life-saving emergency surgeries/or transfusion. ii. These Centers shall be under the active direction and personal supervision of a qualified Medical Officer, processing the qualifications and experiences specified in condition (i) of Rule 122-G. iii. Each blood unit shall be tested before use for freedom from HIV I and II antibodies, hepatitis B surface antigen, malarial parasites and other tests specified under the monograph "Whole Human Blood" in current edition of Indian Pharmacopoeia. iv. These Centers shall have adequate infrastructure facilities for storage and transportation of blood. v. The blood collected and tested by such Centers shall be transfused by the Center itself and may be made available for use of other peripheral Armed Forces hospitals or Centers during operational circumstances.

Schedule F (Part XII B) under the Drugs and Cosmetics Rules, 1945

REQUIREMENTS FOR THE FUNCTIONING AND OPERATION OF A BLOOD CENTRE AND/OR FOR PREPARATION OF BLOOD COMPONENTS

I. BLOOD CENTERS/BLOOD COMPONENTS

A. **GENERAL**
1. **Location and Surroundings:** The blood centre shall be located at a place which shall be away from open sewage, drain, public lavatory or similar unhygienic surroundings.
2. **Building:** The building(s) used for operation of a blood centre and/or preparation of blood components shall be constructed in such a manner so as to permit the operation of the blood center and preparation of blood components under hygienic conditions and shall avoid the entry of insects, rodents and flies. It shall be well lighted, ventilated and screened (mesh), wherever necessary. The walls and floors of the rooms, where collection of blood or preparation of blood components or blood products is carried out, shall be smooth, washable and capable of being kept clean. Drains shall be of adequate size and connected directly to a sewer, shall be equipped with traps to prevent back siphon-age.
3. **Health, Clothing and Sanitation of Staff:** The employees shall be free from contagious or infectious diseases. They shall be provided with clean overalls, headgears, footwears and gloves, wherever required. There shall be adequate, clean and convenient handwashing and toilet facilities.

B. ACCOMMODATION FOR A BLOOD CENTRE

A blood centre shall have an area of 100 square meters for its operations and an additional area of 50 square meters for preparation of blood components. It shall be consisting of a room each for:

1. Registration and medical examination with adequate furniture and facilities for registration and selection of donors
2. Blood collection (air-conditioned)
3. Blood component preparation (this shall be air-conditioned to maintain temperature between 20°C to 25°C)
4. Laboratory for blood group serology (air-conditioned)
5. Laboratory for blood transmissible diseases like hepatitis, syphilis, malaria, HIV-antibodies (air-conditioned)
6. Sterilization-cum-washing
7. Refreshment-cum-rest room (air-conditioned)
8. Store-cum-records
9. Counselling area with adequate privacy
10. Identified Quality Control area with component preparation area may be provided.

Notes:

1. The above requirements as to accommodation and area may be relaxed, in respect of testing laboratories and sterilization-cum-washing room, for reasons to be recorded in writing by the Licensing Authority and/or the Central License Approving Authority, in respect of blood centres operating in hospitals, provided the hospital concerned has a pathological laboratory and a sterilization-cum-washing room common with other departments in the said hospital.
2. Refreshments to the donor after phlebotomy shall be served so that he is kept under observation in the Blood Centre.

C. PERSONNEL

Every blood centre shall have following categories of whole time competent technical staff:

a. Medical Officer, possessing the qualifications specified in condition (i) of Rule 122-G.
b. Blood Centre Technician(s) possessing:
   (i) Diploma in Medical Laboratory Technology (DMLT) or Transfusion Medicine or Blood Bank Technology after 10+2 with one year experience in the testing of blood and/or its components in licensed Blood Centre; or
   (ii) Degree in Medical Laboratory Technology (MLT) or Blood Bank Technology with six months' experience in the testing of blood and/or its components in licensed Blood Centre; or

(iii) B.Sc. in Hematology and Transfusion Medicine with 6 months' experience in the testing of blood and/or its components in licensed Blood Centre; or

(iv) M.Sc. in Transfusion Medicine with 6 months' experience in the testing of blood and/or its components in licensed Blood Centre; or

(v) Post Graduate Diploma in Medical Laboratory Technology (PGDMLT)/Post Graduate Diploma in Medical Laboratory Science (PGDMLS) with six month's experience in the testing of blood and/or its components in licensed Blood Centre.

c. Registered Nurse(s)

d. Technical supervisor (where blood components are manu-factured), possessing:

(i) Diploma in Medical Laboratory Technology or Transfusion Medicine or Blood Bank Technology after 10+2 with 1 year experience in the testing of blood or its components or both in licensed Blood Centre; or

(ii) Degree in Medical Laboratory Technology or Blood Bank Technology with 6 month's experience in the testing of blood or its components or both in licensed Blood Centre; or

(iii) B.Sc. in Hematology and Transfusion Medicine with 6 months' experience in the testing of blood or its components or both in licensed Blood Centre; or

(iv) M.Sc. in Transfusion Medicine with 6 months' experience in the testing of blood or its components or both in licensed Blood Centre; or

(v) Post Graduate Diploma in Medical Laboratory Technology or Post Graduate Diploma in Medical Laboratory Science with 6 months' experience in the testing of blood or its components or both in licensed Blood Centre; or

(vi) Post Graduate Diploma in Transfusion Technology (PGDTT) approved by the Central Government or State Government with experience of 6 months in testing of blood or its components or both in licensed Blood Centre.

Blood Centre organizing blood donation camps shall have following whole time or part time counselling staff (Counsellor or Medical Social Worker) possessing:

(a) Master's degree in social work, sociology, psychology with 6 months of experience; or

(b) Degree in Science or Health Science with 1 year of experience; or

(c) Person with 10+2 having 3 years of experience in the field of counselling in the blood centres collecting blood <3,000 units per annum can share counsellor or medical social worker within the institution.

Notes:

1. The requirements of qualification and experience in respect of Technical Supervisor and Blood Centre Technician shall apply in the cases of persons who are approved by the Licensing Authority and/ or Central License Approving Authority after the commencement of the Drugs and Cosmetics (Amendment) Rules, 1999.

2. As regards the number of whole time competent technical personnel, the blood centre shall comply with the requirements laid down in the Directorate General of Health Services Manual.

3. It shall be responsibility of the licensee to ensure thorough maintenance of records and other latest techniques used in blood banking system that the personnel involved in blood banking activities for collection, storage, testing and distribution are adequately trained in the current Good Manufacturing Practices/ Standard Operating Procedures for the tasks undertaken by each personnel. The personnel shall be made aware of the principles of Good Manufacturing Practices/Standard Operating Procedures that affect them and receive initial and continuing training relevant to their needs.

D. **MAINTENANCE**

The premises shall be maintained in a clean and proper manner to ensure adequate cleaning and maintenance of proper operations. The facilities shall include:

1. Privacy and thorough examination of individuals to determine their suitability as donors.

2. Collection of blood from donors with minimal risk of contamination or exposure to activities and equipment unrelated to blood collection.

3. Storage of blood or blood components pending completion of tests.

4. Provision for quarantine, storage of blood and blood components in a designated location, pending repetition of those tests that initially give questionable serological results.

5. Provision for quarantine, storage, handling and disposal of products and reagents not suitable for use.

6. Storage of finished products prior to distribution or issue.

7. Proper collection, processing, compatibility testing, storage and distribution of blood and blood components to prevent contamination.

8. Adequate and proper performance of all procedures relating to plasmapheresis, plateletpheresis and leukapheresis.

9. Proper conduct of all packaging, labelling and other finishing operations.

10. Provision for safe and sanitary disposal of:
    i. Blood and/or blood components not suitable for use, distribution or sale.
    ii. Trash and items used during the collection, processing and compatibility testing of blood and/or blood components.

E. **EQUIPMENT**

Equipment used in the collection, processing, testing, storage and sale/distribution of blood and its components shall be maintained in a clean and proper manner and so placed as to facilitate cleaning and maintenance. The equipment shall be observed, standardized and calibrated on a regularly scheduled basis as described in the Standard Operating Procedures Manual and shall operate in the manner for which it was designed so as to ensure compliance with the official requirements (the equipment) as stated below for blood and its components.

Equipment that shall be observed, standardised and calibrated with at least the following frequencies:

S. No.	Equipment	Performance	Frequency	Frequency of calibration
1	Temperature recorder	Temperature recorder	Daily	As often as necessary
2	Refrigerated centrifuge	Observe speed and temperature	Each day of use	As often as necessary
3	Hematocrit centrifuge	....	....	Standardise before initial use, after repair or adjustments and annually
4	General lab. centrifuge	....	....	Tachometer, every 6 months
5	Automated typing blood	Observe controls for correct results	Each day of use	....
6	Haemoglobinometer	Standardize against cyanmethemoglobin standard	–ditto–	....
7	Refractometer or Urinometer	Standardize against distilled water	–ditto–	....

Continued

Continued

S. No.	Equipment	Performance	Frequency	Frequency of calibration
8	Blood container weighing device	Standardize against container of known weight	–ditto–	As often as necessary
9	Water bath	Observe temperature	–ditto–	–ditto–
10	Rh view box (wherever necessary)	–ditto–	–ditto–	–ditto–
11	Autoclave	Observe temperature	Each day of use	As often as necessary
12	Serologic rotators	Observe controls for correct results	–ditto–	Speed as often as necessary
13	Laboratory thermometers	....		Before initial use
14	Electronic thermometers	....	Monthly	....
15	Blood agitator	Observe weight of the first container of blood filled for correct results	Each day of use	Standardize with container of known mass or value before initial use, and after repairs or adjustments
16	Standard Certified Weight(s)	....	....	Once in a year
17	Equipment for Transfusion Transmitted Infection (TTI) laboratory like ELISA Plate Reader if ELISA is used or Chemiluminescence Immunoassay (CLIA) or Enzyme-linked Fluorescence Assay (ELFA)	....	Each run Each day of Use	Once in a year
18	Micropipettes if ELISA is used	....	....	Once in a year

F. **SUPPLIES AND REAGENTS**

All supplies and reagents used in the collection, processing, compatibility testing, storage and distribution of blood and blood components shall be stored at proper temperature in a safe and hygienic place, in a proper manner and in particular:

i. All supplies coming in contact with blood and blood components intended for transfusion shall be sterile, pyrogen-free, and shall not interact with the product in such a manner as to have an adverse effect upon the safety, purity, potency or effectiveness of the product.

ii. Supplies and reagents that do not bear an expiry date shall be stored in a manner that the oldest is used first.

iii. Supplies and reagents shall be used in a manner consistent with instructions provided by the manufacturer.

iv. All final containers and closures for blood and blood components not intended for transfusion shall be clean and free of surface solids and other contaminants.

v. Each blood collecting container and its satellite container(s), if any, shall be examined visually for damage or evidence of contamination prior to its use and immediately after filling. Such examination shall include inspection for breakage of seals, when indicated, and abnormal discoloration. Where any defect is observed, the container shall not be used or, if detected after filling, shall be properly discarded.

vi. Representative samples of each lot of the following reagents and/or solutions shall be tested regularly on a scheduled basis by methods described in the Standard Operating Procedures Manual to determine their capacity to perform as required:

S. No.	Reagents and solutions	Frequency of testing along with controls
1	Anti-human serum	Each day of use
2	Blood grouping serums	Each day of use
3	Lectin	Each day of use
4	Antibody screening and reverse grouping cells	Each day of use
5	Hepatitis test reagents	Each run
6	Syphilis serology reagents	Each run
7	Enzymes	Each day of use
8	HIV I and II reagents	Each run
9	Normal saline (LISS and PBS)	Each day of use
10	Bovine albumin	Each day of use

G. **GOOD MANUFACTURING PRACTICES (GMPs)/STANDARD OPERATING PROCEDURES (SOPs)**

Written Standard Operating Procedures shall be maintained and shall include all steps to be followed in the collection, processing, compatibility testing, storage and sale or distribution of blood and/ or preparation of blood components for homologous transfusion, autologous transfusion and further manufacturing purposes. Such procedures shall be available to the personnel for use in the areas concerned. The Standard Operating Procedures shall inter alia include:

1. a. Criteria used to determine donor suitability.
   b. Methods of performing donor qualifying tests and measurements including minimum and maximum values for a test or procedure, when a factor in determining acceptability;
   c. Solutions and methods used to prepare the site of phlebotomy so as to give maximum assurance of a sterile container of blood;
   d. Method of accurately relating the product(s) to the donor;
   e. Blood collection procedure, including in-process precautions taken to measure accurately the quantity of blood drawn from the donor;
   f. Methods of component preparation, including any time restrictions for specific steps in processing.
   g. All tests and repeat tests performed on blood and blood components during processing;
   h. Pretransfusion testing, wherever applicable, including precautions to be taken to identify accurately the recipient blood components during processing;
   i. Procedures of managing adverse reactions in donor and recipient reactions;
   j. Storage temperatures and methods of controlling storage temperatures for blood and its components and reagents;
   k. Length of expiry dates, if any, assigned for all final products;
   l. Criteria for determining whether returned blood is suitable for reissue;
   m. Procedures used for relating a unit of blood or blood component from the donor to its final disposal;
   n. Quality control procedures for supplies and reagents employed in blood collection, processing and re-transfusion testing;
   o. Schedules and procedures for equipment maintenance and calibration;
   p. Labelling procedures to safeguard its mix-ups, receipt, issues, rejected and in-hand;

q. Procedures for plasmapheresis, plateletpheresis and leukapheresis if performed, including precautions to be taken to ensure reinfusion of donor's own cells.

r. Procedures for preparing recovered (salvaged) plasma if performed, including details of separation, pooling, labelling, storage and distribution;

s. All records pertinent to the lot or unit maintained pursuant to these regulations shall be reviewed before the release or distribution of a lot or unit of final product. The review or portions of the review may be performed at appropriate periods during or after blood collection processing, testing and storage. A thorough investigations, including the conclusions and follow-up, of any unexplained discrepancy or the failure of a lot or unit to meet any of its specification shall be made and recorded;

2. A licensee may utilize current Standard Operating Procedures, such as the Manuals of the following organizations, so long as such specific procedures are consistent with, and at least as stringent as, the requirements contained in this Part, namely:

   i. Directorate General of Health Services Manual.

   ii. Other Organizations' or individual blood centre's manuals, subject to the approval of State Licensing Authority and Central License Approving Authority.

H. CRITERIA FOR BLOOD DONATION

Note: For details, please refer to Annexure 6.1 of Chapter 6 on DONOR Health Check-up.

I. GENERAL EQUIPMENT AND INSTRUMENTS

1. For Blood Collection Room

   i. Donor beds, chairs and tables: These shall be suitably and comfortably cushioned and shall be of appropriate size.

   ii. Bedside table

   iii. Sphygmomanometer and Stethoscope

   iv. Recovery beds for donors

   v. Refrigerators, for storing separately tested and untested blood, maintaining temperature between 2°C to 6°C with digital dial thermometer, recording thermograph and alarm device, with provision for continuous power supply

   vi. Weighing devices for donor and blood containers.

2. For Haemoglobin Determination

   i. Copper sulphate solution (specific gravity 1.053)

   ii. Sterile lancet and impregnated alcohol swabs

   iii. Capillary tube (1.3 × 1.4 × 96 mm for Pasteur pipettes)

     iv. Rubber bulbs for capillary tubings

     v. Sahli's hemoglobinometer/Colorimetric method

3. **For Temperature and Pulse Determination**

     i. Clinical thermometers

     ii. Watch (fitted with a seconds-hand) and a stop-watch.

4. **For Blood Containers**

     a. Only disposable PVC blood bags shall be used (closed system) as per the specifications of IP/USP/BP.

     b. Anticoagulants: The anticoagulant solution shall be sterile, pyrogen-free and of the following composition that will ensure satisfactory safety and efficacy of the whole blood and/or for all the separated blood components.

          i. Citrate Phosphate Dextrose Adenine solution (CPDA) or citrate Phosphate Dextrose Adenine-1 (CPDA-1) –14 mL solution shall be required for 100 mL of blood.

Note 1:

     i. In case of single/double/triple/quadruple blood collection bags used for blood component preparations, CPDA blood collection bags may be used.

     ii. Acid Citrate Dextrose solution (ACD with Formula-A). IP- 15 mL solution shall be required for 100 mL of blood.

     iii. Additive solutions such as SAGM, ADSOL, and NUTRICEL may be used for storing and retaining Red Blood Corpuscles up to 42 days.

Note 2: The licensee shall ensure that the anticoagulant solutions are of a licensed manufacturer and the blood bags in which the said solutions are contained have a certificate of analysis of the said manufacturer.

5. **Emergency Equipment/Items**

     i. Oxygen cylinder with mask, gauge and pressure regulator.

     ii. Five percent glucose or normal saline.

     iii. Disposable sterile syringes and needles of various sizes.

     iv. Disposable sterile IV infusion set.

     v. Ampoules of adrenaline, noradrenaline, mephentine, betamethasone or dexamethasone, metoclopramide injections.

     vi. Aspirin

6. **Accessories**

     i. Such as blankets, emesis basins, haemostats, set clamps, sponge forceps, gauze, dressing jars, solution jars, waste cans.

     ii. Medium cotton balls, 1.25 cm adhesive tapes.

     iii. Denatured spirit, tincture iodine, green soap or liquid soap.

     iv. Paper napkins or towels.

     v. Autoclave with temperature and pressure indicator.

vi. Incinerator

vii. Stand-by generator

7. **Laboratory Equipment**

i. Refrigerators for storing diagnostic kits and reagents, maintaining a temperature between 4°C to 6°C (± 2°C) with digital dial thermometer having provision for continuous power supply.

ii. Compound microscope with low and high power objectives.

iii. Centrifuge table model.

iv. Water bath: having range between 37°C to 56°C.

v. Rh viewing box in case of slide technique.

vi. Incubator with thermostatic control.

vii. Mechanical shakers for serological tests for syphilis.

viii. Hand lens for observing tests conducted in tubes.

ix. Serological graduated pipettes of various sizes.

x. Pipettes (Pasteur).

xi. Glass slides.

xii. Test tubes of various sizes/micrometre plates (U or V type)

xiii. Precipitating tubes 6 mm × 50 mm of different sizes and glass beakers of different sizes.

xiv. Test tube racks of different specifications.

xv. Interval timer electric or spring wound.

xvi. Equipment and materials for cleaning glass wares adequately.

xvii. Insulated containers for transporting blood, between 2°C to 10°C temperatures, to wards and hospitals.

xviii. Wash bottles.

xix. Filter papers.

xx. Dielectric tube sealer.

xxi. Plain and EDTA vials.

xxii. Chemical balance (wherever necessary).

xxiii. ELISA reader with printer, washer and micropipettes.

J. **SPECIAL REAGENTS**

i. Standard blood grouping sera Anti-A, Anti-B and Anti-D with known controls. Rh typing sera shall be in double quantity and each of different brand or if from the same supplier each supply shall be of different lot numbers.

ii. Reagents for serological tests for syphilis and positive sera for controls.

iii. Anti-human globulin serum (Coombs serum)

iv. Bovine albumin 22% enzyme reagents for incomplete antibodies.

v. ELISA or Rapid or RPHA test kits for hepatitis and HIV I and II.

vi. Detergent and other agents for cleaning laboratory glass wares.

K. TESTING OF WHOLE BLOOD

    i. It shall be responsibility of the licensee to ensure that the whole blood collected, processed and supplied conforms to the standards laid down in the Indian Pharmacopoeia and other tests published, if any, by the Government.

    ii. Freedom from HIV antibodies (AIDS) test. Every licensee shall get samples of every blood unit tested before use, for freedom from HIV I to HIV II antibodies either from laboratories specified for the purpose by the Central Government or in his own laboratory. The results of such testing shall be recorded on the label of the container.

    iii. Each blood unit shall also be tested for freedom from hepatitis B surface antigen and hepatitis C virus antibody, VDRL and malarial parasite and results of such testing shall be recorded on the label of the container.

Notes:

a. Blood samples of donors in plot tube and the blood samples of the recipient shall be preserved for 7 days after issue.

b. The blood intended for transfusion shall not be frozen at any stage.

c. Blood containers shall not come directly in contact with ice at any stage.

L. RECORDS

The records which the licensee is required to maintain shall include inter alia the following particulars, namely:

1. **Blood Donor Record:** It shall indicate serial number, date of bleeding, name, address and signature of donor with other particulars of age, weight, haemoglobin, blood grouping, blood pressure, medical examination, bag number and patient's detail for whom donated in case of replacement donation, category of donation (voluntary/replacement) and deferral records and signature of Medical Officer In-charge.

2. **Master Records for Blood and its Components:** It shall indicate bag serial number, date of collection, date of expiry, quantity in mL. ABO/Rh Group, results for testing of HIV I and HIV II antibodies, Malaria, VDRL, Hepatitis B surface antigen and Hepatitis C virus antibody and irregular antibodies (if any), name and address of the donor with particulars, utilization issue number, components prepared or discarded and signature of Medical Officer In-charge.

3. **Issue Register:** It shall indicate serial number, date and time of issue, bag serial number, ABO/Rh Group, total quantity in mL, name and address of the recipient, group of recipient, unit/institution, details of crossmatching report, and indication for transfusion.

4. **Records of Components Supplied:** Quantity supplied; compatibility report, details of recipient and signature of issuing person.

5. Records of ACD/CPD/CPD-A/SAGM bags giving details of manufacturer, batch number, date of supply, and results of testing.

6. **Register for Diagnostic Kits and Reagents Used:** Name of the kits/reagents, details of batch number, date of expiry and date of use.

7. Blood centre must issue the crossmatching report of the blood to the patient together with the blood unit.

8. Transfusion adverse reaction records.

9. Records of purchase, use and stock in hand of disposable needles, syringes, blood bags, shall be maintained.

Note: The above said records shall be kept by the licensee for a period of five years.

M. LABELS

The labels on every bag containing blood and/or component shall contain the following particulars, namely:

1. The proper name of the product in a prominent place and in bold letters on the bag.

2. Name and address of the blood center.

3. License number.

4. Serial number.

5. The date on which the blood is drawn and the date of expiry as prescribed under Schedule P to these rules.

6. A coloured label shall be put on every bag containing blood. The following color scheme for the said labels shall be used for different groups of blood:

Blood group	Colour of the label
O	Blue
A	Yellow
B	Pink
AB	White

7. The results of the tests for hepatitis B surface antigen and hepatitis C virus antibody, syphilis, freedom from HIV I and HIV II antibodies and malarial parasite.

8. The Rh group.

9. Total volume of the blood, the preparation of blood, nature and percentage of anticoagulant.

10. Keep continuously temperature at 2°C–6°C for whole human blood and/or components as contained under III of Part XII B.
11. Disposable transfusion sets with filter shall be used in administration equipment.
12. Appropriate compatible crossmatched blood without a typical antibody in recipient shall be used.
13. The contents of the bag shall not be used if there is any visible evidence of deterioration like haemolysis, clotting or discoloration.
14. The label shall indicate the appropriate donor classification like "Voluntary Donor" or "Replacement Donor" in no less prominence than the proper name.

Notes:
1. In the case of blood components, particulars of the blood from which such components have been prepared shall be given against item numbers (5), (7), (8), (9) and (14).
2. The blood and/or its components shall be distributed on the prescription of a Registered Medical Practitioner.

II. BLOOD DONATION CAMPS

A blood donation camp may be organized by:
a. A licensed designated Regional Blood Transfusion Center; or
b. A licensed Government blood centre; or
c. The Indian Red Cross Society; or
d. A licensed blood centre run by registered voluntary or charitable organizations recognized by State or Union Territory Blood Transfusion Council; or
e. A private hospital blood centre

Notes:
i. "Designated Regional Blood Transfusion Center" shall be a centre approved and designated by a Blood Transfusion Council constituted by a State Government (in accordance with procedure laid down by the National Blood Transfusion Council in this regard) to collect, process and distribute blood and its components to cater to the needs of the region and that Centre has also been licensed and approved by the Licensing Authority and Central License Approving Authority for the purpose.
ii. The designated Regional Blood Transfusion Center, Government blood center and Indian Red Cross Society shall intimate within a period of seven days, the venue where blood camp was held and details of group-wise blood units collected in the said camp to the Licensing Authority and Central License Approving Authority.

For holding a blood donation camp, the following requirements shall be fulfilled/complied with, namely:

(A) **Premises, Personnel, etc.**

    a. Premises under the blood donation camp shall have sufficient area and the location shall be hygienic so as to allow proper operation, maintenance and cleaning.

    b. All information regarding the personnel working, equipment used and facilities available at such a camp shall be well-documented and made available for inspection, if required, and ensuring:

        i. Continuous and uninterrupted electrical supply for equipment used in the camp;

        ii. Adequate lighting for all the required activities;

        iii. Handwashing facilities for staff;

        iv. Reliable communication system to the central office of the controller/organizer of the camp;

        v. Furniture and equipment arranged within the available place;

        vi. Refreshment facilities for donors and staff;

        vii. Facilities for medical examination of the donors;

        viii. Proper disposal of waste.

(B) **Personnel for Outdoor Blood Donation Camp**

To collect blood from 50 to 70 donors in about 3 hours or from 100 to 120 donors in 5 hours, the following requirements shall be fulfilled/complied with:

    i. One Medical Officer and two nurses or phlebotomists for managing 6–8 donor tables;

    ii. Two counsellors or medical social workers;

    iii. Three blood centre technicians;

    iv. Two attendants;

    v. Vehicle having a capacity to seat 8–10 persons, with provision for carriage of donation goods including facilities to conduct a blood donation camp.

(C) **Equipment**

    1. BP apparatus

    2. Stethoscope

    3. Blood bags (single, double, triple, quadruple)

    4. Donor questionnaire

    5. Weighing device for donors

    6. Weighing device for blood bags

    7. Artery forceps, scissors

    8. Stripper for blood tubing

    9. Bed sheets, blankets/mattress

10. Lancets, swap stick/toothpicks
11. Glass slides
12. Portable Hb meter/copper sulphate method or any other quantitative method can be used for determination of haemoglobin estimation
13. Test tube (big) and 12 × 100 mm (small)
14. Test tube stand
15. Anti-A, Anti-B and Anti-AB Anti-sera and Anti-D.
16. Test tube sealer film
17. Medicated adhesive tape
18. Plastic waste basket
19. Donor cards and refreshment for donors
20. Emergency medical kit
21. Insulated blood bag containers with provisions for storing between 2°C and 10°C
22. Dielectric sealer or portable tube sealer
23. Needle destroyer (wherever necessary).

III. PROCESSING OF BLOOD COMPONENTS FROM WHOLE BLOOD BY A BLOOD CENTER

The blood components shall be prepared by blood centers as a part of the blood center services. The conditions for grant or renewal of license to prepare blood components shall be as follows:

(A) **Accommodation**

i. Rooms with adequate area and other specifications, for preparing blood components depending on quantum of workload shall be as specified in item B under the heading "I. BLOOD CENTERS/ BLOOD COMPONENTS" of this Part.

ii. Preparation of blood components shall be carried out only under closed system using single, double, triple or quadruple plastic bags except for preparation of Red Blood Cells Concentrates, where single bags may be used with transfer bags.

(B) **Equipment**

i. Air conditioner
ii. Laminar air flow bench
iii. Suitable refrigerated centrifuge
iv. Plasma Expressor or Automated Extractor or Multi Head Tube Sealer
v. Clipper and clips and or dielectric sealer
vi. Weighing device
vii. Dry rubber balancing material
viii. Artery forceps, scissors

ix. Refrigerator maintaining a temperature between 2°C to 6°C, a digital dial thermometer with recording thermograph and alarm device, with provision for continuous power supply

x. Platelet agitator with incubator (wherever necessary).

xi. Deep freezers or Snap Freezer maintaining a temperature between –30°C to –40°C and –75°C to –80°C;

xii. Refrigerated water bath for plasma thawing

xiii. Insulated blood bag containers with provisions for storing at appropriate temperature for transport purposes

xiv. Cryobath and any better equipment or technology

(C) **Personnel**

The whole time competent technical staff meant for processing of blood components (that is Medical Officer, Technical Supervisor, Blood Centre Technician and Registered Nurse) shall be as specified in item C, under the heading "I. BLOOD CENTERS/BLOOD COMPONENTS" of this part.

(D) **Testing Facilities**

General: Facilities for A, B, AB and O groups and Rh (D) grouping. Hepatitis B surface antigen and hepatitis C virus antibody, VDRL, HIV I and HIV II antibodies and malarial parasites shall be mandatory for every blood unit before it is used for the preparation of blood components. The results of such testing shall be indicated on the label.

(E) **Categories of Blood Components**

1. **Concentrated Human Red Blood Corpuscles:** The product shall be known as "Packed Red Blood Cells" that is Packed Red Blood Cells remaining after separating plasma from human blood which also include modified packed red blood cells including semi-packed red blood cells, washed red blood cells, leucoreduced red blood cells, irradiated red blood cells and frozen red blood cells.

Types of Red Cell components:

(i) Saline washed red cells: Red cells washed with sterile normal saline by centrifugation at 2–8°C

(ii) Leucodepleted red cells: Shall be prepared by a method known to reduce leucocytes in the final component to less than 5×10^8 when intended to prevent febrile reactions and to less than 5×10^6 when required to prevent alloimmunisation or cytomegalovirus infection. For achieving a level of less than 5×10^6 leucocyte filters are necessary.

(iii) Irradiated red cells: Prepared by gamma cell or X-irradiation at 25 Gy to prevent graft versus host disease due to proliferation of lymphocytes.

(iv) Frozen Packed Red Blood Cells: Cryoprotective substance may be added to the Packed Red Blood Cells for extended storage between –80°C to –196°C.

(v) Packed red cell aliquot prepared for transfusion to paediatric patients by technique to preserve sterility.

The quality control criteria for validation of the processes should be as follows: One percent of Packed Red cells may be tested of which at least 75% of the packed red cells shall conform to following quality control criteria:

(a) Volume:
   250 mL +/– 10% from 450 mL bag
   150 mL +/– 10% from 350 mL bag

(b) Hematocrit:
   65–70% when stored in CPDA-1 solution
   50–60% when stored in SAGM solution

(c) Culture: Sterile

General requirements

a. **Storage:** Immediately after processing, the packed red blood Cells shall be kept at a temperature maintained between 2°C and 6°C.

b. **Inspection:** The component shall be inspected immediately after separation of the plasma, during storage and again at the time of issue. The product shall not be issued if there is any abnormality in colour or physical appearance or any indication of microbial contamination.

c. **Suitability of Donor:** The source blood for packed red blood cells shall be obtained from a donor who meets the criteria for blood donation as specified in item H under the heading "I. BLOOD CENTERS/BLOOD COMPONENTS" of this part.

d. **Testing of whole blood:** Blood from which packed red blood cells are prepared shall be tested as specified in item K relating to Testing of Whole Blood under the heading "I. BLOOD CENTRES/BLOOD COMPONENTS" of this part.

e. **Pilot Samples:** Pilot samples collected in integral tubing or in separate pilot tubes shall meet the following specifications:

   i. One or more pilot samples of either the original blood or of the packed red blood cells being processed shall be preserved with each unit of packed red blood cells which is issued

   ii. Before they are filled, all pilot sample tubes shall be marked or identified so as to relate them to the donor of that unit or packed red blood cells.

   iii. Before the final container is filled or at the time the final product is prepared, the pilot sample tubes accompanying a unit of packed red blood cells shall be attached in a tamper-proof manner that shall conspicuously identify removal and reattachment.

iv. All pilot sample tubes, accompanying a unit of packed red blood cells, shall be filled immediately after the blood is collected or at the time the final product is prepared, in each case, by the person who performs the collection of preparation.

f. **Processing**

i. **Separation:** Packed red blood cells shall be separated from the whole blood:

a. If the whole blood is stored in ACD solution within 21 days, and

b. If the whole blood is stored in CPDA-I solution, within 35 days, from the date of collection. Packed red blood cells may be prepared either by centrifugation done in a manner that shall not tend to increase the temperature of the blood or by normal undisturbed sedimentation method. A portion of the plasma, sufficient to ensure optimal cell preservation, shall be left with the packed red blood cells.

ii. **Packed Red Blood Cells Frozen:** Cytophylactic substance may be added to the packed red blood cells for extended manufacturer's storage not warmer than –65°C provided the manufacturer submits data to the satisfaction of the Licensing Authority and Central License Approving Authority, as adequately demonstrating through in vivo cells survival and other appropriate tests that the addition of the substance, the material used and the processing methods result in a final product meets the required standards of safety, purity and potency for packed red blood cells, and that the frozen product shall maintain those properties for the specified expiry period.

iii. **Testing:** Packed red blood cells shall conform to the standards as laid down in the Indian pharmacopoeia.

2. **Platelets Concentrates:** The product shall be known as "Platelets Concentrates" that is platelets collected from one unit of blood and resuspended in an appropriate volume of original plasma.

Types of Platelets:

i. Platelet Rich Plasma: Plasma which is rich in platelets and separated from whole blood

ii. Random Donor Platelet Concentrate

(a) Prepared from platelet-rich plasma

(b) Prepared from Buffy Coat

    iii. Pooled Platelets
        (a) Prepared by pooling of 6 units of random donor platelet, preferably ABO or Rh type matched are pooled in to one bag of "Pooled Platelets"

General requirements

i. **Source:** The source material for platelets shall be platelet-rich plasma or buffy coat which may be obtained from the whole blood or by plateletpheresis.

ii. **Processing:**

    a. Separation of buffy coat or platelet-rich plasma and platelets and resuspension of the platelets shall be in a closed system by centrifugal method with appropriate speed, force and time.

    b. Immediately after collection, the whole blood or plasma shall be held in storage between 20°C to 24°C. When it is to be transported from the venue of blood collection to the processing laboratory, during such transport action, the temperature as close as possible to a range between 20°C to 24°C shall be ensured. The platelet concentrates shall be separated within 6 hours after the time of collection of the unit of whole blood or plasma.

    c. The time and speed of centrifugation shall be demonstrated to produce an unclamped product, without visible haemolysis, that yields a count of not less than 3.5×10^{10} and 4.5×10^{10}, i.e. platelets per unit from a unit of 350 mL and 450 mL blood respectively. One percent of total platelets prepared shall be tested, of which, 75% of the units shall conform to the above said platelets count.

    d. The volume of original plasma used for resuspension of the platelets shall be determined by the maintenance of the pH of not less than 6 during the storage period. The pH shall be measured on a sample of platelets which has been stored for the permissible maximum expiry period at 20–24°C.

    e. Final containers used for platelets shall be colourless and transparent to permit visual inspection of the contents. The caps selected shall maintain a hermetic seal to prevent contamination of the contents. The container material shall not interact with the contents, under the normal conditions of the storage and use, in such a manner as to have an adverse effect upon the safety, purity, potency, or efficacy of the product. At the time of filling, the final containers shall be marked or identified by number so as to relate it to the donor.

iii. **Storage:** Immediately after resuspension, platelets shall be placed in storage not exceeding a period of 5 days, between 20°C to 24°C, with continuous gentle agitation of the platelet concentrates maintained throughout such storage.

iv. **Testing:** The units prepared from different donors shall be tested at the end of the storage period for:

   a. Platelet count;

   b. pH of not less than 6 measured at the storage temperature of the unit;

   c. Measurement of actual plasma volume;

   d. One percent of the total platelets shall be tested for sterility;

   e. The tests for functional viability of the platelets shall be done by swirling movement before issue;

   f. If the results of the testing indicate that the product does not meet the specified requirements, immediate corrective action shall be taken and records maintained.

v. **Compatibility Test:** Compatible transfusion for the purpose of variable number of red blood cells, A, B, AB and O grouping shall be done if the platelets concentrate is contaminated with red blood cells.

Preparation of pooled platelet concentrate: One single unit of random donor platelets is not enough to provide adequate haemostatic dose in an adult patient. Therefore, up to 6 units of random donor platelets, preferably ABO or Rh type matched are pooled into one bag of "Pooled Platelet Concentrate". The pooled platelets may be prepared by pooling buffy coats and then processed into one unit of pooled buffy coats—pooled platelet concentrate. Alternatively, pooling can be done after preparation of random donor platelets by platelet-rich plasma method or buffy coat method. If the pooling is done in an open system (using spikes for pooling), the shelf-life of the pooled platelets will be 6 hours, while for closed system (using sterile connecting device) the expiry date will be that of the platelet unit having the shortest expiry date. The labelling requirements for the final pooled product shall remain same as any other platelet product except that the final pack should have a unique pool number or donation numbers of all contributing units.

The platelet content in the pooled product should be $\geq 2 \times 10^{11}$/unit. Modified platelet component includes: leucodepleted, irradiated, washed platelets or platelets suspended in additive solution.

3. **Granulocyte Concentrates**
   (i) Granulocyte concentrates are prepared either by pooling multiple units of buffy coat or by apheresis as described under apheresis section. The same shall be stored at 20–24°C and used within a maximum period of 24 hours.
   (ii) Pooled granulocytes shall meet the same Quality Control requirements as that for apheresis granulocytes. (at least 1×10^{10})
   (iii) Group specific tests/HLA test wherever required shall be carried out

4. **Fresh Frozen Plasma**: Plasma frozen within 6 hours after blood collection and stored at a temperature not warmer than –30°C, shall be preserved for a period of not more than one year.
   The quality control criteria for validation of the processes should be as follows:
   Volume: 180–220 mL from 350 mL bag
   220–300 mL from 450 mL bag
   Factor VIII: At least 70 iu/bag
   Excess and expired plasma may be issued for fractionation to the licensed fractionation centre in the Country with justification to be recorded in writing.

5. **Cryoprecipitate:** Concentrate of anti-hemophiliac factor shall be prepared by thawing FFP at 4°C in a cold room or blood center refrigerator or 4–10°C in a cryobath. The –80°C deep freezer should be used for faster freezing of plasma for preparation of cryoprecipitate.
   The quality control criteria for validation of the processes should be as follows:
   Volume: 15–20 mL
   Fibrinogen: At least 150 mg/bag
   Factor VIII: At least 80 iu/bag

   Preparation of pooled cryoprecipitate: One single unit of cryoprecipitate is not enough to provide adequate haemostatic dose in an adult patient. Therefore, multiple units of cryoprecipitate may be pooled in one bag. If the pooling is done in an open system (using spikes for pooling), the shelf-life of the pooled cryoprecipitate will be 6 hours.
   The labelling requirements for the final pooled product shall remain same as any other cryoprecipitate product except that the final pack should have a unique pool number or donation numbers of all contributing units.

   a. **Storage:** Cryoprecipitate shall be preserved at a temperature not higher than –30°C and may be preserved for a period of not more than one year from the date of collection.

b. **Activity:** Anti-hemophiliac factor activity in the final product shall be not less than 80 units per bag. One percent of the total cryoprecipitate prepared shall be tested, of which seventy five percent of the unit shall conform to the said specification

(F) **Apheresis Using a Cell Separator**

General requirements:

(a) **Accommodation**: An air-conditioned area of 10 square meters shall be provided for apheresis/therapeutic procedures in the blood centre.

(b) **Equipment**:
   i. Cell separator
   ii. Dielectric tube sealer
   iii. Other emergency equipment/items
      – Oxygen cylinder with mask, gauge and pressure regulator.
      – Five percent glucose or normal saline.
      – Disposable sterile syringes and needles of various sizes.
      – Disposable sterile IV infusion sets.
      – Ampoules of adrenaline, noradrenaline, mephentine, betamethasone or dexamethasone, metoclopramide injections.
      – Aspirin

(c) **Criteria for selection of donors:** At least 48 hours must elapse between successive apheresis and not more than twice in a week. For haematopoietic stem cells the procedures can be done daily.

Types of Apheresis:

1. Plasmapheresis
2. Plateletpheresis for harvesting platelet concentrate (Single Donor Platelets)
3. Leucapheresis for harvesting:
   – Granulocyte concentrate
   – Lymphocytes
   – Mononuclear cells
4. Erythrocytapheresis—red cell apheresis including double unit red cell collection
5. Haematopoietic stem cells (Peripheral Blood Stem Cells)

1. **Plasmapheresis:** The total serum protein shall be 6 g/dL before the first plasmapheresis procedure.
   In repeated plasmapheresis:
   a. It should be tested before the third procedure if done within four weeks and it shall be 6 g/dL.
   b. The quantity of plasma separated from the blood of donor shall not exceed 500 mL per sitting and once in a fortnight or shall not exceed 1,000 mL per month.

2. **Plateletpheresis (Single Donor Platelets):**
   i. Plateletpheresis shall not be carried out on donors who have taken medication containing aspirin within 3 days prior to donation
   ii. Platelet count, WBC counts, differential count may be carried out.

   The term plateletpheresis includes platelets collected by apheresis, using a cell separator and the product is called single donor platelets and includes washed single donor platelets, modified single donor platelets (with replacement of compatible plasma), leucoreduced single donor platelets and double single donor platelets collected from single donor. Single donor platelets should have a platelet count of $\geq 3 \times 10^{11}$/unit.
   i. Storage: Shall be kept up to 5 days between 20°C to 24°C with continuous agitation.
   ii. Apheresis platelet concentrates should contain minimum of 3×10^{11} platelets in 75% of the units tested amongst 1% of monthly production or 4 platelet concentrates per month, whichever is higher.
   iii. The pH must be 6 or higher at the end of permissible storage period.

3. **Leucapheresis:** This procedure includes collection of granulocytes (Granulocytapheresis), lymphocytes or peripheral blood stem cells or haematopoietic stem cells for treatment of traditional conditions followed by their preservation.

4. **Erythropheresis:** This is the collection of 2 units of red cells from a single donor meeting specified requirements.

5. **Therapeutic Plasmapheresis and Cytapheresis:** Therapeutic apheresis activity is allowed in the blood centre attached to the hospital having apheresis facilities under the responsibility of Registered Medical Practitioner (RMP) who has obtained the consent of patient and record of which shall be maintained and signed by the RMP and blood center medical officer.

   This shall be done only at the written request of the patient's physician. Patient's informed consent shall be taken. Records of the procedure shall be maintained. Provisions for emergency care shall be available by the patient's physician.

Storage Conditions, Expiry of Blood, Blood Components and Blood Products as per Schedule P of the Drugs and Cosmetics Act, 1940, and Rules, 1945

S. No.	Name of drug	Expiry (Months)	Storage conditions
1.	Anti-hemophilic human globulin	12	In a cool place
2.	Dried plasma	60	At temperature not exceeding 25°C
3.	Dried normal human serum	60	At temperature not exceeding 25°C
4.	Frozen plasma	60	In deep freeze
5.	Liquid plasma	24	In cold place
6.	Liquid normal human serum albumin	60	In cold place
7.	Whole human blood –		
	a. Collected in ACD solution	21 days	At temperature between 4°C and 6°C
	b. Collection in CPDA solution	35 days	At temperature between 4°C and 6°C

Note:

1. The term "cool place" means 'place having a temperature between 10°C and 25°C'.
2. The term "cold place" means 'place having a temperature not exceeding 8°C'.

Storage Conditions, Expiry of Blood and Blood Components as per WHO Guidelines

S. No.	Name of drug	Expiry (Months)	Storage conditions
1.	Concentrated RBC	35 days	2–6°C
2.	Platelet concentrate	Max. 5 days	20–24°C in agitator
3.	FFP	7 years	–65°C or below
4.	FFP/Cryoprecipitate	24 months	–40° to –64°C
5.	-do-	12 months	–30° to –39°C
6.	-do-	6 months	–25° to –29°C
7.	-do-	3 months	–2° to –24°C

Surplus Plasma Exchange

INTRODUCTION

Surplus plasma is the volume of the plasma that exceeds the volume of plasma being actively utilized by the blood center. In other words, surplus plasma is that which remains unutilized after consumption at the blood center. This extra (unutilized) blood plasma can be issued or transferred to other blood centers or to fractionators for fractionation.

Blood plasma is the major blood component prepared from safe blood collected/obtained from voluntary nonremunerated blood donors at a well-maintained and licensed blood center facility. Plasma is rich in proteins such as albumin, globulins, and coagulation factors. All such proteins and coagulation factors are separated by a process called plasma fractionation. The products so obtained are called plasma-derived medicinal products (PDMPs).

Plasma has limited usefulness in its raw form as it is usually indicated in coagulopathies due to single or multiple factor deficiency. It is also indicated in therapeutic plasma exchange as a replacement fluid to make up for lost coagulation factors and maintain colloid oncotic pressure. It is one of those important components of the blood, which is the raw material for the production of PDMPs. Following are examples of PDMPs:

- Albumin
- Coagulant proteins such as factor VIII (FVIII)
- Immunoglobulins such as intravenous immunoglobulin (IVIg)
- Hyperimmune products from specialized source plasma hepatitis B immunoglobulin (HBIg), tetanus immunoglobulin (Ig), etc.

Currently, about 30 distinct protein products approved by World Health Organization (WHO) can be isolated from human plasma.

The main plasma protein therapeutics and their respective clinical indications are given in **Table 1**.

S. No.	Products	Main indication
		Table 1: Main plasma-derived medicinal products (PDMPs) and their clinical indications.
Albumin		
1.	Human serum albumin	Volume and protein replacement
Blood coagulation factors		
2.	Factor VIIIa	Hemophilia A
3.	Prothrombin complex concentrate (PCC/PPSB)	Complex liver diseases; warfarin or coumarin derivatives reversal
4.	Factor IX	Hemophilia B
5.	Factor VII	Factor VII deficiency
6.	Factor VII	Factor VII deficiency
7.	von Willebrand factor	von Willebrand factor deficiency (type 3 and severe forms of type 2)
8.	Factor XI	Hemophilia C (factor XI deficiency)
9.	Fibrinogen	Fibrinogen deficiency
10.	Factor XII	Factor XII deficiency
11.	Activated PCC	Hemophilia with anti-factor VIII (or factor IX) inhibitors
Protease inhibitors		
12.	Antithrombin	Antithrombin III deficiency
13.	Alpha-1 antitrypsin	Congenital deficiency of alpha-1 antitrypsin with clinically demonstrable panacinar emphysema
14.	C1-inhibitor	Hereditary angioedema
Anticoagulants		
15.	Protein C	Protein C deficiency/thrombosis
16.	Fibrin sealant (fibrin glue)	Topical hemostatic/healing/sealing agent (surgical adjunct)

Continued

Continued

S. No.	Products	Main indication
Intramuscular immunoglobulins (IMIg)		
17.	Normal (polyvalent)	Prevention of hepatitis A (also rubella and other specific infections)
18.	Hepatitis B	Prevention of hepatitis B
19.	Tetanus	Treatment or prevention of tetanus infection
20.	Anti-Rho (D)	Prevention of hemolytic disease of the newborn
21.	Rabies	Prevention of rabies infection
22.	Varicella/zoster	Prevention of chickenpox infection
Intravenous immunoglobulins (IVIg)		
23.	Normal (polyvalent)	• Replacement therapy in immune deficiency states • Immune modulation in immune disorders
24.	Hepatitis B	Prevention of hepatitis B virus (HBV) infection (e.g., liver transplant)
25.	Anti-Rho (D)	Prevention of hemolytic disease of the newborn
26.	IVIG M (Immuno-globulin M-enriched human intravenous immunoglobulin)	Septic shock; binding of endotoxins

These plasma-derived medicines are essential and lifesaving in many conditions, e.g., acute hypovolemia conditions such as burns and trauma, autoimmune disorders, infections, congenital deficiencies, and coagulopathies.

Presently, albumin and IVIg are mainly two plasma products being manufactured from domestic (Indian) plasma in the country. Therefore, many other plasma products required for various life-threatening clinical manifestations are imported into the country. This makes such products costly, unavailable when needed, that too with short shelf life. Now, India is sought after as medical tourism destination due to changing disease patterns, improved clinical diagnostic facilities, and affordability.

The following fractionation plants/centers are presently functional in India:
1. PlasmaGen BioSciences Pvt Ltd (Bangalore, India)
2. Reliance Life Sciences (Bangalore, India)

3. Biocon Ltd (Bangalore, India)
4. Intas Pharmaceuticals Ltd (Ahmedabad, India)
5. Bharat Serums and Vaccines Ltd (Mumbai, India)
6. Virchow Biotech (Hyderabad, India)
7. Fusion Healthcare (Hyderabad, India)
8. Hemarus (Hyderabad, India)

Since in most of the licensed blood centers except tertiary care health centers, blood plasma produced is in excess, therefore the Government of India has framed "National Policy for Access to Plasma Derived Medicinal Products from Human Plasma for Clinical/Therapeutic Use" in 2014. The main objectives of the policy are as follows:

- Governments to promote the supply and use of safe and adequate quantities of plasma-derived medicines for clinical/therapeutic use.
- Ensure adequate resources to develop and organize the plasma/PDMPs mobilization across the country.
- Appropriate regulatory and legislative measures to govern activities related to plasma-derived products.
- Promoting research and development in the areas of blood components, plasma fractions, and plasma-derived products.
- Strengthen the quality systems of Blood Transfusion Services for the plasma collection, transport, processing, manufacture, and distribution of PDMPs.

The Drugs and Cosmetics Rules, 1945 and National Standards for Blood Centers and Blood Transfusion Services 2022 (2nd Edition) issued by the Government of India permit transfer of excess and expired plasma for fractionation to the licensed fractionation centers within the country with justification to be recorded in writing.

GUIDELINES FOR EXCESS TRANSFER OF PLASMA (Annexure 81.1)

Blood centers having surplus plasma are permitted by the Government of India to supply it to domestic fractionators to meet the demand of the Indian market, and blood products obtained from Indian plasma are sold to the domestic market. It will not be exported until domestic demand is met. In order to increase the availability of lifesaving medicines, the Government of India has set a "cashless" exchange value of ₹1,600 per liter for surplus plasma available in blood centers. The modalities of exchange value include:

- Buyback of plasma-derived products of equivalent value for clinical use by needy patients at the institution wherein the blood center is located.
- Receipt of equipment/consumables for strengthening of blood centers.

- Any other modality approved by the National Blood Transfusion Council (NBTC): An agreement as per mutually agreed terms and conditions approved by the respective State Blood Transfusion Council (SBTC) is to be signed by the blood centers and also the fractionators before sending plasma for fractionation. It has been made obligatory for all the blood centers to take informed consent of all donors for allowing utilization of their blood/plasma for fractionation and derivation of essential plasma-derived medicines.

PROCEDURE FOR TRANSFER OF SURPLUS PLASMA

1. Sign an agreement [memorandum of understanding (MOU)] **(Annexure 81.2)** with the fractionator as per mutually agreed terms and conditions approved by the SBTC/NBTC. Send a copy of the agreement to respective SBTC.
2. The representative of the fractionator will visit along with packing material and thermocol boxes in the blood center for taking surplus plasma.
3. Blood center to hand over each unit of surplus plasma unit (ID wise) along with blood group, date of collection, transfusion trans-mitted infections (TTI) status, and volume wise as per format **(Annexure 81.3)**.
4. The representative will put each unit in bubble wrap packing and pack such units in the thermocol boxes, and dry ice will be added on top of the packed plasma units.
5. Certificate of testing and quality of plasma units is also prepared **(Annexure 81.4)**.
6. Total volume of the surplus plasma in liters is calculated and the invoice is raised **(Annexure 81.5)**.
7. Nonreturnable gate pass is prepared and an e-way bill is generated online. (Format of e-way bill is in **Annexure 81.6**).
8. Surplus plasma packed in boxes, certificate of testing and quality, e-way bill, invoice, and nonreturnable gate pass are handed over to the representative for transportation to the fractionator's facility. The representative also brings the document certifying that "this shipment/parcel/boxes contain processed and tested plasma—a component which is prepared from whole blood and it is perishable/temperature sensitive. The fractionator is sending this plasma to its licensed blood product manufacturing facility for fractionation."
9. The fractionator releases the exchange value of surplus plasma as per the signed agreement.

ANNEXURE 81.1

GUIDELINES FOR SUPPLY OF SURPLUS PLASMA BY LICENSED BLOOD CENTRES TO INDIGENOUS FRACTIONATORS IN THE COUNTRY ISSUED VIDE DO NO. S-12016/01/2012-NACO (NBTC) DATED 28 OCT 2015 BY NATIONAL AIDS CONTROL ORGANISATION, MINISTRY OF HEALTH AND FAMILY WELFARE, GOVT. OF INDIA.

1. The fractionators must undertake to fulfil needs of Indian market first and none of products recovered from the Indian plasma should be exported before fulfiling domestic demand.
2. Uniform exchange value of ₹ 1600/- (Rupee Sixteen hundred only) per litre of plasma was agreed upon.
3. All blood centres must ensure taking informed consent of the blood donor for allowing the use of his blood for fractionation, and derivation of essential plasma medicines therefrom.
4. The modalities for use of exchange value would be finalized by the respective State Blood Transfusion Councils and would be primarily directed toward ensuring availability of plasma-derived products to patients requiring them. These would include buyback of plasma-derived products of equivalent value for clinical use by needy patients accessing care at the institution where the blood centre exchanging the plasma is located. Receipts of equipment or consumables for strengthening of blood centres capacity and improving component recovery, storage, and utilization. Any other modality approved by NBTC.
5. Blood Component Separation Units would directly enter into an Agreement with the fractionators, as per mutually agreed terms and conditions approved by respective SBTC before sending plasma for fractionation.
6. Feedback would be provided by fractionators to NBTC/respective SBTC in order to provide evidence of the quality of the plasma being fractionated, so as to enable corrective and preventive action.
7. NBTC would review the fractionators periodically so as to prevent any misuse of this strategy.

ANNEXURE 81.2

Format of Agreement (MOU)

This Agreement is for transfer of surplus human plasma (herein referred to as **"AGREEMENT"**) entered on this date_____by and between:

M/s. _____having drug mfg. license no. _____ valid up

to _____ at (address) _____ (hereinafter referred

to as **"Blood Centre", (Party 1)** which expression unless repugnant to the context or otherwise include its successors, assigns and legal representatives) of the One Part.

AND

_____ a company incorporated under the Companies Act,

1956, having its registered office at _____

Hereinafter referred to as Party 2, which expression unless repugnant to the context or otherwise include its successors, assigns and legal representatives) of the Other Part.

Blood Centre and _____ are hereinafter individually or

collectively referred to as the "Party" or the "Parties".

Whereas

a. Party 1 Blood Centre is engaged in running and operating a blood centre duly licensed under the Drugs and Cosmetics Act 1940 and Rules 1945, which promotes, encourages and conducts programs for donation of blood and is also engaged in the enhancement of blood component usage including improvement in standards of blood centreing.

b. Party 2 is a research based leading healthcare manufacturing company engaged in research, development, manufacturing, marketing and distribution of pharmaceutical products nationally as well as internationally.

c. Blood centre componentizes the donated human blood and after servicing the need patients with the required blood components, there is excess plasma component which remain unutilized. Blood centre is interested in supplying excess and unutilized plasma as and when available with it to suitable plasma fractionation centre/ company which is in need of the same, through proper arrangement.

d. Party 1 _____ has approached the Party 2 _____

to procure noncontaminated and good quality surplus fresh frozen plasma component to which blood centre has agreed to supply under the terms and conditions hereinafter appearing below.

Now, therefore, in reliance upon the mutual promises and consideration, the adequacy whereof is hereby acknowledged and the following undertakings and representations, the parties agree and covenant as under:

ARTICLE I: DEFINITIONS AND INTERPRETATION

1. As used in this Agreement, the following terms shall mean and be interpreted to convey the meanings ascribed thereto in this Article 1:
   a. "Affiliate" shall mean with respect to a Party, any entity or person, that directly or indirectly through one or more intermediaries, controls, is controlled by or is under common control with such Party. The term "control" shall mean either the ownership, directly or indirectly, of (i) fifty percent (50%) or more of the voting stock or equity shares or other ownership interest or with a right to elect the majority of directors or equivalent governing body of such entity or person or (ii) power to direct or cause the direction of the management, policies or decisions of an entity or person whether through ownership of voting securities, control or otherwise.
   b. "Agreement" shall mean this Agreement and possible corrections or modifications thereafter, executed between the Parties;
   c. "Confidential Information" shall have the meaning as defined in Article VI.
   d. "Effective Date" shall mean the date of this Agreement,
   e. "FFP" or "fresh frozen plasma" is plasma separated from whole blood and stored and frozen at or below −30°C within 6 hours of blood collection.
   f. "CPP" or "cryo-poor plasma" is the plasma collected as the supernatant after cryoprecipitate is separated.
   g. "Third Party" shall mean any person or entity other than: (i) Party-1......(ii) Party-2........., and in their respective Affiliates.
2. No provision of this Agreement shall be interpreted adversely against a Party solely because that Party was responsible for drafting that particular provision.
3. This Agreement has been drawn up in English. In the event of any discrepancy between the English text of this Agreement [or any Agreement resulting therefrom or relating thereto] and any translation thereof, the English language version shall prevail. The English language version shall also prevail for interpretation purposes.
4. The words "include", "included," or "including" are used to indicate that the matters listed are not a complete enumeration of all listed items. Unless the context requires otherwise, words denoting the singular shall include the plural and vice versa. Words denoting one gender shall include another gender, unless the context requires otherwise.

ARTICLE II: OBLIGATIONS OF BLOOD CENTRE

1. The quality of plasma supplied by blood centre to Party-2 shall adhere to the criteria mentioned below and shall be in accordance with the applicable statutory requirements including Drugs and Cosmetics Act and Rules 1945 made thereunder.

   Criteria:
   a. Blood centre shall be fully responsible for quality testing of plasma for HIV I and II, HBsAg, HCV, Syphilis and Malaria.
   b. Blood centre shall supply only good quality plasma which is non-positive of aforesaid diseases.
   c. Blood centre shall provide test results/donor report in hard and soft copy for all plasma supplied to Party-2.
   d. Blood centre shall provide required information in formats shared by Party including epidemiology data.
   e. Haemolysed plasma: Party-2 shall duly notify the receipt of any Haemolysed plasma from blood centre. The equivalent volume of plasma should be replenished by blood centre as FOC in next plasma pick up. Alternatively, the equivalent amount shall be adjusted from payment/future pick-ups.
   f. Blood centre shall arrange to provide the plasma bags in proper condition and at required temperature at blood centre.
   g. Blood centre shall maintain the record of donors of all the plasma supplied to Party-2......for a minimum period of 5 (five) years from the date of donation.
   h. Blood centre shall provide tested, qualified and packed plasma to Party-2.
   i. Blood centre shall maintain all regulatory approvals and necessary licenses, registrations and authorizations etc., throughout the term and provide copies of such licenses and approvals to Party-2 for verification as and when required by Party-2.

ARTICLE III: OBLIGATIONS OF PARTY-2

1. Party-2 shall ensure that the plasma is stored and transported to the designated place under the required temperature as laid down under the requisite guidelines. Once plasma is handed over to Party-2 thereafter, the responsibility of transporting it in an appropriate/suitable condition shall solely lie on Party-2.
2. Party-2 shall give a copy of all required regulatory approvals and necessary licenses, registrations and authorizations etc., to blood centre for verification, as and when required by blood centre.

ARTICLE IV: SUPPLY OF QUALITY PLASMA

1. *Plasma volume calculation*: The volume of plasma in each bag will be calculated by the following formula:

   Volume of plasma in bag = (Weight of filled plasma bag − weight of empty plasma bag)/1.03

   (Here 1.03 is specific gravity of plasma)
2. Supply of FFP should be within 6 (six) months from the date of collection.

ARTICLE V: FINANCIALS AND PAYMENT TERMS

The parties hereby duly acknowledge the letter no DO No. S-12016/01/2012-NACO (NBTC) dated 28th October 2015 (latest letter No. IM1 10|2/07/2022/NBTC Dated 14th June 2022) and agreed to abide by the conditions issued by NACO from time to time including the conditions mentioned in the letter for supply of surplus plasma and shall arrange for the pickup of plasma from blood centre. Freight and octroi expenses arising on account of transportation of plasma shall be solely borne by Party-2.

The parties have agreed to the following for supply and exchange of surplus plasma. Blood centre shall supply the plasma at the following exchange value:

Fresh frozen plasma (FFP) @ .... per liter

Blood centre will supply the plasma to Party-2 and raise invoices from time to time on the rates mentioned above. Payment will be made through NEFT/RTGS/cheque within 21 days from the submission of invoice.

Party-2 shall provide the payment directly to vendor account supplying reagents and consumables as per requirements of Party-1 in kind in lieu of the plasma being supplied by the blood centre.

ARTICLE VI: CONFIDENTIALITY

Party-2 and blood centre shall maintain utmost secrecy of all IPs, data, particulars method, formulas, details drawings and other confidential proprietary information (confidential information) of other party during and after the completion of the term.

This confidential information shall be utilized by the parties for the purpose of this agreement only and the same shall not be divulged, disclosed, or communicated to any third party without prior written permission of Party-2 or blood centre as the proprietors of such confidential information, as the case may be.

However, restrictions as to confidentiality shall not be applicable to such information which are:

- In a public domain at the time of disclosure or thereafter enters the public domain without any breach on the part of any parties to this agreement.
- The receiving party is already in a possession of such information.
- Is independently developed by receiving party without use or reference to the confidential information disclosed by the disclosing party.
- Is disclosed to a party by third party who to the best of such party's knowledge is without any obligation towards the other party.
- Is required to be disclosed under the applicable laws or under statutory requirements, provided the receiving party provides the disclosing party with reasonable prior written notice of such disclosure and makes a reasonable effort to obtain, or to assist the disclosing party to enable the other party in obtaining, a protective order preventing or limiting the disclosure.

ARTICLE VII: TERM

This agreement shall be valid for_____years from date of signing by the parties. This agreement may be further extended for such term and on such terms and conditions as may be mutually agreed upon by the parties. Any party to this agreement may cancel or terminate this agreement before the expiry of the initial term as mentioned above, by giving 6 (six) months advance notice in writing to this effect to the other party and upon such termination, the terms of this agreement shall be of no effect whatsoever, except for rights and covenants that by their very nature survive termination.

ARTICLE VIII: EXCLUSIVITY

Notwithstanding anything to the contrary elsewhere in the Agreement, the Parties hereby agree and acknowledge that the Blood centre shall exclusively supply the Plasma to Party-2_____during the Term

of this agreement. Party-2 is however free to procure surplus plasma from any other blood centre on such terms and conditions as it may deem fit and proper.

ARTICLE IX: REPRESENTATIONS, WARRANTIES, AND INDEMNITIES

1. Blood centre hereby represents and warrants to Party-2 that:
   a. It is duly registered entity entitled to supply plasma.
   b. It shall obtain and maintain at its cost all licenses, registrations and authorizations as are necessary to supply plasma.
   c. The collection, storage, processing, testing, and dispatching of plasma owned or possessed by it shall be in compliance at all times during the period of supply, with all applicable statutory requirements in force.
   d. It has all requisite power and authority to execute, deliver and perform this Agreement and the terms and conditions contained herein, and each of its obligations are enforceable against it in accordance with the terms of this Agreement.
   e. The execution, delivery, and performance of this Agreement does not in any way conflict or violate any provision of law, rule, judgment, order or any other contract applicable to such party.
   f. It has no outstanding commitments, liabilities or obligations, contractual or otherwise, which would in any material respect conflict with or impede its ability and right to enter into this Agreement or fulfil any and all of its obligations hereunder or to conduct the business contemplated hereby.
   g. It is not subject to any existing, pending or threatened litigation or other proceeding which could have a material adverse effect on its ability to fulfil its undertakings and obligations in terms of this Agreement.

2. Party-2 hereby represents and warrants to blood centre that:
   a. It is duly registered entity entitled to procure plasma.
   b. It shall obtain and maintain at its cost all licenses, registrations and authorizations as are necessary to supply plasma.
   c. It has all requisite power and authority to execute, deliver and perform this Agreement and the terms and conditions contained herein, and each of its obligations are enforceable against it in accordance with the terms of this Agreement.
   d. The execution, delivery and performance of this Agreement does not in any way conflict or violate any provision of law, rule, judgment, order or any other contract applicable to such Party.
   e. It has no outstanding commitments, liabilities or obligations, contractual or otherwise, which would in any material respect conflict with or impede its ability and right to enter into this Agreement or fulfil any and all of its obligations hereunder, or to conduct the business contemplated hereby.

It is not subject to any existing, pending or threatened litigation or other proceeding which could have a material adverse effect on its ability to fulfil its undertakings and obligations in terms of this Agreement.

3. Blood centre shall indemnify, defend and hold harmless- Party-2, its Affiliates and their respective officers, directors, employees and agents from and against any and all liabilities, damages, losses, actions, proceedings, judgments, decrees, costs or expenses (including reasonable attorney's fees and expenses) on account of:

   a. Any breach of any terms and conditions of this Agreement, warranties and covenants;
   b. Negligence arising due to supply of plasma of inappropriate quality as provided in clause 2(a) of this Agreement;
   c. Failure of the plasma to comply with the criteria and quality as provided in clause 2(a) of this Agreement.
   d. Failure to supply the plasma as per the terms of the Agreement.

4. Party-2 shall indemnify, defend and hold harmless blood centre and their Affiliates and their respective officers, directors, employees and agents from and against any liability, damage, loss, cost or expense (including reasonable attorney's fees and expenses) on account of:

   a. Any breach of any of the terms and conditions of this Agreement, warranties and covenants;
   b. Negligence

ARTICLE X: FORCE MAJEURE

If any party is prevented from the performance of their respective obligations (in whole or in part) for reasons of force majeure, viz., acts of God, acts of public enemy, terror attacks, war, riot, insurrection, embargo, earthquake, floods etc., then such party must provide a written notice of happening of any such eventuality to the other party within 7 (seven) days from both the date of occurrence and cessation of such force majeure event. The affected party shall not be liable for non-fulfilment or delayed performance due to the force majeure event and the period of force majeure shall be excluded accordingly, in case the affected party has made best efforts to mitigate the damages/loss. Provided, however that, such events should have a material adverse effect on the affected Party's performance of its obligations under this Agreement.

ARTICLE XI: MISCELLANEOUS AMENDMENT AND WAIVER

This Agreement may be amended, modified or supplemented only by a written instrument executed by each of the parties and no waiver of any provision(s) of this Agreement shall be effective unless set forth in a written instrument executed by the party waiving such provision.

Entire Agreement

This Agreement constitutes the whole agreement between the parties relating to the subject matter hereof and supersedes any prior agreements or understandings relating to such subject matter.

Severability

If any provision of this Agreement or the application thereof to any person or circumstance shall be invalid or unenforceable to any extent, the remainder of this Agreement and the application of such provision to persons or circumstances other than those as to which it is held invalid or unenforceable, shall be valid and enforceable to the fullest extent permitted by law. Any invalid or unenforceable provision of this Agreement shall be replaced with a provision which is valid and enforceable and most nearly reflects the original intent of the unenforceable provision.

Assignment

Neither party will assign or transfer any rights or obligations under this Agreement without the prior written consent of the other party, except that a party may assign this Agreement without such consent to its successor in interest by way of merger, acquisition or sale of all or substantially all of its assets. Subject to the foregoing, this Agreement shall inure to the benefits of and be binding upon the successors and permitted assigns of the parties.

Survival

Such clauses which by its very nature should survive the expiry and termination of this Agreement shall survive such termination or expiry.

Relationship

Nothing in this Agreement shall create or be deemed to create any relationship between the parties including but not limited to partnership or principal and agent or employer and employee or joint venture, nor authorize either Party to enter into any commitment for or on behalf of the other party.

Dispute Resolution

Save where expressly stated to the contrary in this Agreement, any dispute, difference, or controversy of whatever nature howsoever arising under, out of or in relation to this Agreement, between the parties and so notified in writing by either Party to the other (the "Dispute") in the first instance shall be attempted to be resolved amicably. If the dispute is not resolved amicably, it shall be decided by reference to arbitration by 3 (three) arbitrators. Each party shall appoint 1 (one) arbitrator and the third shall be nominated by the said two arbitrators. The arbitration shall be held in accordance with The Arbitration and Conciliation Act, 1996 and amendments or statutory modifications or re-enactments thereto. The arbitrators shall give a reasoned award. The award by a majority of the arbitrators rendered in writing shall be final and binding on both the parties. The fee and other expenses of the arbitrator nominated by respective party shall be borne by the party nominating the arbitrator. The fee and other expenses of the third arbitrator and other arbitration expenses shall be shared equally by both the parties. The arbitration proceedings shall be held in English language. The venue of such arbitration shall be _____ .

The Arbitrator shall not have the power to award punitive damages, attorney's fees and/or any other losses, expenses, claim or damages, which are excluded by this Agreement.

The arbitration proceedings, including any outcome, shall be confidential. Nothing in this clause will preclude any party from seeking interim or provisional relief from a court of competent jurisdiction, including a temporary restraining order, preliminary injunction or other interim equitable relief, concerning a dispute either prior to or during any arbitration if necessary to protect the interests of such Party or to preserve the status quo pending the arbitration proceeding. The arbitrator's award shall be final and binding and shall be enforceable through any Court with competent jurisdiction.

Governing Law

This Agreement shall be construed and interpreted in accordance with and governed by the laws of Union of India.

Notices

Any notice required to be given hereunder shall be in writing and shall be effectively served (i) if delivered personally, upon receipt by the other party; (ii) if sent by prepaid courier service, airmail or registered mail, within five (5) days of being sent; or (iii) if sent by facsimile or other similar means of electronic communication (with confirmed receipt), upon receipt of transmission notice by the sender. Any notice required to be given hereunder shall be sent to the addresses referred below:

To _____

Address: _____

_____

Contact No: _____

To _____

Address: _____

Contact No.: _____

Either party shall not use the brand name, logo, mark or any other intellectual property in any manner whatsoever, without a prior written approval from the other Party.

Neither party shall make or permit any person to make any public announcement concerning this Agreement without the prior written consent of the other Party.

This Agreement may be signed in two counterparts, each of which when signed and dated shall constitute an original of this Agreement but all the counterparts shall together constitute the same Agreement.

Executed on the Day/ Month/Year

_____   _____

_____   _____

WITNESS 1:

_____   _____

WITNESS 2:

_____   _____

ANNEXURE 81.3

Name & Address of blood centre: _____

Box ID: _____

Material: FFP

S. No.	Donor ID	Donation Date	Blood Group	HBsAg	HIV I and II	HCV	Syphilis	Malaria	Vol. in mL
1									
2									
3									
4									
5									
6									
7									
8									
9									
10									
11									
12									
13									
14									
15									
16									
17									
18									
19									
20									
21									
22									
23									
24									
25									
26									
27									
28									
29									
30									

Total No. of units: _____

Total Volume (In litres): _____

The plasma units mentioned above have been componentized and stored as per provisions under the Drugs and Cosmetics Act, 1940 and Rules 1945. These units have been individually tested and found nonreactive for HBSAg, HIV I and II, HCV, Malaria and Syphilis.

Signature: _____

Date and Stamp: _____

ANNEXURE 81.4

Name & Address of blood centre: _____

License No.: _____

Certificate of Testing and Quality

Plasma Type: _____

No. of Boxes: _____

Total No. of units: _____

Total Volume of Plasma: _____

Date of Donation: From: _____   To: _____

We certify that the above-mentioned plasma has been collected in the licensed blood centre facilities under the Drugs and Cosmetics Act, 1940 and Rules 1945.

The plasma units in this shipment were prepared and inspected for compliance with Drugs and Cosmetics Act, 1940 and Rules 1945. The following tests have been performed individually on all mentioned units of plasma in accordance to Indian laws and consignee requirements.

Test and generation	Test kit name	Manufacturer	Generation of virology kit	Results	Lot No. of kit	Date of expiry of kit
HBsAg						
Anti-HCV						
Anti-HIV I and II						
Syphilis						
Malaria Parasite						
ID NAT						

The plasma supplied is human plasma for fractionation, obtained from whole blood donation, collected from healthy and voluntary donors in India. The whole blood was collected in triple/quadruple bags and plasma was obtained following the provisions under the Indian Laws.

Plasma was recovered from Whole Blood in less than 6 hours of donation and after centrifugation and separation, frozen by cooling at −30°C or below within one hour.

The storage temperature is routinely at a temperature of −20°C or below, after taking into consideration the expected variances to account for normal defrost cycles, loading and unloading etc.

Hereby, we certify that as per the guidelines of Drugs and Cosmetics Act, 1940 and Rules 1945, all the units have been found to be free from HIV I and II antibodies, Hepatitis B surface antigen, Hepatitis C virus antibodies, Malaria Parasite and Syphilis. All units are nonreactive (NEGATIVE) by NAT testing.

Authorized Signatory   **Date and Stamp**

ANNEXURE 81.5

Name of Institution: _____

Address: _____

_____

GSTIN: _____

Customer Details		Invoice Details	
Name	--	Invoice No.	--
Address	--	Invoice Date	--
GSTIN	--	Invoice Type	Integrated
Phone number	--		

S. No.	Material Description	HSN/SAC	Rate	GST Rate	Qty.	Gross Amount	Net Amount
1.	FFP, PLASMA	3002	–	0%	–	–	–

Summary	Amount
Gross Amount	
IGST	
R/off	
Net Amount	

Amount in Words	–

Terms and Conditions	Bank Details	
• Payment is requested by crossed ordered Cheque/DD in favour of M/s_____ or made by NEFT/RTGS • Goods once handed over cannot be taken back or replaced • Subject jurisdictions _____ court only	_____ _____	For _____ _____ Stamp and Signatures of Authorized Signatory

ANNEXURE 81.6

Sample Format of E-way Bill Generated

E-way Bill

QR CODE

---

1. E-Way Bill Details:

E-way bill No.:_____ Generated Date: _____ Generated by: _____

Valid up to: _____ Mode: _____ Approx. Distance: _____

Type: Outwards-Others-Plasma   Document Details: Challan No: _____

Transaction type: Regular

---

2. Address Details:

From	To
GSTIN: _____ _____	GSTIN: _____ _____
Dispatch from: _____ _____	Ship to: _____ _____

---

3. Goods Details:

HSN: Product name and Desc.   Quantity:_____   Taxable Amount ₹ _____

Tax Rate (C+S+I + Cess Non. Avol.) Code

3002   FFP plasma and FFP plasma   _____ LTR _____

NE+NE+NE+0.000+0.00

Total Taxable Amt: _____ CGST Amt: _____ SGST Amt. _____ IGST Amt: _____

CESS Amt: _____ CESS non adol Amt: _____

---

4. Transportation Details:

Transporter ID and Name: _____

Transporter Doc. No. and Date: _____

---

5. Vehicle Details:

Mode: _____ Vehicle/Trans: _____ From:_____ Entered Date:_____

Entered By:_____ CEWS No. (If any): _____ Multi Vehi. Info (If any)_____

Road   _____   _____   _____

Barcode

Process for Grant/Renewal of License for Blood Center under Drugs and Cosmetics Act, 1940 and Rules,1945

NEED FOR BLOOD CENTER LICENSE

A blood center is an accredited licensed facility in an organization (private or public hospital or other establishment) that performs all or part of its operations, including the collection, processing, storage, and distribution of blood drawn or received from another licensed blood center and for preparation, storage, and distribution of blood/blood components and apheresis.

Human "blood" is included in the definition of "drug" in Section 3(b) of the Drugs and Cosmetics Act, 1940, which means and includes whole human blood, collected from a donor and mixed with an anticoagulant for its preservation. "Blood component" is also a drug, prepared, obtained, derived, or separated from a unit of blood drawn from a donor. "Apheresis" refers to the process of aseptically withdrawing blood from a donor, after separating plasma or platelets or leukocytes, is re-transfused simultaneously into the same donor. "Blood donor" refers to a person who voluntarily donates his/her blood after he/she has been declared fit after medical examination, for donating blood, on fulfilling criteria as per the Drugs and Cosmetics Act and Rules without accepting any consideration in return in any form but does not include a professional or a paid donor.

Schedule X-B of the Drugs and Cosmetics Act/Rules provides requirements for the functioning and operation of a blood center and/ or preparation of blood components. It provides mandatory testing of blood for blood transmissible diseases—human immunodeficiency virus (HIV) I and HIV II antibodies, hepatitis B surface antigen, hepatitis C virus antibodies, venereal disease research laboratory (VDRL) and malaria testing, adequate testing procedures, requirement for storage and labeling requirements, and quality control of blood and blood components. Further, the Drugs and Cosmetics Rules 1945 also stipulate the qualifications and experience for blood center personnel, maintenance of complete and accurate records, etc.

The blood centers require a manufacturing license on Form 28-C, which is issued after a joint inspection by a team of officers from the Central Drugs Authority [Central Drugs Standard Control Organization (CDSCO)], State Drugs Control/Licensing Authority (SLA), and a blood center expert as per provisions under the Act. The manufacturing license is prepared and signed by the concerned State Licensing Authority (SLA) and approved by the Drugs Controller General (India), who is the Central License Approving Authority (CLAA) under the Drugs and Cosmetics Rules, 1945.

PROCEDURE FOR OBTAINING LICENSE TO OPERATE BLOOD CENTER

Applications for grant or renewal of manufacturing licenses for the operation of blood centers or the preparation of human blood components are made by government-run blood centers, Indian Red Cross Society, hospital, charitable trust, or voluntary organization to the SLA as well as CLAA. Blood center run by charitable trust or voluntary organization must be approved by the respective State/UT Blood Transfusion Council according to the procedures established for that purpose by the respective State Blood Transfusion Council and the National Blood Transfusion Council.

Norms/guidelines for the issue of no objection certificate (NOC) by the State/UT Blood Transfusion Councils for grant/renewal of blood centers licenses were issued by the Government of India (GOI) vide letter D.O. No. S-12016/1/2014-NBTC dated September 21, 2015 **(Annexure 82.1)** so as to bring transparency and uniformity in blood center licensing procedure across different states. Therefore, the requirement of NOC for grant/renewal of blood center license should be checked with the respective State Blood Transfusion Council.

The requirement of accommodation for a blood center, personnel, equipment, criteria for blood donation, processing of blood components, good manufacturing practices, testing and storage facility, standard operating procedures, and validation of equipment, etc., is provided under Part X-B of the Drugs and Cosmetics Rules, 1945. Application form, fees to be paid along with application for grant/renewal of license by the applicant, and conditions of license have been provided under Drugs and Cosmetics Rules, 1945 from Rules 122F to 122P.

MANDATORY REQUIREMENTS

- Applicant/licensee will provide and maintain adequate staff, plant, and premises for proper operation of the blood center for processing whole human blood and the preparation of its components and/or blood products.
- Applicant/licensee must maintain staff, premises, facilities, and equipment in accordance with Rule 122G under Drugs and Cosmetics Rules, 1945. Licensee must maintain necessary records and registers as set forth in Schedule F, Part XII-B and XII-C under Drugs and Cosmetics Rules, 1945.
- Licensee must test whole human blood, its components and blood products in his own laboratory and maintain records and registers in respect of such tests as specified in Schedule F, Part XII-B and Part XII-C under Drugs and Cosmetics Rules, 1945. Records and registers shall be retained for 5 years from the date of manufacture.

VARIOUS STEPS INVOLVED IN PROCESSING OF APPLICATION FOR GRANT/RENEWAL OF LICENSE FOR BLOOD CENTER

Step 1

The applicant has to submit application on Form 27-C along with the following documents to the respective SLA. A copy of the said application must be submitted to the concerned zonal/subzonal office of the CDSCO and local drug office. The application can also be submitted online in states having such facility.

1. Application on duly filled Form 27-C **(Annexure 82.2)**
2. Proof for depositing requisite license fee of ₹ 7,500/- (original treasury challan or receipt of any other mode of depositing fee) under correct head of account for 10 items and ₹ 300/- per item exceeding 10 items
3. NOC from respective State or UT Blood Transfusion Council (if required)
4. Constitution of the blood center with names and addresses of the proprietor/partners/directors/trustee. Copy of memorandum of article/trust deed/partnership deed to be attached wherever applicable
5. Affidavit by proprietor/partners/director(s)/managing director/ managing trustee [specimen of affidavits **(Annexure 82.3)**] duly attested by notary
6. Certified copy of ownership/tenancy agreement for the premises

7. Power of attorney in favor of authorized signatory [specimen of power of attorney **(Annexure 82.4)**] duly attested by notary for submitting application for grant/renewal of license on behalf of the applicant.

8. Specific resolution of Board of directors/trustees, etc., relating to the opening of the blood center (if not already included in memorandum of association)

9. Original layout showing section-wise blood center premises including the dimensions, total area in metric system, and location of various sections, doors, windows, etc., according to the requirements of Drugs and Cosmetics Rules, 1945. The suggested site plan of the blood center is at **Annexure 82.5**

10. List of technical personnel appointed with their appointment/ joining letters

11. Attested photocopies of qualifications, experience and approval certificates of medical officer, technical supervisor, blood center technicians, counselor, and registered nurse. A relieving letter from previous employer from where resigned if applicable

12. Affidavits [sample **Proforma of affidavits (Annexures 82.6 to 82.8)**] duly attested by notary from blood center staff regarding full-time work, responsibilities, and not drawing blood from professional donors of Medical officer, Laboratory Technician and Nurse.

13. Details of all machinery and equipment installed for blood collection/processing, giving full details, namely invoices, make, capacity, material of which it is made, and whether it is automatic or manual, etc.

14. List of blood/blood components to be processed and method for their preparation, duly signed by an authorized person/medical officer

15. Specimen formats of all the records/registers to be maintained as per the Drugs and Cosmetics Rules, 1945

16. Specimen labels, consent form for donors including for apheresis as per the Drugs and Cosmetics Rules, 1945

17. List of reference books and literature provided

18. Standard operating procedures (SOPs) and various procedures for blood centers duly signed by authorized person/medical officer

19. Document related to arrangement for biomedical waste management under the Biomedical Waste (Management and Handling) Rules, 1996

20. List of voluntary donors

21. Provisions of transport and other facilities for outside blood donation camps if required as per the Drugs and Cosmetics Act, 1940 and Drugs and Cosmetics Rules, 1945

Step 2

After receipt of the application, the SLA/CLAA scrutinizes the application for its completeness in all aspects. Any deficiencies/discrepancies identified by the SLA/CLAA must be communicated to the applicant for compliance. Further action shall be taken once compliance with the deficiencies/discrepancies is received from the applicant. If the application is found suitable after compliance, it will be processed for the inspection of the premises, facilities, and competence of the technical staff by the SLA/CLAA.

Step 3

After prior notice to the applicant, a joint inspection of the proposed blood center will be conducted according to the format specified in **Annexure 82.9**. If the inspection reveals shortcomings/discrepancies, the applicant shall be intimated to rectify the same and submit compliance report to the SLA/CLAA.

Step 4

A verification of compliance with shortcomings/discrepancies identified during first inspection is done by the authorities (SLA/CLAA).

Step 5

The SLA, upon recommendation of the inspection team, will prepare/sign license in triplicate on Form 28-C and forward it to CLAA, New Delhi for his/her countersignatures.

Step 6

1. Upon receipt of the countersigned license on Form 28-C from CLAA, the SLA will issue the applicant a license to operate blood center under intimation to CLAA. If the application is rejected, the SLA/CLAA will intimate to the applicant.
2. The applicant can inform the SLA within 6 months of rejection of the application of license, that the conditions laid down have been satisfied and deposits inspection fees of ₹250/-, the SLA shall, after getting it inspected, grant/renew license.

The whole procedure for obtaining the license to operate blood center has been summarized in flowsheet diagram given in **Annexure 82.10**.

IMPORTANT NOTES

- Change in technical staff to be intimated to the SLA/CLAA/Local FDA office forthwith.
- In case of change in constitution of the firm/company, application for grant of new license for operation of blood center to be submitted forthwith to the SLA/CLAA/Local FDA office. The applicant is required to obtain new license within 3 months of change of constitution.
- In case of change of the premises of licensed blood center, new license for the new site is to be obtained prior to shifting to the new site.
- The validity of the license is 5 years. Renewal application is to be submitted before the expiry date. However, it can be submitted with late fees of ₹ 1,000/- per month up to maximum 6 months after expiry.
- In case of any alteration in building/machinery, the SLA/CLAA/Local FDA office needs to be intimated.
- In case of blood donation camp outside blood center premises, details to be sent to SLA/CLAA within 7 days.
- Prior permission for holding such outside camps should be obtained as per state guidelines issued by the State Blood Transfusion Council (SBTC).
- Any transfer of blood/blood components must be intimated to the concerned SLA or CLAA as the case may be.
- Any transfer of surplus plasma should be done under intimation to SLA as per the guidelines from the National AIDS Control Organisation (NACO) as well as respective state.

PROCESS FOR RENEWAL OF LICENSE

The Blood Center License holder need to apply for renewal of its License by submitting application on Form 27-C along with other documents (same as for grant of license) before its expiry (or within 6 months of its expiry after payment of late fee) to the SLA with copy to CLAA/Local FDA office. The license shall continue to be in force, until orders on his application are communicated to him.

The process of renewal of License is almost similar to that for grant of License (joint inspection of the facility of licensee by the officers of SLA/CLAA etc.).

Note: This chapter describes the general procedure for the guidance of its readers regarding Grant/Renewal of License to operate Blood Center, however, there might be variations in the procedure being adopted by various State/UTs, for which readers are advised to comply with the local requirements also.

ANNEXURE 82.1

DOCUMENT- 7

GUIDELINES FOR ISSUANCE OF "NOC" FOR NEW BLOOD BANK, RENEWAL OF LICENSE, CRITERIA'S FOR DESIGNATION BLOOD BANK AS RBTC

एन. एस. कंग, भा.प्र.से
अपर सचिव
NAVREET SINGH KANG, IAS
Additional Secretary

भारत सरकार
स्वास्थ्य एवं परिवार कल्याण मंत्रालय
राष्ट्रीय एड्स नियंत्रण संगठन
Government of India
Ministry of Health & Family Welfare
National AIDS Control Organisation

D. O. No. S-12016/1/2014-NBTC
Dated : 21st September, 2015

My Dear Secretary,

You would be aware that the Government of India had adopted the National Blood Policy in April 2002, which sought a comprehensive, efficient and a total quality management approach within a nation-wide system, to ensure access to adequate and safe blood supply. The National Blood Transfusion Council (NBTC) has also been set up to oversee and coordinate the functioning of blood transfusion services through the State/UT Blood Transfusion Councils, who are responsible for overall implementation of an organized blood transfusion service through a network of Regional Blood Transfusion Centres and other blood banks.

2.   In the past, clarifications has been sought by various States regarding the procedure to be adopted for allowing establishment of new blood banks, renewal thereof, and grant of status of Regional Blood Transfusion Centres etc. The matter was accordingly considered by the NBTC in its meeting on 05.08.2015 and the norms for the above have been approved. These norms are detailed in the enclosure and include

A. Norms for setting up of blood banks;
B. Norms for grant of no objection certificate for licensing of new blood banks and renewal of license of existing blood banks;
C. Norms for grant of status of Regional Blood Transfusion Centre; and
D. Norms for grant of permission for conducting voluntary blood donation camps.

3.   These have been approved so as to bring clarity and uniformity in the practice and procedure across different States. It may be ensured that the State Blood Transfusion Council in your State adopts and implements the same.

4.   Action taken in this regard may be intimated to undersigned within a month of receipt of this communication.

With regards,

Yours sincerely,

(N. S. KANG)

To
Principal Secretary (Health)
All States

6th Floor, Chandralok Building, 36 Janpath, New Delhi -110001, Telefax : 011-23325331/ 23351700
E-mail : nacoasdg@gmail.com

NORMS FOR STATE BLOOD TRANSFUSION COUNCIL AS APPROVED BY GOVERNING BODY OF NATIONAL BLOOD TRANSFUSION COUNCIL

A. **Norms for set up of New Blood Banks**

Every district should have at least one blood bank, but clustering of blood banks in urban/ semi-urban areas should be avoided. New blood banks need to be set up based on geographic location and population demand only.

B. **Norms for grant of 'No objection certificate' (NOC) by the SBTC**

B1. **For New Blood Bank License:**

1. A registered voluntary or charitable organizations, which is registered in the, territory of Union of India or Union Territory, as the case may be under any such law which is at the time of enforcement of this rule in force.

2. The aforesaid organization must be atleast two years old and should not be a family society or trust.

3. The objectives mentioned in the Memorandum of Association must include the activities related to health care delivery system or blood transfusion services.

4. The activities undertaken by the organization must showcase social accountability and be reflected in the annual Audited Statement of accounts of the last two year (i.e. before the submission of application).

5. The organization should submit undertaking to ensure annual blood collection - more than 2000 units per year with nearing 100% contribution from Voluntary blood donor, preferably collected from outdoor blood donation camps.

6. The organization should submit undertaking to appoint Medical Social Worker (MSW) and Counselor with the blood bank for arranging Voluntary Blood Donation (VBD) camps and Pre and Post Test counseling respectively.

7. The organization should submit undertaking to establish blood component separation facility of its own or a storage facility for components within a period of two years from receiving license to operate blood bank.

8. The organization should submit undertaking to abide with the guidelines of - SBTC/NBTC issued from time to time, including the guidelines for processing charges for blood and blood components.

Note:

c. The Organization should submit undertaking on the letter head expressing willingness to abide with aforesaid conditions.

d. The SBTC should process the application within thirty days from the date of its receipt in the office; failing which NOC shall be deemed granted to the organization.

B2   For Renewal Blood Bank License:

1. The compliance to point no. 1-4 of norms at B1 (No objection certificate (NOC) for New Blood Bank License) shall be ensured.

2. The organization should submit photocopy of license and application months before the expiry of validity period of license.

3. The organization should submit Annual blood collection report wherein the total blood collection (Jan-Dec) is shown with voluntary contribution to total collection along with number of blood donation camps conducted. (The annual blood collection should be more than 2000 units per year with nearing 100% contribution from Voluntary blood donor, preferably collected from outdoor blood donation camps. The condition may be relaxed for rural, tribal, hilly region, desert, island and Armed Forces)

4. The organization should submit the proof and details of appointment of Medical Social Worker (MSW) and Counselor with the blood bank for arranging Voluntary Blood Donation (VBD) camps and Pre and Post Test counseling respectively along with the training certificates.

5. The organization should submit Annual report indicating blood component separation facility has been established either of its own or a storage facility, wherein the components were sourced from RBTC approved by SBTC.

6. The organization should submit details of processing charges collected by the blood bank after 12th February 2014. The SBTC should verify, if charges collected are subsidized or at par with guidelines issued by NBTC.

Note :

c)   The Organization should submit undertaking on the letter head expressing willingness to abide with aforesaid conditions.

d)   The SBTC should process the application within thirty days from the date of its receipt in the office; failing which NOC shall be deemed granted to the organization.

C. Norms for grant of 'Regional Blood Transfusion Center' (RBTC) status to blood banks.

RBTC is a blood bank approved by the SBTC taking into consideration the regional needs of blood & blood components and the ability of RBTC in terms of premises, personnel and equipment to cater to the same.   A center will be designated as RBTC only after SBTC formally networks it with blood bank/ blood storage centers in the region and establishes two way linkages for exchanges of blood and blood components.

1. The blood bank should be licensed and provide round the clock service

2. The blood bank should have minimum collection of 2000 per annum with voluntary contribution nearing to 90%. (The criteria for minimum collection may be relaxed in rural, tribal, hilly region, desert, island and Armed Forces).

3. The Blood bank should have component separation facility. Alternatively, Blood bank should provide undertaking to establish component separation facility within two years' time frame.

4. The blood bank should have adequate facilities to store and transport blood and blood components at required temperature and ambient conditions.

5. The blood bank should have minimum TTI screening by ELISA facility for atleast 80% collected unit and should be practicing tube method for blood grouping and cross matching. (The criteria for minimum testing may be relaxed in -rural, tribal, hilly region, desert, island and Armed Forces).

6. The blood bank should be capable of imparting periodic training to staff attached with Blood Storage Center for blood grouping, cross matching, storage, identifying haemolysis and record keeping.

7. All equipment in the blood bank should be under AMC/CMC and calibrated at the time of applying for RBTC Status and subsequent renewal every year as mandated under Drugs and Cosmetic Act.

8. All records books should be available with the Blood Bank as stipulated in the Drugs and Cosmetics Act 1940 and Rules 1945 there upon.

9. The blood bank should have computer and trained staff to maintain database of donor, blood and products and inventory of demand and supplies made on daily basis.

10. The blood bank must update its stock status of blood availability blood group wise online with NBTC website.

Note:

The RBTC status accorded will be initially for a period of two years only. However, it would be renewed based on the performance and fulfillment of all aforesaid conditions for a further period of five years and at five years interval thereafter.

D. Norms for grant of permission to conduct voluntary blood donation camps:

Drugs and Cosmetics Act, 1940 and rules 1945 thereupon under Schedule f= Part XII B has permitted following types of licensed Blood Banks to collect blood by conducting voluntary blood donations camps.

1. Government Blood Bank.
2. Indian Red Cross Society Blood Bank.
3. Regional Blood Transfusion Centers designated by SBTC.
4. Blood Banks managed by registered voluntary or charitable trust organizations recognized by BTC.

However, to ensure 100% blood collection from voluntary non remunerated blood donors in the country, it was decided to permit hospital based private blood banks also to conduct blood donation camps. The DCGI was requested to examine the same and introduce a suitable amendant to the act.

Note: Subsequent to this letter dated 21.9.2015, the Government of India, vide gazette notification number G.S.R.-328 (E) Dated 3rd April 2017 permitted 'private hospital blood center' also to conduct blood donation camps.

ANNEXURE 82.2

Form 27-C
(See rule 122-F)

APPLICATION FOR GRANT/RENEWAL* OF LICENSE FOR THE OPERATION OF A BLOOD CENTER FOR PROCESSING OF WHOLE BLOOD AND/OR* PREPARATION OF BLOOD COMPONENTS

1. I/We_____, of M/s _____ hereby apply for the grant of license/renewal of license number _____dated _____to operate a Blood Center, for processing of whole blood and/or* for preparation of its components on the premises situated at _____.

2. Name(s) of the item(s):
   1. Whole Human Blood IP
   2.
   3.

3. The name(s), qualification and experience of competent Technical Staff are as under:
   (a) Name(s) of Medical Officer.   _____
   (b) Name(s) of Technical Supervisor.   _____
   (c) Name(s) of Registered Nurse.   _____
   (d) Name(s) of Blood Center Technician. _____

4. The premises and plant are ready for inspection/will be ready for inspection on_____.

5. A license fee of rupees 6,000/- and an inspection fee of rupees 1,500/- has been credited to the Government under the Head of Account _____ (receipt enclosed).

_____
                                                          Signature

Dated _____   **Name and Designation**

*Delete, whichever is not applicable.

Note:

1. The application shall be accompanied by a plan of the premises, list of machinery and equipment for collection, processing, storage and testing of whole blood and its components, memorandum of association/constitution of the firm, copies of certificate relating to educational qualifications and experience of the competent technical staff and documents relating to ownership or tenancy of the premises.

2. A copy of the application together with the relevant enclosures shall also be sent to the Central Licence Approving Authority and to the concerned Zonal/Sub-Zonal Officers of the Central Drugs Standard Control Organization.

ANNEXURE 82.3

Proforma of Affidavit to be submitted by Proprietor/Partners/Director(s)/Managing Director/ Managing Trustee

I_____ S/o; W/o; D/o Shri _____, Age _____, and Resident of _____ declare solemnly on oath as under:

1. That I am proprietor/partner/Managing Director/Managing Trustee/ Principal Medical Officer of _____ (Complete Address of Blood Center) _____ by whom an application for grant of license for the operation of a Blood Center for processing of Whole Human Blood and preparation of Blood Components has been made on Form Nos. 27-C to the Licensing Authority under the provisions of Drugs and Cosmetics Act, 1940 and Rules, 1945.

2. That following are the other Partners/Directors/Trustees of the firm:

S. No.	Name(s)	Age	Residential address

3. That the building in which manufacturing activities are proposed are taken on rent/lease from _____ /are own premises/ Government Building which are adapted as per Schedule F, Part XII-B/C of the said Rules.

4. That adequate qualified competent technical staff has already been appointed. Details of the qualified technical personnel including their affidavits have been attached with the application.

5. That I will be responsible for the conduct of day-to-day activities of the firm for the purpose of Section 34 of the said Act as well as other prevailing enactments established by Government of India.

6. That undersigned will ensure that no professional donor is bled in the Blood Center.

Witness No. 1 _____
(Signature, Name and Address)

Witness No. 2 _____
(Signature, Name and Address)

_____
(DEPONENT)
Name

VERIFICATION

I, _____ verify that the contents of para 1 to 6 of this affidavit are true to the best of my knowledge and belief.

Date: _____

Place: _____

_____
(DEPONENT)
Name

ANNEXURE 82.4

Proforma of Affidavit for Power of Attorney to be Executed by Partners/Managing Director

I, _____ S/o; W/o; D/o Shri _____, age _____, Resident of _____ declare solemnly on oath as under:

1. That I am Partner/Managing Director of M/s _____, (Complete Address of manufacturing site) _____ by whom an application for grant of license for operation of Blood Center has been made to the State Licensing Authority/Central License Approving Authority under Drugs & Cosmetics Rules 1945.

2. That Shri _____ S/o: W/o; D/o _____ Age _____ Resident of _____ is authorized to sign and submit documents on behalf of the firm to the State Licensing Authority/Central License Approving Authority under Drugs and Cosmetics Rules 1945_____.

3. That the signatures of Shri _____ are hereby attested as under:

Signatures of Shri _____

Witness No. 1 _____
(Signature, Name and Address)

Witness No. 2 _____
(Signature, Name and Address)

_____
(DEPONENT)
Name

VERIFICATION

I, _____ verify that the contents of para 1 to 3 of this affidavit are true to the best of my knowledge and belief.

Date: _____

Place: _____

_____
(DEPONENT)
Name

ANNEXURE 82.5

Suggested Site Plan of Blood Center

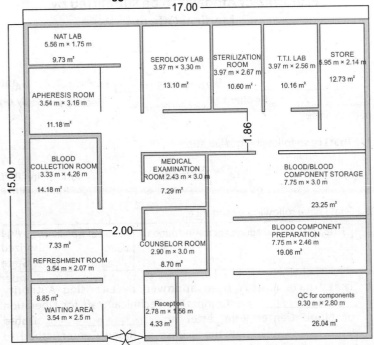

Details of carpet area for blood center

S. No.	Area name	Unit	Total area
	Blood center		
1	Reception area	Sqm.	4.33
2	Waiting area	Sqm.	8.85
3	Refreshment room	Sqm.	7.33
4	Blood collection room	Sqm.	14.18
5	Storeroom	Sqm.	12.73
6	Washing and sterilization room	Sqm.	10.6
7	Serology lab	Sqm.	13.10
8	TTI lab	Sqm.	10.16
9	NAT lab	Sqm.	9.73
10	Medical examination	Sqm.	7.29
11	Counselor room	Sqm.	8.7
	Total		107.00
	Component area		
13	Quality control	Sqm.	26.04
14	Blood component preparation	Sqm.	19.06
15	Blood component storage	Sqm.	23.25
	Total		68.35
	Apheresis area		
16	Apheresis room	Sqm.	11.18

ANNEXURE 82.6

Proforma of Affidavit to be submitted by Medical Officer

I, _____ S/o; W/o; D/o Shri _____, Age _____, Resident of _____ declare solemnly on oath as under:

1. That I have following qualification:

   S. No.   Qualification   University

2. That I have following experience:

S. No.	Name and address of the institution	Period of working with dates

3. That I have already been approved by Licensing Authority _____ as Competent Technical staff for Operation of Blood Center vide letter no. _____ Dated _____ on the license of Blood Center issued to _____ bearing Licence No. _____ granted on _____ Under Drugs and Cosmetics Rules 1945

4. That I am Registered with Medical Council _____ at No. _____ on _____. That I have got adequate knowledge and experience in blood group serology and methodology and medical principles involved in blood and its components.

5. That I have joined as whole time employee in _____ (Complete Address of Blood Center) _____ on _____ and will inform the Licensing Authority _____ as soon as I resign from this institution.

6. That I was working previously with _____, (Complete Address of Blood Center) _____ up to _____ and have informed the Licensing Authority _____ on _____ regarding my resignation from this institution.

7. That I will be responsible for the operation of Blood Center for the purpose of Section 34 of the said Act as well as other prevailing enactments established by Government of India.

8. That undersigned will ensure that no professional donor is bled in the Blood Center

Witness No. 1 _____
(Signature, Name and Address)

Witness No. 2 _____
(Signature, Name and Address)

_____
(DEPONENT)

VERIFICATION

I, _____ verify that the contents of para 1 to 8 of this affidavit are true to the best of my knowledge and belief.

Date: _____

Place: _____

_____
(DEPONENT)
Name

ANNEXURE 82.7

Proforma of Affidavit for Blood Center Technician

I, _____ S/o Shri _____, Age _____, and Resident of _____ declare solemnly on oath as under:

1. That I have following qualification:

S. No.	Qualification	University

2. That I have following experience:

S. No.	Name and address of the institution	Period of working with dates

3. That I have already been approved by Licensing Authority _____ as Competent Technical staff for operation of Blood Center vide letter no. _____ Dated _____ on the licences of Blood Center issued to _____ bearing Licence No. _____ granted on _____

4. That I am Registered with State Technical Board/Council of _____ at No. _____ on _____.

5. That I have joined as whole time in Blood Center, _____ _____ on _____ and will inform the Licensing Authority as soon as I resign from this institution.

6. That I was working previously with _____, (Complete Address of Blood Center) _____ up to _____ and have informed the Licensing Authority _____ on _____ regarding my resignation from this institution.

7. That I will be responsible for the operation of Blood center for the purpose of Section 34 of the said Act as well as other prevailing enactments established by Government of India.

8. That undersigned will ensure that no professional donor is bled in the Blood Center.

Witness No. 1 _____
(Signature, Name and Address)

Witness No. 2 _____
(Signature, Name and Address)

_____
(DEPONENT)
Name

VERIFICATION

I, _____ verify that the contents of para 1 to 8 of this affidavit are true to the best of my knowledge and belief.

Date: _____

Place: _____

_____
(DEPONENT)
Name

ANNEXURE 82.8

Proforma of Affidavit to be submitted by Registered Nurse

I, _____ S/o; W/o; D/o Shri _____, Age _____, Resident of _____ declare solemnly on oath as under:

1. That I have following qualification:

    S. No.   Qualification   University

2. That I have following experience:

S. No.	Name and address of the institution	Period of working with dates

3. That I have already been approved by Licensing Authority _____ as Competent Technical staff for Operation of Blood Center vide letter no. _____ Dated _____ on the license of Blood Center issued to _____ bearing License No. _____ granted on _____

4. That I am Registered with Nursing Council _____ at No. _____ on _____.

5. That I have joined _____ (Complete Address of Blood Center) _____ on _____ and will inform the Licensing Authority as soon as I resign from this institution.

6. That I was working previously with _____ (Complete Address of Blood Center) _____ up to _____ and have informed the Licensing Authority _____ on regarding my resignation from this institution.

7. That I will be responsible for the operation of Blood Center for the purpose of Section 34 of the said Act as well as other prevailing enactments established by Government of India

8. That undersigned will ensure that no professional donor is bled in the Blood Center

Witness No. 1 _____
(Signature, Name and Address)

Witness No. 2 _____
(Signature, Name and Address)

_____
(DEPONENT)
Name

VERIFICATION

I, _____ verify that the contents of para 1 to 8 of this affidavit are true to the best of my knowledge and belief.

Date: _____

Place: _____

_____
(DEPONENT)
Name

ANNEXURE 82.9

Central Drugs Standard Control Organization
Blood Center Inspection Check List
(Use separate sheets, if necessary)

Name of Institution		Date of Inspection		
Address of the Institution				
Telephone No.: Fax No.: E-mail:				
License number and date of issue				
Inspected By				
Institution represented by				
Purpose of inspection				
Type of Institution	Government	Charitable/ Voluntary	Red Cross	Others (specify)
Constitution Details	Limited			
Products				
Technical staff	Number	Present/ Absent		
Doctor				
Technical Supervisor				
Technicians				
Registered Nurse				
Counsellor				

A	Total Collection	Year		
	(last two calendar years)	Voluntary		
		Replacement		
		Professional		
		Total		
	Distribution	Used in own hospital		
		Issued to others		
		Discarded		
B	**Premises**	Total area		
	Details of areas	**Comments**		
1	Registration, Medical Examination Waiting area/ Reception			
2	Blood collection (A/C ?)			
3	Serology lab. (A/C ?)			
4	Transmissible Diseases lab. (A/C ?)			
5	Sterilization & washing			
6	Refreshment & Rest room (A/C)			
7	Store & Records room			
8	Blood issue area			
9	Components preparation & Storage area		Central conditioned	
10	Apheresis area			
	Comments on Area			
C	Standard Books?	Yes/No/NA		
1	(Obtain list)			
2	Blood center manual	Yes/No/NA		
3	Standard operating procedures	Yes/No/NA		
a	Criteria to determine donor suitability	Yes/No/NA		
b	Method of donor selection	Yes/No/NA		

Continued

Continued

c	Preparation of phlebotomy site	Yes/No/NA	
d	Product to donor traceability	Yes/No/NA	
e	Collection procedures, precautions etc.	Yes/No/NA	
f	Method of components preparation	Yes/No/NA	
g	Test methods	Yes/No/NA	
h	Pre-transfusion testing	Yes/No/NA	
i	Adverse reaction management	Yes/No/NA	
j	Storage temperature & its control	Yes/No/NA	
k	Expiry date assignment	Yes/No/NA	
l	Returned blood management	Yes/No/NA	
m	QC for reagents & supplies	Yes/No/NA	
n	Maintenance, calibration & validation of equipment	Yes/No/NA	
o	Labelling procedures	Yes/No/NA	
p	Apheresis procedures	Yes/No/NA	
q	Any other SOPs	Yes/No/NA	
D	Procedure for disposal of blood (expired, clotted, improperly collected, HIV + etc.)	Yes/No/NA	
E	Donor education/ Motivation material	Yes/No/NA	
F	Donor selection	Yes/No/NA	
1	Donor record	Yes/No/NA	
2	Selection/rejection manual	Yes/No/NA	

Continued

Continued

3	**Donor record details**		
a	Age	Yes/No/NA	
b	Interval between donations	Yes/No/NA	
c	Last pregnancy/delivery/Abortion	Yes/No/NA	
d	Immunization details	Yes/No/NA	
e	Recent drug intake	Yes/No/NA	
f	Major surgery	Yes/No/NA	
g	Malaria	Yes/No/NA	
h	Jaundice	Yes/No/NA	
i	Other viral infection	Yes/No/NA	
j	Fever & common cold	Yes/No/NA	
k	History–Cancer, TB, Diabetes, Drug addiction, etc.	Yes/No/NA	
l	Alcohol intake	Yes/No/NA	
m	Transfusion history	Yes/No/NA	
4	**Donor Examination**	Yes/No/NA	
a	Weight	Yes/No/NA	
b	Venipuncture site	Yes/No/NA	
c	Hemoglobin	Yes/No/NA	
d	Blood pressure	Yes/No/NA	
e	Pulse	Yes/No/NA	
f	Temperature	Yes/No/NA	
G	**Collection of Blood**		
a	Preparation of phlebotomy site	Yes/No/NA	
b	Type and amount of anticoagulant used	Yes/No/NA	
c	Amount of blood collected (random wt.)	Yes/No/NA	
d	Blood collected in bags/bottles	Yes/No/NA	
e	Pediatric bags?	Yes/No/NA	
f	Is mixing done during collection? How?	Yes/No/NA	

Continued

Continued

g	Is new bag used in case of 2nd puncture?	Yes/No/NA	
h	How are sample tubes labeled?	Yes/No/NA	
i	Emergency kit available?	Yes/No/NA	
H	**Storage of Blood**		
a	Temperature recording graph preserved?	Yes/No/NA	
b	Alarm system checks done?	Yes/No/NA	
c	Physical verification done? Frequency?	Yes/No/NA	
d	How is blood transported? Outside, to wards?	Yes/No/NA	
I	**Blood Testing**		
a	Sterility testing	Yes/No/NA	
b	Hemoglobin estimationmethod	Yes/No/NA	
c	Method for ABO grouping	Yes/No/NA	
d	Procedure for grouping	Yes/No/NA	
e	Method of pooled cell preparation	Yes/No/NA	
f	Du test done on D- samples?	Yes/No/NA	
g	Test for unexpected antibodies done?	Yes/No/NA	
h	Hepatitis test done? Describe method and name of kit manufacturer	Yes/No/NA	
i	Syphilis test done? Describe method and name of kit manufacturer	Yes/No/NA	
j	HIV test done? Describe method and name of kit manufacturer	Yes/No/NA	

Continued

Continued

k	HCV test done? Describe method and name of kit manufacturer	Yes/No/NA	
l	Malaria test done? Describe method	Yes/No/NA	
m	Donor informed in case of +ve results?	Yes/No/NA	
n	In case of HbsAg/ HIV +ve results Donor deferred permanently	Yes/No/NA	
o	Are HbsAg/HIV +ve donors followed up?	Yes/No/NA	
J	**Testing of Reagents, etc.**		
a	Antisera tested?	Yes/No/NA	
b	Method of antisera testing	Yes/No/NA	
c	CPDA solution testing	Yes/No/NA	
K	**General Equipment and Instruments**		
a	Refrigerators for blood storage Type & capacity & number		Yes/No/NA
b	Temperature recorder in refrigerator		Yes/No/NA
c	Audible alarm system in refrigerator		Yes/No/NA
d	Balance for bag weighing		Yes/No/NA
e	Autoclave with temp. and pressure display		Yes/No/NA
f	Incinerator		Yes/No/NA
g	Emergency power supply (generator)		Yes/No/NA
h	Donor beds, chairs, tables		Yes/No/NA
i	Bedside table		Yes/No/NA
j	Sphygmomanometer & stethoscope		Yes/No/NA
k	Recovery bed for donors		Yes/No/NA
l	Donor weighing scale		Yes/No/NA

Continued

Continued

L	**Emergency Equipment**	
a	Oxygen cylinder, mask, gauge and pressure regulator	Yes/No/NA
b	5% dextrose or normal saline inj.	Yes/No/NA
c	Sterile disposable syringes and needles (various sizes)	Yes/No/NA
d	Sterile disposable IV sets	Yes/No/NA
e	Adrenaline, Noradrenaline, Mephentine, Betamethasone (or dexamethasone), Metoclopramide injections	Yes/No/NA
M	**Accessories**	
a	Blankets, emesis basins, hemostats, set clamps, sponge forceps, gauze, dressing jars, waste cans etc.	Yes/No/NA
b	Medium cotton balls, 1.25 cm adhesive tapes	Yes/No/NA
c	Denatured spirit, Tinc. Iodine, green or liquid soap	Yes/No/NA
d	Paper napkins or towels	Yes/No/NA
N	**Laboratory Equipment**	
a	Refrigerator for kits and reagents storage Refrigerator make and capacity Temperature display provided	Yes/No/NA Yes/No/NA
b	Compound microscope with low- & high-power objectives	Yes/No/NA
c	Table centrifuge	Yes/No/NA
d	Water bath- 37–57°	Yes/No/NA
e	Rh viewing box	Yes/No/NA
f	Incubator with thermostat	Yes/No/NA
g	Mechanical shakers for serological test for syphilis	Yes/No/NA
h	Hand lens	Yes/No/NA
i	Serological graduated pipettes of various sizes	Yes/No/NA
j	Pasteur pipettes	Yes/No/NA
k	Glass slides	Yes/No/NA
l	Test tubs of various sizes/microplates	Yes/No/NA
m	Precipitating tubes (6 × 50 mm) of various sizes	Yes/No/NA
n	Test tube racks	Yes/No/NA
o	Interval timer	Yes/No/NA
p	Material and equipment for glassware cleaning	Yes/No/NA
q	Blood transporting containers	Yes/No/NA
r	Wash bottles	Yes/No/NA

Continued

Continued

s	Filter papers	Yes/No/NA
t	Dielectric tube sealer	Yes/No/NA
u	Plain and EDTA vials	Yes/No/NA
v	Chemical balance	Yes/No/NA
w	Elisa reader with printer, washer and micropipettes	Yes/No/NA
x	Colorimeters/hemoglobinometer (strike off which is not applicable) for hemoglobin determination	Yes/No/NA

O	**Records and Reports**		
			Comments on records, if any
a	Blood stock register	Yes/No/NA	
b	Blood donor record	Yes/No/NA	
c	Issue register	Yes/No/NA	
d	Record of blood bags	Yes/No/NA	
e	Crossmatching records	Yes/No/NA	
f	Register of diagnostic reagents and kits	Yes/No/NA	
g	Adverse reaction records	Yes/No/NA	
h	Stock register of other consumable articles	Yes/No/NA	
i	Are records destroyed?	Yes/No/NA	
j	Labels of blood containers as per Schedule F of the D & C Act	Yes/No/NA	
P	**Outdoor Camps**		
a	Eligible to hold outdoor camps	Yes/No/NA	
b	Average number of camps held per month	Yes/No/NA	
c	Vehicle available?	Yes/No/NA	
d	How are blood bags transported	Yes/No/NA	
e	Proof sanitary conditions of camps	Yes/No/NA	
f	Detailed statement of blood collected in camps	Yes/No/NA	

PROCESSING OF BLOOD COMPONENTS FROM WHOLE HUMAN BLOOD

Q	ACCOMMODATION/PREMISES		COMMENTS
1	Area provided for component preparation.		
2	Is an additional 10-sq. meter area provided for apheresis procedures.		
a	Is blood component room air-conditioned?	Yes/No/NA	
b	Is blood component room well lighted?	Yes/No/NA	
c	Are walls and floors smooth & washable?	Yes/No/NA	
d	Are overall hygienic conditions maintained in the premises?	Yes/No/NA	
e	Comments on Area: The plan of premise is already approved.		
R	**PERSONNEL**	YES/NO	Comment
	Whether Technical Supervisor with adequate basic qualification and experience is available with the blood center. Name, Qualifications & Experience		
S1	**Equipment**		Make/Model/Capacity
(i)	Air Conditioner	Yes/No/NA	
(ii)	Laminar air flow bench	Yes/No/NA	
(iii)	Suitable refrigerated centrifuge	Yes/No/NA	
(iv)	Plasma expresser	Yes/No/NA	
(v)	Clipper and clips and/or dielectric sealer	Yes/No/NA	
(vi)	Weighing device	Yes/No/NA	
(vii)	Dry rubber balancing material	Yes/No/NA	
(viii)	Artery forceps, scissors	Yes/No/NA	

Continued

Continued

(ix)	Refrigerator maintaining a temperature between 2°C to 6°C, a digital dial thermometer with recording thermograph and alarm device, with provision for continuous power supply.	Yes/No/NA	
(x)	Platelet agitator with incubator (wherever necessary)	Yes/No/NA	
(xi)	Deep freezers maintaining a temperature between –30°C to –40°C and –75°C to –80°C	Yes/No/NA	
(xii)	Refrigerated water bath for plasma Thawing.	Yes/No/NA	
(xiii)	Insulated blood bag containers with provisions for storing at appropriate temperature for transport purposes.	Yes/No/NA	
(xiv)	Whether components are prepared only in a closed system using single, double, triple or quadruple plastic bags.	Yes/No/NA	
S2	**Equipment (Good Manufacturing Practice, GMP)**		**COMMENTS**
1	Are equipment located in logical sequence and permit effective cleaning?	Yes/No/NA	
2	Are equipment calibrated/ validated periodically?	Yes/No/NA	
T	**PREPARATION OF BLOOD COMPONENTS**		
1.	Concentrated Human RBC's (Packed Red Blood Cells)		COMMENTS
a	Whether SOP is available for preparation of PRC? Specify: Source material Method RPM Time	Yes/No/NA	

Continued

Continued

b	Is blood collected from suitable donor? (Check the donor record).	Yes/No/NA	
c	Are the packed red cells confirmed to the standard of IP 2022	Yes/No/NA	
d	How the pilot tubes/samples are numbered?	Yes/No/NA	
e	Whether pilot tube is attached in a tamper-proof manner to the unit?	Yes/No/NA	
f	Who is responsible for filling of pilot samples?	Yes/No/NA	
g	Whether pilot samples are filled immediately after the blood is collected or at the time the final product is prepared?	Yes/No/NA	
h	Whether expiry is assigned as per norms? (specify the period)	Yes/No/NA	
2.	**Platelets concentrates**		**COMMENTS**
a	Whether SOP is available for preparation of platelets concentrates? Specify: Source material Method RPM Time	Yes/No/NA	
b	Whether the whole blood/ source material is stored at 20–24°C after collection, before processing to platelet concentrates?	Yes/No/NA	
c	Whether platelet concentrates are separated within 6 hours after the time of collection whole blood/source material	Yes/No/NA	

Continued

Continued

d	Whether platelet concentrates are tested: Platelet count (Note the count) pH (not less than 6) measurement of plasma volume sterility (1% of total platelets prepared shall be tested for sterility), 'functional viability' (swirling movement)	Yes/No/NA	
e	Whether compatibility test prepared on every unit before issue	Yes/No/NA	
f	Whether platelet yield is calculated (1% of total platelets prepared shall be tested of which 75% of units shall confirm to standards)	Yes/No/NA	
3.	**Fresh frozen plasma**		**COMMENTS**
a	Whether SOP is available for preparation of FPF? Specify: Source material Method RPM Time	Yes/No/NA	
b	Whether deep freezers capable of maintaining temp. between 75°C to 80°C and –30°C to –40°C are available	Yes/No/NA	
c	Whether the source material/ human blood stored at 4°C till processed	Yes/No/NA	
d	Whether thawing facilities are provided (note the thawing temperature)	Yes/No/NA	
e	Lag time between collecting of blood and processing of FFP (check records)	Yes/No/NA	

Continued

Continued

4.	**Apheresis procedure**		**COMMENTS**
a	Whether cell separator facility is provided?	Yes/No/NA	
b	Whether donor is certified fit for apheresis? (check the record)	Yes/No/NA	
c	Time allowed between successive apheresis on a single donor	Yes/No/NA	
d	Whether protein estimation of donor carried out if serial apheresis is to be conducted.	Yes/No/NA	
e	Whether inquiries about aspirin intake made before platelet apheresis.	Yes/No/NA	
f	Whether RBC's are re-transfused during platelet apheresis or plasmapheresis. If not, what precautions are taken?	Yes/No/NA	
g	Whether following tests are carried out before apheresis procedures:		
	Name of the test Acceptance criteria		
	(i) Hemoglobin/Hematocrit (ii) Platelet count (iii) WBC count (iv) Differential count (v) Serum protein		COMMENTS
h	How much quantity of plasma is to be collected (Plasma apheresis)		
	DURATION (I) Single sitting (II) Per months		COMMENTS
U	**Storage of blood components**		

S. No.	BLOOD COMPONENT	TEMPERATURE	DURATION/ EXPIRY PERIOD
1.	FFP		
2.	Platelet concentrate		
3.	Red cell concentrate		
4.	Whole human blood		
5.	Cryoprecipitate		

Continued

Continued

	Apheresis procedure		COMMENTS
a	Whether cell separator facility is provided?	Yes/No/NA	
b	Whether donor is certified fit for apheresis (Check record)	Yes/No/NA	
c	Time allowed between successive apheresis on a single donor	Yes/No/NA	
d	Whether protein estimation of donor carried out if serial apheresis is to be conducted	Yes/No/NA	
e	Whether inquiries about aspirin intake made before platelet apheresis	Yes/No/NA	
f	Whether RBC's are re-transfused during platelet apheresis or Leukapheresis. If not, what precautions are taken?	Yes/No/NA	
g	**Whether following tests are carried out before apheresis procedures**		
	Name of Test	Acceptance Criteria	
	• Hemoglobin/Hematocrit	$\geq$ 12.5 g/dL	
	• Platelet count	$\geq$ 1.5 lac/cubic mm	
	• WBC count	4 to 11000/cubic mm	
	• Differential count	As per norms	
	• Serum proteins	NLT 6 g/dL	
h	**How much quantity of plasma is to be collected (Plasma Apheresis)**		
	DURATION (i) Single sitting	Not exceeding 500 mL/sitting	
	(ii) Per months	Not exceeding 1000 mL/month	
V	**Records and labels**	**YES/NO**	**COMMENTS**
1	Whether details of quantity supplied, compatibility report, details of receipts and signature of issuing person mentioned in the component record.	Yes/No/NA	

Continued

Continued

2	Whether master record for component and issue register is mentioned as per norms	Yes/No/NA		
3	Whether labels for components are prepared as per norms	Yes/No/NA		
4	Whether all details on labels are filled by the responsible person on the final container	Yes/No/NA		
W	**Total no. of components prepared with their final disposition**			
Year	**Item**	**Final disposition**		**Total processing**

ANNEXURE 82.10

Flow Sheet Diagram for Establishing Blood Center

Location and Surroundings Away from open sewage, drain, public lavatory or similar unhygienic surroundings	**Building(s)** Hygienic and avoid the entry of insects, rodents and flies, well-lighted, ventilated and screened mesh, floors and walls shall be smooth washable and drains of adequate size and traps to be provided	**Accommodation: Blood Center** • 100 m² for whole human blood • 50 m² for components • 10 m² for apheresis • Along with ancillary areas

NOC from SBTC NOC from respective State Blood Transfusion Council (if required)	**Infrastructure Facility** Personnel, Machinery, Equipment and Instruments, Reagents and Kits, etc, and documentation/ SOPs as specified under Rule 122-G and Schedule F-II	**Layout Plan** Site Plan of Blood Center premises showing location of various sections like donor room, refreshment room, laboratories, etc., with dimensions of area of each section in metric system

Step 1 Statutory Application Application on Form 27-C along with requisite fees and relevant documents to respective State Licensing Authority (SLA) Copy to concerned Zonal/Subzonal Office of the CDSCO and local Drug Office	**Step 2 Scrutiny of Application** SLA/CLAA scrutinizes the application to ensure its completeness. In case the application is found in order, processing is done for the joint inspection of the premises, facilities for mfg. and testing and competence of the technical personnel	**Step 3 Joint Inspection** Joint inspection is carried out by representative of CDSCO, SLA and Blood Center Expert. Re-inspection can be done in case of shortcoming/ discrepancies (during first inspection) for verification of compliance thereof

Step 6 Issue of License SLA then issue the License to the applicant for operation of Blood Center after receiving countersigned license from CLAA	**Step 5 Preparation of License** On receipt of the recommendation of the Joint Inspection Team, the SLA prepare/sign license on Form 28-C and forward to CLAA, New Delhi, for countersignatures	**Step 4 Verification of Deficiencies** Verification for compliance of shortcoming/ discrepancies observed during first inspection, is done

CHAPTER 83

Voluntary Blood Donation Camps

INTRODUCTION

Voluntary blood donors are the best source of appropriately secured, trusted, and safe supply of quality blood and blood components from low-risk population. Voluntary nonremunerated blood donors include those persons, who give their blood, plasma, or other blood components with free consent without any payment for it, either in the form of cash or in-kind, which could be considered a substitute for money. This includes time off work, other than reasonably needed for the donation and travel. Tokens of love, affection, refreshments, and reimbursement of the travel costs are compatible with voluntary, nonremunerated blood donation. Gift of blood by such donors voluntarily constitutes one of the most perfect examples of altruism in action. The purpose of voluntary blood donation is to wipe off the scarcity of blood and ensure safe and quality blood and blood components round the clock to the ailing mankind. This will help the medical fraternity to safeguard interests of human suffering, even in the far-flung remote areas of the country.

Healthy, committed, responsive, and motivated voluntary blood donors are the backbone of blood transfusion services throughout the world. As per the Hon'ble Supreme Court Judgment, professional blood donation was prohibited in the country with effect from January 1, 1998, and it is an offense under the Drugs and Cosmetics Rules, 1945 now to create a situation of near total voluntary blood donation program in the country and phasing out even the replacement donor system.

"National Voluntary Blood Donation Day" is celebrated on October 1st of every year across the country to raise awareness and promote voluntary blood donation. Concept of voluntary blood donation initiative can be traced back to 1942, during the time of World War II, when the first blood center was established in Kolkata. Blood donation agencies organize workshops and seminars to educate people about the benefits of donating blood throughout the country. With a huge population of youth, blood donation drives are conducted by public as well as private hospitals and government/nongovernment organizations at college/school campuses. The Government of India launched an initiative called *e-RaktKosh* (*Rakt*: Blood, *Kosh*: Repository), a web-based system in 2016 that composes all blood centers in the state into a single network, providing information about blood donation camps and the availability of human blood in blood centers/hospitals. A mobile application for the *e-RaktKosh* portal was launched in 2020 to improve accessibility. As per the statistics, India presently requires around 1.45 crore blood units every year. Presently, around 70% of human blood is collected through voluntary blood donation, and rest 30% is through replacement donation through more than 4,000 licensed blood centers in the country, which calls for greater awareness generation among the common public.

WHERE ONE CAN DONATE BLOOD

Any person interested to donate his/her blood can donate either in a licensed blood center or outside in blood donation camps as per provisions under the Drugs and Cosmetics Rules, 1945.

Blood Centers

Blood center is a licensed establishment under the Drugs and Cosmetics Rules, 1945, where any person can walk in voluntarily any time round the clock at their own convenience to donate blood, if found medically fit after medical examination. The blood center can also organize an in-house blood donation camp in its licensed premises on prefixed dates with the organizers and blood center in charge.

Outdoor Blood Donation Camps

Organizers such as educational/religious institutions, industrial and commercial houses, etc., can organize blood donation camps in their premises or at other suitable sites on a fixed day in coordination with State Blood Transfusion Council (SBTC) following provisions of Drugs and Cosmetics Rules, 1945 to collect desired number of blood units.

REQUIREMENT FOR BLOOD DONATION CAMP

Staff to be Provided by the Blood Center

For collection of 50–70 units in about 3 hours or 100–120 units in 5 hours, the following staff is needed:
- One blood transfusion/medical officer and two nurses or phlebotomists for managing six to eight donor tables

- Two blood center counselors or medical social workers
- Three blood center technicians
- Two attendants
- Vehicle with capacity to sit 8–10 persons and carriage of donation goods, including facilities to conduct blood donation camp

Equipment

Details of equipment required for the outside blood donation camp are given below:

List of equipments required for blood donation camp outside blood center

- BP apparatus
- Stethoscope
- Blood bags (single, double, triple, quadruple)
- Donor Questionnaire
- Weighing device for donors
- Weighing device for blood bags
- Donor cards and refreshments for donors
- Stripper for blood tubing
- Bedsheets, blankets/mattresses
- Lancets, swap sticks/toothpicks
- Portable Hb meter/copper sulfate method or any other quantitative method can be used for determination of hemoglobin estimation
- Test tube (big) and 12 × 100 mm (small)
- Dielectric sealer or portable tube sealer
- Needle destroyer (wherever necessary)
- Refrigerated/insulated boxes to carry blood bags
- Armrest, hand sponges
- Artery forceps, scissors, tongue depressors, kidney trays, etc.

- Infusion stand
- Needle cutter
- Markers, donor identification stickers
- Glass slides
- Test tube stand
- Test tube sealer film
- Plastic waste basket
- Medicated adhesive tape
- Artery forceps, scissors
- Tube sealer
- Emergency medical kit
- Antiseptic solution
- Dry ice or coolant
- Insulated blood bag containers with provisions for storing between 2 and 10°C
- Anti-A, anti-B, and anti-AB antisera and anti-D
- Sphygmomanometer
- Blood mixer machine
- HemoCue/hemoglobinometer
- Linens, mattresses, pillows
- Bins for collecting infectious and noninfectious waste materials
- Oxygen cylinder
- Sodium hypochlorite solutions

(BP: blood pressure; Hb: hemoglobin)

Accessories to be Provided by Organizers

- Venue for the voluntary blood donation camp should be dust/dirt free and clean, well-lighted, ventilated, and spacious with hand-washing facilities/toilets for staff as well as donors.
- Voluntary blood donation camp should be organized in sites of public assembly, namely educational institutions, youth groups, offices, factories, etc.
- Continuous, uninterrupted electric supply for the equipment used in the blood camp
- Sufficient cots, tables, chairs for registration, medical examination, and blood donation
- Clean drinking water with disposable glasses and refreshment area
- Volunteers for registration of donor, medical examination, and refreshment
- Banners regarding blood donations at the entrance, registration, and donation areas, etc., to guide the members of the blood donation camp and donors
- Communication plan according to a good strategy such as displaying posters and distributing informative leaflets at the public places well in advance for motivation of the blood donors

ORGANIZATION OF OUTDOOR VOLUNTARY BLOOD DONATION CAMP

Phase 1: Prior to Camp

- The blood centers need to estimate their requirement of blood units based on the availability of blood units in their stock for a particular period to avoid wastage of blood.
- Blood centers must discuss their requirement of blood units with the blood camp organizers and request them to arrange camp.
- Blood donor organization to coordinate with various schools/colleges/universities, industries, religious bodies, etc., for organizing camps regarding sites, dates, etc., and venue is fixed with the number of units required and list of committed donors.
- Blood centers are to seek prior permission from SBTC/local authority as per the state policy.
- Blood center staff are to visit the venue to ensure its suitability.
- Information, education, and communication (IEC) materials are to be provided to the organizers.

Phase II: During the Camp

- Blood center team arrives at the venue of blood camp well before the time.
- Ensure that the venue is neat, clean, dust free with adequate furniture, and desired room temperature maintained with the help of heaters or air conditioners and with IEC material displayed.
- Blood center team should reach the venue in time to start the camp on time.
- After registrations, donors should be subjected to screening/medical examination.
- Overcrowding should be avoided during the blood donation process.
- Blood donors should be made comfortable in the blood donation camps by ensuring adequate seating arrangement.
- Blood donation area must be with adequate lighting, ventilation, and desired temperature.
- Bleeding procedures should be as per mandatory standards under the Drug and Cosmetics Rules, 1945.
- There must be appropriate provision for donor refreshments.
- There must be arrangement for maintenance of cold chain.
- There must be necessary arrangement for management of donor reactions.
- Entry of other persons to the area should be restricted.
- Efforts should be made to wind up the camp at the stipulated time.
- Discarded blood bags/tubing/needles/and other consumables should be segregated separately for disposal as per biosafety protocols and waste management.
- Needles, lancets, and syringes should be destroyed with the needle cutter prior to their disposal.
- The blood donation camp area must be cleaned with suitable disinfectant (sodium hypochlorite: Working area and phenyl or bleaching powder: Floor) after the camp is over.
- Collected blood units should be transferred to the blood center under cold chain maintenance.

Phase III: After the Camp

All voluntary blood donors should be given thank-you letters as well as blood group cards either individually or through their particular organization. Blood donors should be kept in touch regularly through birthday cards, anniversary cards, etc. Collected blood units must be subjected to all mandatory tests such as malaria, human immunodeficiency virus (HIV), hepatitis B surface antigen (HBsAg), hepatitis C virus (HCV), and syphilis and information be given to donors, if necessary. Express your thanks and gratitude to the organizer for arranging the camp.

PATH OF THE DONOR

The donor needs to pass through various steps in the voluntary blood donation camp, which includes the waiting area, at which donors enter and then pass through the donor registration area, where the registration work is done. The donor then proceeds to the area where his/her hemoglobin test is done and then to the medical officer for his/her medical examination. He/she then enters the blood donation site or bleeding area if accepted as donor. After donating blood, he/she leaves the blood donation area and goes to the refreshment area, where food and liquid refreshment are served. Donors are also observed post donation period by the staff present there. Finally, the donors leave the blood donation camp.

Activities to be Carried Out During Outside Voluntary Blood Donation Camp

1. *Registration*: Name, father's name, age, address, telephone number, etc., of the blood donor are recorded at the registration counter of the blood donation camp, and the questionnaire is given to donors to access their present and past health status so as to identify a suitable donor whose blood will be safe. Precounselling of the blood donors is also done during registration process.
2. *Hemoglobin test*: Blood donor's hemoglobin is checked in the blood donation camp itself and by a blood center technician before the donor is declared fit to ensure that he/she is not suffering from anemia and can safely donate a unit of blood.
3. *Medical examination*: Medical officer records the medical history of the donor to ascertain about his/her suitability as donor, and he will examine donors. Donor's weight, blood pressure, pulse, and temperature are recorded. Only good health, mentally alert, and physically fit persons are accepted as blood donors.
4. *Donation of blood*: After declaring fit as donor by the medical officer, the identity of the donor is crosschecked with the donor form, and entries are made in the donor register. Appropriate blood bag is selected and inspected for any defects such as suspended particles, discoloration, and pressure is applied to check for any leaks. Anticoagulant and additive solution are inspected for appropriate volume, color, and particulate contaminants and back tube number is entered in the donor register. Prepare bag level with donor identity, unit number, blood group, and date of bleeding on the blood bag. Pass the donor and the blood bag to the phlebotomist.

   A phlebotomist will recheck the identity of donor and verify with the bag and donor form. Blood is withdrawn with the help of a sterile and disposable kit after cleaning the blood donor's arm with an antiseptic solution. Blood collection process normally takes only 5–8 minutes.

Strip the donor tubing completely as possible into the bag, starting at seal. Work quickly to prevent blood from clotting in the tube. Invert blood bag several times to mix it thoroughly, and then allow tube to refill with anticoagulated blood from the bag. Repeat this procedure.

After phlebotomy, care of donor is very important. Apply pressure with sterile gauze over the point of insertion of the needle and apply bandage after bleeding stops. Keep the donor under observation for some time. Communicate with the donor to divert his attention and keep him/her comfortable. Cool and friendly environment will keep the donor comfortable.

5. *Refreshment*: After blood donation, the donor is allowed to sit in the refreshment area and served with some light refreshments and it must be ensured that he remains in the refreshment room for at least 15 minutes. The donor is advised to increase water consumption during the day and refrain from smoking for half an hour. A hearty goodbye with a request to donate again after 3 months will inspire him/her to become a regular donor. Problem, if any, faced by donor in camp be handled with tender, love, care, and compassion.

The donor should be made to understand that refreshment has nothing to do with immediate recuperation of blood loss during blood donation. A piping hot or cold drink and light refreshment are offered in the refreshment area in a relaxed mood and also to observe the donor in the donation camp (postdonation) for some time. Whatever be the refreshment, they should be served neatly and nicely with a smile. This is the last stage of the camp; it leaves a permanent impression in the mind of the donors. Talking with the donor throughout all the stages is extremely important as it helps them to feel friendly, happy, and also to get rid of their fear (if first-time donors).

Blood center technicians should be aware of any reaction during the entire process and keep necessary kits ready for resuscitation. When any reaction occurs to a donor, motivator, or medical social worker, they should remain calm and try not to get other donors upset and call the medical officer-in-charge and also ensure the prevention of the donor from falling down. Placing the donor on the bed or floor with a pillow under the feet helps in subsiding minor reactions. Doctors should check the donor in all such cases. In case of bleeding from the site of venepuncture, giving pressure with cotton wool, folding the arm with a cotton wool pad in between, and raising the folded hand a little upward help in stopping such bleeding. Once the bleeding stops, the venepuncture site may be sealed again.

Serious complication of blood donation is syncope (fainting or vasovagal syndrome), which may be caused by the sight of blood (psychological) or due to withdrawal of blood (neurophysiological).

6. *Segregation of biomedical waste*: Discarded blood bag tubing/needles must be segregated for disposal as per biosafety protocols and waste management and should never be left unattended. Needles, lancets, and syringes should be destroyed with the needle cutter. The entire area should be cleaned with a disinfectant (sodium hypochlorite or bleaching powder) after the camp is over.

CHECKLIST FOR THE BLOOD DONATION CAMP

The blood center staff should ensure that the procedures given in **Table 1** are followed.

Table 1: Checklist for the procedures to be followed during blood donation camps.				
Procedure carried out	**SOP no.**	**Yes/No**	**Signature of MO**	**Signature of LT**
Predonor counseling				
Donor selection				
Donor screening				
Preparation of phlebotomy				
Blood collection				
Postdonation counseling				
Donor reaction management				
Storage of blood in the camp				
Transport of blood				
Segregation and disposal of biomedical waste				
(LT: laboratory technician; MO: medical officer; SOP: standard operating procedure)				

Note: Draft performa for reporting of blood units collected during outside voluntary blood donation camp to SBTC/State Drug Regulatory Authorities is enclosed as **Annexure 83.1**.

CONCLUSION

The purpose of holding a blood donation camp is also to motivate people to donate blood to promote voluntary blood donation apart from blood collection. Holding blood donation camps are fantastic, best, and safe for the patients/recipients as well as for blood donors. Efforts must be made to motivate the public to donate blood during such blood donation camps by various communication means, including the oral communication, which is the most effective method of recruiting donors. Sensitize about the need for blood, shortage of blood, ease of blood donation, and myth about blood donation to the public. Hospital staff, especially clinicians, can actively contribute in motivating relatives and friends of patients/donors to donate blood and to become regular voluntary blood donors. Blood center staff should be courteous, interested, cheerful, and friendly, as well as professional and efficient. With increase in population and development of more advanced medical and surgical procedures, the need for blood is ever increasing. Only voluntary blood donors can help to maintain an adequate supply of safe and quality blood as well as blood components to save precious lives of those who are in need. Holding a voluntary blood donation camp efficiently and regularly will ensure adequate round the clock availability of blood during emergency situations. By donating blood, one gives a second chance of life to someone unknown, most of the time. Blood donation is a divine experience as blood donors become part of an exceptional group dedicated to alleviate the human suffering. Donating blood may reduce the risk of heart disease and stimulate the generation of red blood cells. There is no substitute for human blood, as one unit of blood saves three lives which can only be acquired from a generous blood donor.

ANNEXURE 83.1

Suggested Performa for Reporting Blood Units Collected During Outside Voluntary Blood Donation Camps to Regulatory Authorities

Name and Address of Blood Center: _____

Drug License No.:_____

Date of holding outside Blood Donation Camp:_____

Timings of outside Blood Donation Camp held:_____From_____
to_____.

Location/site of Blood Donation Camp (with Complete Postal Address):_____

Permission from Local Authority (if required):_____

Organizer of the Blood Donation Camp:_____

_____

Any other organisation/blood Center (Red Cross etc.) joined:_____

_____

Name, Qualification and other details of Person under whose Supervision the Camp Organised:_____

Details of Technical Persons who were Present during the Camp

S. No.	Technical persons	Name	Approved or not	Signatures
1.	Medical Officer			
2.	Technical Supervisor			
3.	Laboratory Technician			
4.	Staff Nurse			
5.	Counsellor			
6	Misc.			

Total blood donors screened:_____M_____F_____

No. of donors deferred:_____M_____F_____

No. of donor reactions:_____M_____F_____

No. of blood units under collected:_____

Units of blood collected during the camp:_____M_____F_____

Storage of these blood units during the camp:_____

Facility of transport of blood units provided:_____

Details of Blood Units Collected

S. No.	Blood group	No. of blood units	(Age/M/F)
1.			
2.			
3.			
4.			
Total			

Note:
- Attach some snaps of the blood donation facilities provided during the camp with storage and transportation facility.
- Copy of the permission letter from the local authority (if required)
- Well ventilated clean/dust free area with temperature control facilities (not exceeding 25°C)
- Time between collection and centrifugation for component preparation should not exceed 6 hours.
- After collection blood should be stored at 2–10°C in especially designed boxes. In case the temperature is over 10°C, the units should be discarded.

Processing Charges for Blood Centers (Private as well as Public Sector)

Provisions under Rules 122-P of the Drugs and Cosmetics Rules, 1945 provide that *"no licensee shall neither collect blood from any professional donor or paid donor nor shall he prepare blood components and/or manufacture blood products from blood drawn from such a donor"* suggesting that blood is not "manufactured for sale" purpose but for supply and distribution thereof. However, to compensate the service providers for the expenses incurred on processing and testing during the process of blood collection, testing, storage, and compatibility testing, the Government of India has provided guidelines for recovery of such expenses by the blood centers in the public as well as private sector from the patients.

The guidelines for recovery of processing charges for blood and blood components were released by the Department of AIDS Control, Ministry of Health and Family Welfare, Government of India on February 12, 2014, which subsequently have been validated periodically. The revised guidelines for recovery of processing charges for the year 2022 are to be effective from the date of issue of letter NO F.No. IM 11012/07/2022/NBTC dated June 14, 2022, of the Directorate General of Health Services, Ministry of Health and Family Welfare, Government of India, Room No. 560, 'A' Wing, Nirman Bhawan, New Delhi-110 108 (copy of this letter enclosed as **Annexure 84.1**).

The charges for services provided by blood centers may have variations due to differences in market availability of skilled manpower, items, and other ancillary requirements from state to state and sector to sector. The Government of India arrived at present processing charges for blood and blood components after considering the average of these factors. These guidelines are indicative in nature, and the concerned department of the State is authorized to take its own decisions.

The processing charges may be subsidized by the State government/ State Blood Transfusion Council (SBTC) for the blood centers in the government sector/Government of India-supported blood centers. The SBTCs may constitute an expert subcommittee to assess the additional testing/services being included in the processing charges required to enhance blood safety.

It is mandatory for all blood centers (government supported and nongovernment supported) to provide blood/blood component free of cost to the following patients, who require repeated blood transfusion as a lifesaving measure:

- Thalassemia
- Hemophilia
- Sickle cell anemia
- Any other blood dyscrasia requiring repeated blood transfusion

Processing charges for blood and blood components for below poverty line (BPL) patients accessing blood from nongovernment-supported blood centers shall be in compliance with the charges decided by the respective State government/SBTC. Processing charges for blood/blood components should be displayed prominently in the blood center premises for the benefit of the recipients.

Note: It has been observed that these guidelines for processing charges framed and issued by the Government of India prescribe the processing fees and testing charges, including specialized test charges, depending upon the tests being carried out by the blood center. But these charges do not include charges for the screening of the donor prior to blood donation for apheresis and also the charges where the blood bag or blood collection kit is wasted due to various unavoidable reasons. In such cases, it is suggested that the blood center may approach SBTC to allow for recovery of such processing charges of apheresis donors.

ANNEXURE 84.1

DR ANIL KUMAR
MD
Addl. DDG
Telefax: +91 11 23061329
E-mail: dr.anilkumar@nic.in

सत्यमेव जयते

Directorate General of Health Services
Ministry of Health & Family Welfare Government of India
Room No. 560, 'A' Wing, Nirman Bhawan, New Delhi-110 108

F.No. IM 11012/07/2022/NBTC

14th June, 2022

To

    The Director/Member Secretaries of
    All States Blood Transfusion Councils

Subject: Revised Guidelines-2022 for Recovery of Processing Charges for Blood and Blood Components-reg.

Sir/Madam,

1. The Guidelines for Recovery of Processing Charges for Blood and Blood components were released by the Department of AIDS control, Ministry of Health and Family Welfare, Government of India on 12th February 2014, which subsequently have been validated periodically.

2. National Blood Transfusion Council (NBTC) in its 30th Governing Body meeting held on 17th February, 2021 accorded approval to set up a Technical Working Group (TWG) to review existing Processing Charges for Blood and Blood Components including exchange value for Surplus Plasma. The recommendations of the TWG were endorsed by the Chairman of Technical Resource Group (TRG) of NBTC. After having considered the said recommendations, the revised guidelines for processing charges have been finalized and approved by the competent authority of the Ministry of Health and Family Welfare, Government of India.

3. The revised guidelines for recovery of Processing Charges for the year 2022, to be effective from the date of issue of this letter are as follows:

3.1 TABLE 1: PROCESSING CHARGES FOR GOVERNMENT BLOOD CENTERS

S. No.	Blood/Components	Processing Charges (in Rupees)
1	Whole Blood	1,100
2	Packed Red Cells	1,100
3	Fresh Frozen Plasma	300
4	Platelet concentrate	300
5	Cryoprecipitate	200

3.2 TABLE 2: PROCESSING CHARGES FOR NON-GOVERNMENT BLOOD CENTERS

S. No.	Blood/Components	Processing Charges (in Rupees)
1	Whole Blood	1,550
2	Packed Red Cells	1,550
3	Fresh Frozen Plasma	400
4	Platelet concentrate	400
5	Cryoprecipitate	250

3.3 TABLE 3: PROCESSING CHARGES OF OTHER TESTS, COMPONENTS & PROCESSES (Government and Non-Government)

Following charges are for individual tests, components and various processes which are specialized in nature but are not part of routine blood processing. As was part of recommendation of 2014 guidelines, the charges of specialized tests, processes and components per unit of blood can be divided amongst other components from same unit.

S. No.	Other Blood Tests, Components & Processes	Processing Charges (in Rupees)
1	NAT	1,200
2	Chemiluminescence	500*
3	ELISA Anti-HIV 1/2 (4th GEN)	50*
4	ELISA HBsAg (4th Gen)	50*
5	ELISA Anti-HCV (4th Gen)	150*
6	Anti-HBc	250
7	Antibody Screening (Donor)	300

Continued

Continued

S. No.	Other Blood Tests, Components & Processes	Processing Charges (in Rupees)
8	Leukofiltration- RBC	1,000
9	Leukofiltration Platelet	1,500
10	Grouping Crossmatching/ Automation	280*
11	Grouping Crossmatching/Semi Automation	120*
12	Phenotyping for Extended Serology	500
13	Irradiation	1,000
14	Bacterial Detection	400
15	Platelets (apheresis)	11,000

*No charges should be added as an additional, which are already factored in processing charges.

3.4 TABLE 4: SURPLUS PLASMA EXCHANGE VALUE IN GOVERNMENT AND NON-GOVERNMENT BLOOD CENTERS

S. No.	Component	Exchange Value for Surplus (Excess) Plasma
1	Surplus Plasma (exchange value)	1,600/Litre

4. The TWG has only considered the revision of processing charges in respect of items given under **Tables 1, 2 and 3** and exchange value as given under **Table 4**. For the rest part, the guidelines as issued in 2014 will continue to be applicable and for ease of reference are reproduced below from point No. 4.1 to 4.7.

4.1 TABLE 5: THE ADDITIONAL PROCESSING CHARGES FOR BLOOD COMPONENTS USING QUADRUPLE BAGS BY BUFFY COAT METHOD ARE RECOMMENDED AS UNDER:

S. No.	Component	Additional Processing Charge for Blood Components using Quadruple Bags by Buffy Coat Method (in Rupees)
1	Red Cell	150
2	Platelet	150
3	Plasma	100

4.2 The charges for services being provided by blood centres may have variations due to difference in market availability of skilled manpower, items and other ancillary requirements which may vary from State to State and sector to sector. However, it is necessary that the costs of blood are recouped by the blood centres. Accordingly, an average of these factors has been considered while arriving at the overall processing charges for blood and blood components. The Guidelines are indicative in nature and the concerned department of the State may take its own decisions.

4.3 The processing charges may be subsidized by the State Government/State Blood Transfusion Council for the blood centres in the Government sector/Government of India supported blood centres. The SBTCs may constitute an expert sub-committee to assess the additional testing/services being included in the processing charges, required to enhance blood safety.

4.4 It is mandatory for all blood centres (Government supported and non-Government supported) to provide blood/blood component free of cost to the following patients, who require repeated blood transfusion as a life saving measure:
- Thalassemia
- Haemophilia
- Sickle Cell Anaemia
- Any other blood dyscrasia requiring repeated blood transfusion.

4.5 State Government/SBTC may additionally decide to provide blood/blood components free of cost to any other category of patients according to the State Government norms.

4.6 Processing Charges for Blood and Blood products for Below Poverty Line (BPL) patients accessing blood from non-Government supported blood centres shall be in compliance with the charges decided by the respective State Government/SBTC.

4.7 Processing Charges for blood/blood components should be displayed prominently in the blood centre premises for benefit of the recipients.

5. These Guidelines would be revised every three years.

Yours sincerely

Kumar

(Dr Anil Kumar)

Copy to:
1. The Project Directors, State AIDS Control Society (SACS), All States/ UTs
2. DCGI, CDSCO, Dte.GHS, Govt. of India.

Copy for information to:
1. Secretary (H&FW), MoHFW, Govt. of India
2. Secretary, Department of Pharma, Govt. of India
3. DGHS, Govt. of India
4. AS and DG, NACO, MoHFW, Govt. of India
5. Chairman NPPA, Department of Pharma, Govt. of India
6. Principal Secretary (Health), All States/UTs

CHAPTER 85

Transfer of Blood/Blood Components

SCOPE AND APPLICATION

This standard operating procedure (SOP) describes the transfer of blood/blood components from one blood center to another blood center (which are licensed under the Drugs and Cosmetics Act, 1940 and Rules, 1945) to avoid wastage of blood/blood components and thereby ensuring judicious use.

RESPONSIBILITY

Management and blood transfusion officers of the recipient blood center as well as supplier blood center share the responsibility to ensure lawful transfer of blood/blood components maintaining cold chain throughout the transfer process.

REQUIREMENTS

- Blood/blood components units to be transferred
- Specially designed blood transport boxes
- Transport vehicle

PROCEDURE

1. Recipient blood center will raise the demand on the specimen request form **(Annexure 85.1)** for inter-blood center transfer of blood/blood components after ensuring adequate storage capacity to store the blood/blood components at mandatory storage temperature.
2. Supplier blood center will prepare the receipt in duplicate format **(Annexure 85.2)** for receiving the request form of recipient blood center for transfer of blood/blood components.

3. Supplier blood center shall prepare details of blood/blood component units to be transferred as per details given in format **(Annexure 85.3)**.

4. Recipient blood center shall acknowledge the receipt of such transferred blood units in duplicate as per format **(Annexure 85.4)**.

5. Supplier blood center can also charge the prescribed processing/testing charges as per National Blood Transfusion Council (NBTC) norms (as given in Chapter 84).

6. Blood/blood components units shall be transferred with the following documents:
   a. Receipt of request form for inter-blood center transfer of blood/blood components
   b. Duly signed issue form for inter-blood center transfer of blood/blood components
   c. Copy of receipt of blood/blood components issued
   d. Receipt and details of processing charges

7. Both the centers will maintain proper inventory of such transfer and receipt of blood/blood components.

8. Supplier blood center shall ensure maintenance of mandatory storage condition of blood/blood components at its blood center as well as during transfer process.

9. Recipient blood center shall issue such transferred blood/blood components to all the patients needing transfusion, not only to its own institution but to other institutions as well.

10. Responsibility for complications, except for those related to crossmatching, will lie on the supplier blood center. However, investigations of any adverse transfusion reaction due to transfusion of such blood/blood components will be the responsibility of the recipient's blood center.

11. Both the blood centers shall maintain the traceability.

12. Both the blood centers shall inform the State Blood Transfusion Council (SBTC)/NBTC about such bulk transfer of blood/blood components.

Note:
- This SOP has been prepared as per guidelines for blood transfer issued vide D.O. No S-12015/04/2015-NBTC dated October 28, 2015, by National AIDS Control Organisation, Ministry of Health and Family Welfare, Government of India (copy attached as **Annexure 85.5**).

   Rules 122-P (xiv-xv) of Drug And Cosmetics Rules, 1945 also provide provisions for transfer of blood/blood components from one blood center to another blood center.

- Packed red blood cell (PRBC) and whole blood units are packed in an insulated container in such a way that ice does not come in direct contact with PRBC/whole blood.
- Temperature in insulated containers can be considered in a range of 2–10°C so long as unmelted ice is present on arrival at the destination.
- Specially designed blood transport boxes with temperature monitoring control should be used for such transfer.

ANNEXURE 85.1

Specimen Request form for Inter-Blood Center Transfer of Blood and Blood Components

Date: .... Time: ....

To
The Blood Center In-Charge
Name and Address of Blood Center (Supplier)

....

....

....

Dear Sir/Madam

Please issue the following tested Blood/Blood Components Units for use in our Blood Center at the required temperature, along with certificate of tests.

S. No.	Blood group	Whole blood/blood components	No. of units

....

Blood Center In-Charge (Recipient)

....

Blood Center Name/Contact Details/ Sign and Seal

ANNEXURE 85.2

Receipt for Receiving the Request Form of Recipient Blood Center for Transfer of Blood/Blood Components

RECEIPT

1. Name of Supplier Blood Center: ....
2. Address: ....
3. Phone No.: ....
4. License No.: ....Validity: ....
5. RBTS: YES/NO ....

Received request dated .... as detailed above.

....

Sign of Blood Center In-Charge (Supplier) with Seal

Date and Time: ....

Note: Fill two copies of this form. One signed copy of each to be retained in supplier blood center and recipient blood center.

ANNEXURE 85.3

Specimen Issue form for Inter-Blood Center Transfer of Blood and Blood Components

Date: ....   Time: ....

To
The Blood Center In-Charge
Name and Address of Blood Center (Recipient)

....

....

....

Dear Sir/Madam

The following units of Blood/Blood Components are issued for use in your Blood Center as per your request dated.............. It is certified that all units below are tested and found nonreactive for TTI (Syphilis, Malaria, HIV, HCV, HBV) and are being transported at requisite temperature. It is further certified that these were stored at the required temperature at this Blood Center.

S. No.	Unit No.	Blood group	Whole blood/ blood compo-nents	Date of collec-tion	Status of testing					Exp. date	Date of testing	Seg-ment No.
					Syph-ilis	Mala-ria	HIV	HCV	HBV			
1												
2												
3												

....

Blood Center In-Charge (supplier)

....

Contact Details, Sign and Seal

ANNEXURE 85.4

Receipt for Acknowledgment of Transferred Blood Units

RECEIPT

1. Name of Recipient Blood Center: ....
2. Address: ....
3. Phone No.: ....
4. License No.: ....Validity: ....
5. RBTS: YES/NO ....

Received Blood/Blood Components as detailed above.

....

Sign of Blood Center In-Charge (Recipient) with Seal

Date and Time: ....

Note: Fill two copies of this form. One signed copy of each to be retained in supplier blood center and recipient blood center.

ANNEXURE 85.5

GUIDELINES FOR BLOOD TRANSFER ISSUED VIDE D.O. NO. S-12015/04/2015-NBTC DATED 28 OCT 2015 BY NATIONAL AIDS CONTROL ORGANISATION, MINISTRY OF HEALTH AND FAMILY WELFARE GOVT. OF INDIA.

1. Transfer shall be allowed between licensed blood center in any sector (Public, NGO and Private).
2. Transfer of blood and components in Bulk shall be permitted across State borders also to ensure the availability at the point of need.
3. All transfers shall be done at the recommended temperature and as per prescribed storage conditions for whole blood and components. The supplier blood center shall be responsible for compliance thereof.
4. The recipient blood center should have capacity to hold the units requested for at appropriate temperature, till the time of utilization.
5. Broad based donor concept should be incorporated in the standard donor form to ensure that the donor agree to his blood unit being utilized beyond the blood center where it is donated.
6. Supplier blood center can levy the prescribed processing/testing charges on the patient/recipient/recipient blood center as per NBTC norms. However, recipient blood center can levy only processing charges for compatibility testing (cross matching) in addition to the charges levied by the supplier blood center, from the patient/recipient for such transferred units.
7. Records of traceability shall be retained throughout the process.
8. Supplier blood center shall be responsible for all complications except for those related to compatibility/crossmatch testing, which will be the responsibility of recipient blood center. Recipient blood center shall report and evaluate all the adverse transfusion reactions including those happening due to blood that has been transferred from supplier blood center.
9. Documents accompanying transfer shall include TTI testing reports and record of transport at appropriate temperature.
10. All recipient blood centers are considered deemed approved to act as functional blood storage centers for the blood and blood components, even though the upper limit of 2,000 units of utilization per annum is not applicable.
11. All blood center/storage units be instructed to issue blood to all patients needing transfusion, not restricting blood units to captive requirement of their institution to which they are attached.
12. Blood center would be informing regarding bulk transfer to SBTC and in case of interstate transfer of blood/blood components to NBTC.

CHAPTER 86

Judicial Pronouncements— Blood Safety

II (2000) CPJ 439
UNION TERRITORY CONSUMER DISPUTES
REDRESSAL COMMISSION, CHANDIGARH
Hon'ble Mr Justice JB Garg, President;
Dr PK Vasudeva and Mrs Devinderjit Dhatt, Members
Jaspal Singh and ANR.—Complainants
Versus
The Post Graduate Institute of Medical Education and Research [PGI],
Chandigarh and ANR.—Respondents Complaint No. 12 of 1997—
Decided on 1.2.2000

Consumer Protection Act, 1986—Sections 2(1) (g), 14(1) (d)—
Medical Negligence—Mismatching of blood—Deficiency in Service—
Compensation—Complainant's wife suffered burn injuries to the extent
of 50%—Admitted to PGI Chandigarh—Patient's blood group was A+,
but was transfused B+ group blood—Kidney damaged due to wrong
transfusion of blood—Mismatching of blood and wrong transfusion
confirmed— PGI Chandigarh liable to pay compensation was held.

After hearing the learned counsel for the parties and perusing the
relevant records with their assistance including evidence of the parties
and other documents on record, Commission come to the conclusion
that there was serious deficiency and negligence on the part of the
PGI and its attending doctor(s)/staff for transfusing wrong blood
group to the patient which caused death of the wife of complainant
no. 1. Mismatching of blood was confirmed by the Senior Resident
in the death summary also. Once the patient was brought to the PGI
or any other Institute of Health Care, the background/history, if any,
for example that the patient was maltreated by the husband, does not
absolve the hospital from its professional obligations. Postgraduate
Institute (PGI), Chandigarh was, therefore, held liable to pay a sum of

₹2.00 lakhs to the complainants out of which 3/4th was ordered to be put in the fixed deposit in favour of minor Amandeep Singh s/o Jaspal Singh, complainant no. 2, and ¼th to be paid to the complainant no. 1 (husband) a Government employee. PGI also to pay costs of ₹5,000/- to the complainants. PGI Authorities however, was given liberty to recover this amount from the erring doctor(s)/staff.

P VERSUS UNION OF INDIA (2001)—KOLKATA HIGH COURT (NEGLIGENCE IN BLOOD TRANSFUSION)

The petitioner, a pregnant lady was admitted for delivery of her child at a hospital under the administrative control of the Indian Navy. After delivery, the petitioner required blood transfusion. A sailor donated fresh blood to hospital, which did not come from the blood bank of the hospital as required under the provisions of the Drugs and Cosmetics Act. The sailor's blood was not tested for HIV at the time of donation. He was later found to be HIV+. It was clear that the petitioner became HIV+ on account of the negligent transfusion of blood to her.

Court felt that since the hospital was under administrative control of the Indian Navy, the Indian Navy had a duty to compensate the petitioner. Correspondence was exchanged between the petitioner and respondent Indian Navy during the pendency of the petition. Finally the respondent made an offer of compensation which included:

a. A Government job at Kolkata or the place where she desired.
b. Accommodation on her appointment on the usual terms and conditions.
c. A sum of ₹10 lakhs from the date of filing of the writ petition @ 18% interest.
d. Medical treatment at the cost of the Government.

Petitioner was agreeable to the offer and Court passed the judgment in terms of compromise arrived at by the parties.

I (2006) CPJ 136 (NC)
NATIONAL CONSUMER DISPUTES
REDRESSAL COMMISSION, NEW DELHI
Hon'ble Mr SN Kapoor, Presiding Member
and Mr BK Taimni, Member
Dr K Vidhyullatha—Appellant
Versus
R Bhagawathy—Respondent
First Appeal No. 379 of 2001—Decided on 25.1.2005

- Consumer Protection Act, 1986—Sections 2(1)(g) and 14(1)(d)—
  Medical Negligence—Wrong blood transfusion after hysterectomy
  operation resulted in intravascular haemolysis and renal failure—
  Opposite party denied treatment to patient—Evidence that on
  developing complications patient was referred to another hospital
  where she had to undergo haemodialysis 8 times—Deficiency in
  service proved on part of OP in transfusing wrong blood—Order of
  Forums below awarding compensation upheld, amount reduced to
  ₹1,00,000 from ₹1,50,000 and interest to 9% from 12%.
- Res ipsa loquitur—Applicability—Complaint regarding wrong blood
  transfusion after hysterectomy operation resulting intra-vascular
  haemolysis and renal failure—Complainant not able to pass urine
  after surgery—Principle *of res ipsa loquitur* attracted—Deficiency in
  service proved.

In Harjot Ahluwalia (minor through his parents) vs. M/s. Spring
Meadows Hospital and Others, II (1997) CPJ 98 (NC), the Hon'ble
Supreme Court has observed: "That the staff attending on the patient
discharge their duties and work on the patient under the control,
guidance and supervision of the consultant/doctor under whose
treatment, care and supervision the patient is admitted." While it is
true as submitted by the learned Counsel for the appellant that the
compensation could not be awarded on the basis of mere allegation.
But amount of compensation in almost all cases is decided on the basis
of fair estimation. While we think that for the mental tension and agony
and acute renal failure, the learned State Commission might have
justifiably estimated the total compensation amounting to ₹1,00,000, for
we take the expenditure of ₹1,000 per day for haemodialysis it would not
exceed ₹15,000 plus overhead expenses ranging from 7,000 to ₹7,500 in
all. We feel that in the aforesaid circumstances, it would be appropriate
to award a sum of ₹1,00,000 in all as compensation with interest @
9% p.a. from the date of complaint till the date of deposit of a sum of
₹1,50,000. The complainant shall be entitled to receive the amount of
₹1,50,000 which is said to have been deposited with the Commission
along with interest which would have accrued thereon and adjust the
same towards the amount payable as aforesaid. With the aforesaid
modification, the appeal was disposed of.

[Equivalent Citation: 2005 (2) CPC 599 (NC)]
IV (2005) CPJ 84 (NC)
NATIONAL CONSUMER DISPUTES
REDRESSAL COMMISSION, NEW DELHI
Hon'ble Mr Justice KS Gupta, Presiding Member;
Mrs Rajyalakshmi Rao, Member
P Kallianikutty Amma and ORS—Complainant
Versus
Unity Health Services (P) Ltd and ORS.—Opposite Parties Original
Petition No. 181 of 1996—Decided on 14.7.2005

Consumer Protection Act, 1986—Section 2(1)(g)—Medical Negligence—
blood transfusion—Alleged, contaminated blood transfused causing
adverse reaction, which ultimately led to death—Allegation not
proved—No evidence produced to show that blood was improperly
stored from time of procurement till time of administration—blood
transfusion took place much before expiry date—Mild adverse reaction
properly attended to in time—Absence of expert evidence in support
of allegations—Medical negligence not proved—Complaint dismissed.

The complaint is not that the blood obtained from the blood
bank was not crossmatched with the patient's blood. The complaint
essentially is that the blood obtained from the blood bank got
contaminated at the Unity Hospital and that the contaminated blood
was administered to the patient causing adverse reaction which
ultimately led to death. The crux of the argument of the opposite parties
is that there was no contamination in the blood and that though there
was a mild adverse reaction to the blood transfusion, it was properly
attended to in time and that the rest of the blood transfusion took place
in an uneventful manner. Their case is that the patient was suffering
from dysfunctional uterine bleeding for at least 14 months before she
came to the Unity Hospital and that septicaemia took place because of
the progression of the disease leading to her death and that there was
no negligence.

We also found that there is no substance in the argument of the
complainant that they had not given consent for blood transfusion. It
has come on record that the husband of the deceased enquired about
the availability of blood from the Royal Hospital from where it was
subsequently obtained. If there was no implied consent, he would not
have gone around making inquiries about the availability of blood for
transfusion.

In addition to all these, as mentioned above, after the death of
the patient, Delhi based brother of the deceased; Shri P Chandra
Shekharan filed a number of complaints before various authorities
alleging negligence and malafides against the opposite parties. Firstly,

on 23.5.1995 he filed a Criminal Complaint No. 246/1995 under Section 304-A of the IPC. This complaint was investigated by the police and recorded by judicial order as closed, as investigation showed that there was no negligence and that the patient died because of septicaemia. Thereafter the Drug Controller, Govt. of Kerala, Thiruvananthapuram was approached on 11.8.1995 alleging that the blood obtained from the Royal Hospital was improperly stored and hence got contaminated. The report of the Drug Controller dated 27.9.1995 clearly held that no evidence has been produced to show that the blood was improperly stored from the time of procurement till the time of administration. As a result, the case of negligence against the opposite parties was not proved. The complaint therefore, was dismissed.

IV (2005) CPJ 261 (NC)
NATIONAL CONSUMER DISPUTES
REDRESSAL COMMISSION, NEW DELHI
Hon'ble Mr Justice MB Shah, President
and Mrs Rajyalakshmi Rao, Member
Supriya Gupta—Complainant
Versus
Trustees of Beach Candy
Hospital and Research Centre—Opposite Party
Original Petition No. 7 of 1997—Decided on 27.10.2005

Consumer Protection Act, 1986—Section 2(1)(g), 21—Medical Negligence—Surgery conducted—Patient contracted Hepatitis 'B'—Alleged, infection has arisen from OP's hospital during blood transfusion at OP's Hospital or due to use of improperly sterilized medical equipment—Absence of evidence in support of allegations—Fresh blood taken from relatives and friends transfused—One unit given from hospital blood bank which was not Hepatitis infected proved—Fresh and disposable cardiac catheters were used on complainant—Infection caused from OP's hospital due to negligent procedure not proved—Complaint dismissed.

M. CHINNAIYAN VERSUS SRI GOKULAM HOSPITAL & QUEEN MARY'S CLINICAL LABORATORY (NATIONAL CONSUMER DISPUTE REDRESSAL COMMISSION, 2006)

Appellant's wife underwent a hysterectomy operation, at the 1st Respondent hospital in 1990 where she was transfused 2 units of blood in the postoperative period which was procured from the 2nd Respondent laboratory in 1990. In mid-1994, the, Appellant's wife developed recurrent loose motions, weight loss, respiratory infection and difficulty in swallowing, etc. On being tested, she was found to be HIV+ and showed symptoms of full-blown AIDS. In July 1995, she developed left-sided hemiparesis, oral candidiasis and TB. Later she was diagnosed with glioma of the brain and died in August 1995.

Her husband filed a complaint before the State Consumer Redressal Forum suing the hospital and pathology laboratory for deficiency of services under the Consumer Protection Act. His complaint was rejected. Aggrieved by this order, he appealed to the National Consumer Dispute Redressal Commission (National Commission). The National Commission held:

a. The 1st respondent gave blood transfusion without obtaining the consent of the patient and that the concerned doctor negligently transfused blood, as he did not inform the Petitioner's wife about the benefits, risks or alternatives of blood transfusion, which amounted to deficiency of service under the Consumer Protection Act.

b. Furthermore, Drugs and Cosmetics Rules, 1945, requires that every licensee of a blood bank gets samples of every blood unit tested for freedom from HIV antibodies, which the 2nd respondent had failed to do.

c. As compensation, the Commission awarded ₹4,00,000 (₹4 lakh) with interest at the rate of 6% p.a. from the date of filing the complaint, which was to be paid jointly and severally by the Respondents and ₹10,000 as costs.

An appeal by one of the respondents to the Supreme Court was dismissed.

(2007) CPJ 395 (NC)
NATIONAL CONSUMER DISPUTES
REDRESSAL COMMISSION, NEW DELHI
Hon'ble Mr Justice KS Gupta, Presiding Member
and Dr PD Shenoy, Member
Susheel Kumar—Petitioner
Versus
Dr Virendra Mahla and ANR.—Respondents
Revision Petition No. 798 of 2007—Decided on 11.7.2007

Consumer Protection Act, 1986—Sections 2(1)(g), 21(b)—Medical Negligence—HIV reports—Patient operated for appendix—blood test taken—Report showed patient HIV-Positive—Further investigations done by other Hospitals—Patient found to be HIV-Negative—Complaint filed for mental agony—Compensation awarded—Order reversed on appeal—Hence revision—Test done by first Hospital (OP) from HIV Niwa Kit of Cadila—Patient advised to co-relate result by Western Blot Technique—Same not done—Harrison's Book of Principles of Internal Medicines referred—No deficiency in service on part of OP—Impugned order upheld.

In the order under challenge the State Commission has quoted two paras from Harrison's Book of Principles of Internal Medicines. Combined reading of these paras would show that the standard screening test for HIV infection is the ELISA, which is an extremely good screening test with a sensitivity of 99.58%; Commercial use of EIA kit by most of the diagnostic laboratories is not optimal with regard to specificity and, therefore, it must be confirmed with a more specific assay. It is not the case of petitioner that test through Western Blot Technique was got done by him after 3.12.2002. Considering the contents extracted above the aforesaid report dated 19.12.2003 does not help the petitioner. To be noted that in aforementioned report dated 10.12.2003 the basis for reaching the conclusion in regard to petitioner being HIV-negative has not been disclosed. In this backdrop, we do not find any merit in the contention advanced by Ms. Aishwarya Bhati, Advocate about respondent being deficient in service for giving the wrong report. There is no illegality or jurisdictional error in the order passed by State Commission warranting interference in revisional jurisdiction under Section 21(b) of the Consumer Protection Act, 1986. Revision petition was, therefore, dismissed.

IV 2007 CPJ 157 (NC)
NATIONAL CONSUMER DISPUTES
REDRESSAL COMMISSION, NEW DELHI
Hon'ble Mr Justice SN Kapoor, Presiding Member
and Mr BK Taimni, Member
Chandigarh Clinical Laboratory—Petitioner
Versus
Jagjeet Kaur—Respondent
Revision Petition No. 1377 of 2003—Decided on 30.8.2007

(i) **Consumer Protection Act, 1986—Section 2(1)(g)—Medical Negligence—Clinical laboratory—Wrong blood test report given—Failure on part of petitioner to take due care to return correct finding—Whether harm caused to patient or not would not be a criteria—Deficiency in service proved—Compensation awarded by Forum affirmed by State Commission—No interference required in revision.**

The complainant Mrs. Jagjeet Kaur was taken to the petitioner laboratory for getting her blood-group checked up and the report was given of her having blood group AB+. The blood-group report was required as she had been advised blood-transfusion, for which she was transferred to GGS Medical College and Hospital, where again blood sample was collected and it gave a report of the complainant's blood belonging to AB (-). It is in these circumstances, a complaint was filed before the District Forum alleging 'medical-negligence' who after hearing the parties and perusal of material on record, directed the petitioner to pay a compensation of ₹25,000 and cost of ₹2,000 to the complainant. Aggrieved by this order, an appeal was filed before the State Commission, which was dismissed, hence this revision petition before us.

We have no doubt that the petitioner is a qualified pathologist but the 'duty of care', required in such case to give a correct finding, which was not given in this case, is a clear instance of medical negligence on the part of the petitioner. The negligence stands proven in this case by the admitted fact that the petitioner gave the report of blood group of the complainant belonging to AB+ whereas in fact it was AB (-) which has not been disputed by the petitioner. Whether harm came to the patient or not would not be a criteria. It is the failure on the part of the petitioner to take due care to return a correct finding, that is at the heart of issue and in which the petitioner completely failed.

In view of above, National Commission did not find any ground to interfere with the well-reasoned order passed by the District Forum and affirmed by the State Commission. The revision petition was, therefore dismissed.

I (2008) CPJ 205 (NC)
NATIONAL CONSUMER DISPUTES
REDRESSAL COMMISSION, NEW DELHI

Hon'ble Mr Justice MB Shah, President and Mrs Rajyalakshmi Rao,
Member
Deo Kumar Singh—Appellant
versus
CBP Sinha (DR.)—Respondent
First Appeal No. 314 of 2004—Decided on 11.12.2007

Consumer Protection Act, 1986—Section 2(1)(g)—Medical Negligence—Wrong blood report—Complainant's wife having blood group Rh Negative reported to be Rh Positive by OP—Pregnancies aborted despite treatment given—Rh factor plays extremely important role during pregnancy—Woman is at risk when she has Negative Rh factor and husband has Positive Rh factor—Complications can be prevented by appropriate medication only when Rh factor of mother is correctly known—Appropriate treatment could not be given due to wrong blood report about Rh factor—Giving report about Rh factors in casual manner has to be condemned—Deficiency in service proved—Compensation granted.

Testing blood type and Rh factor are basic and fundamental aspects of blood test and Pathological Laboratories are required to be extremely careful since the wrong report can make the difference between life and death. Giving the report about these factors in a casual manner has to be condemned since the Rh factor plays an extremely important role in the case of the pregnant woman.

In view of the above discussion, this appeal was allowed. The order of the State Commission was set aside. The respondent was directed to pay a sum of ₹25,000 towards compensation to the complainant, within a period of two months, failing which the amount of ₹25,000 to carry interest at the rate of 9% p.a. In the facts and circumstances of this case, there shall be no order as to costs, as per the orders of commission.

POST GRADUATE INSTITUTE OF MEDICAL EDUCATION AND RESEARCH, CHANDIGARH
VERSUS
JASPAL SINGH

[Civil Appeal No. 7950 of 2002, decided on May 29, 2009]

DK JAIN AND RM LODHA, JJ

1. In this appeal by special leave, the appellant, Post/Graduate Institute of Medical Education and Research, Chandigarh (for short, 'PGI') has challenged the order dated September 29, 2000 passed by the National Consumer Disputes Redressal Commission (for short, "National Commission"). By its order, the National Commission dismissed the appeal filed by PGI under Section 21 of the Consumer Protection Act, 1986 (for short, 'Act, 1986') and affirmed the order passed by the State Consumer Disputes Redressal Commission, Chandigarh (for short, 'State Commission') whereby it directed the PGI to pay compensation in the sum of ₹2 lakhs to the respondents 1 and 2 herein (for short, 'the complainants') and cost of ₹5,000/-.

On March 30, 1996, Smt. Harjit Kaur (wife of complainant no. 1 and mother of complainant no. 2) received accidental burns while making tea on the stove. She sustained 50% TBSA III burns involving upper limbs, part of trunk and most of both lower limbs. Smt. Harjit Kaur was taken to Daya Nand Medical College and Hospital, Ludhiana, immediately where she responded to the treatment well. She remained admitted in Daya Nand Medical College and Hospital up to April 19, 1996. Since the treatment at Daya Nand Medical College and Hospital was expensive, the complainant no. 1 decided to shift his wife to PGI for further treatment. On April 19, 1996, Smt. Harjit Kaur was admitted in PGI, Chandigarh. Dr Varun Kul Shrestha, Senior Resident Doctor, Department of Plastic Surgery attended to her. The condition of Smt. Harjit Kaur started improving at PGI. On May 15, 1995, she was transfused A+ blood which was her blood group. On May 20, 1996, the patient was transfused B+ blood group in the afternoon although her blood group was A+. On the night of May 20, 1996, the urine of the patient was reddish like blood and the attendant nurse was informed accordingly. As to the bad luck of Smt. Harjit Kaur, on the next day, i.e., May 21, 1996 again one bottle of B+ blood group was transfused although her blood group was A+. Because of transfusion of mismatched blood, the condition of Smt. Harjit Kaur became serious; her haemoglobin levels fell down to 5 mg. and urea level went very high. Later on, it transpired that due to transfusion of mismatched blood, the kidney and liver of the patient got deranged. The complainant no. 1 made a written complaint to the Head of the Department of Plastic Surgery for mismatched transfusion of blood to the patient whereupon an inquiry was conducted through senior doctor and wrong transfusion of the blood to the patient was found. The condition of Smt. Harjit Kaur started deteriorating day by day and she ultimately died on July 1, 1996. In the complaint before the State Commission, the complainants alleged that the death of Smt. Harjit Kaur was caused due to the negligence of Dr Varun Kul Shrestha and the medical staff at PGI; that there was negligence in the discharge of service by the PGI and its doctors and they claimed damages to the tune of ₹9 lakhs for the loss of life of Smt. Harjit Kaur.

Although she survived for about 40 days after mismatched blood transfusion but from that it cannot be said that there was no causal link between the mismatched transfusion of blood and her death. Wrong blood transfusion is an error which no hospital/doctor exercising ordinary care would have made. Such an error is not an error of professional judgment but in the very nature of things a sure instance of medical negligence. The hospital's breach of duty in mismatched blood transfusion contributed to her death, if not wholly, but surely materially. Mismatched blood transfusion to a patient having sustained 50% burns by itself speaks of negligence. Therefore, in the facts and circumstances of the case, it cannot be said that the death of Smt. Harjit Kaur was not caused by the breach of duty on the part of the hospital.

2. The State Commission observed:
"That there has been serious deficiency and negligence on the part of the PGI and its attending doctor(s)/staff for transfusing wrong blood group to the patient which caused death of the wife of complainant no. 1. Mismatching of blood has been confirmed by the Senior Resident in the Death Summary also. Once the patient is brought to the PGI or any other Institute of Health Care, the background/history, if any, for example that the patient was maltreated by the husband, does not absolve the Hospital from its professional obligation."

3. Affirming the aforesaid view of the State Commission, the National Commission held thus:
"It is seen that the patient's kidney was damaged and the blood urea level reached to 100 g/%, haemoglobin came down to 5 mg. after the mismatched blood transfusion was given by the Doctor in the said Hospital. It was only after the complainant gave the written complaint to the hospital regarding the wrong transfusion of blood given to the patient, an inquiry was made and it was found correct. The damage

control treatment started only after the written complaint was given by the complainant. Though it is argued by the Counsel for the Appellant that the percentage levels were brought down to normal, it is very clear to us that the internal imbalances of liver and kidney functioning and deteriorating haemoglobin levels started only after the mismatched blood transfusion was given. Though septicaemia has been written as the ultimate cause of death, the patient's health took a nose dive only after wrong blood was given to her and this is clearly negligence on the part of the Doctors of the Hospital which the appellants cannot disown or absolve themselves."

4. The SC upheld the view of the National Commission with the remarks that it does not suffer from any error of law. In the result, the appeal was dismissed with costs ₹20,000/-.

STATE CONSUMER DISPUTES REDRESSAL
COMMISSION UNION TERRITORY, CHANDIGARH
(Consumer Complaint No. 6 of 2011)

Date of Institution 21.01.2011   **Date of Decision 01.03.2012**

Mrs. Suman aged about 30 years w/o Desraj resident of 176, Block J, Colony No. 4, Industrial Area, Chandigarh.

Versus

Government Multi-Specialty Hospital, Sector 16, Chandigarh through its Director Principal.

The facts of the case, in brief, are that in the month of December, 2010, complainant no. 1–Mrs. Suman was pregnant for 9 months and was expecting her baby any day. It was stated that, in order to ensure safe delivery of her baby, under proper medical supervision, she along with her husband Desraj-complainant no. 2, went to Government Multi-Speciality Hospital (hereinafter referred to as GMSH) on 16.12.2010. It was further stated that in GMSH, a medical treatment card was prepared, in the name of Mrs. Suman after taking requisite charges of ₹10/-. It was further stated that the doctor came to the conclusion that complainant no. 1 required blood transfusion, on the same day. She was, therefore, admitted as an in-patient, by Opposite Party No. 1. It was further stated that the team of doctors and technicians consisting of Opposite Parties No. 2, 3 and 4, i.e., Ms Kirti Sood, Dr. Navdeep and Dr. Manpreet respectively were assigned the duties to handle the case of complainant no. 1. It was further stated that the treating doctors directed Sh. Des Raj-complainant no. 2, to arrange a unit of Blood for transfusion, by giving him the requisition slip. It was further stated that the blood unit was arranged, in time, and given to the attending doctors for transfusion. It was further stated that soon after the blood was transfused to complainant no. 1, she started feeling uneasy. It was further stated that her husband-Desraj ran helter-skelter, to inform the doctors/ nurses, but the concerned doctors were not available immediately. It was further stated that after sometime, when the patient was attended to, the concerned Doctor took, it casually and informed that everything would be all right. It was further stated that the condition of complainant no. 1 deteriorated, so much so, that it resulted into the death of the full-term foetus, and failure of the kidney of complainant no. 1. It was further stated that it transpired that the doctors had transfused blood group B+ to Suman, though her blood group was A+. It was further stated that all above facts were accepted and endorsed by Chandigarh Administration itself, on the basis of the inquiry report dated January 3, 2011, submitted by Sub Divisional Magistrate, South, Union Territory, Chandigarh. The relevant conclusions arrived at, by the Inquiry Officer are as under:

The Inquiry Committee implicates the following persons in the commission of this gross medical negligent act:

- **Mrs. Kirti Sood, Lab Technician:** She issued the blood bag without cross-checking for the requisite important details of the patient and more particularly the blood group and later on concealing the facts and tampering with the sample. The possibility of destruction of the sample and the blood requisition form cannot be excluded by the Inquiry Committee.

- **Dr. Navdeep, Intern:** She initiated the transfusion to the patient without checking and re-checking the requisite details of the patient with the details given on the blood bag and started the transfusion on the presumption that the blood bag lying beside the patient is meant for the patient only, violating all the fundamental blood transfusion protocols. Moreover, she failed to inform her seniors regarding the transfusion and showing gross carelessness and insensitivity failed to monitor the patient.

- **Dr. Manpreet, House Surgeon:** The role played by Dr. Manpreet, the House Surgeon is also not a small one. She being wholly responsible for the transfusion of the blood to patients in the labour room, failed to check for the required details on the blood bag with that of the patient's case sheet as soon as the blood bag was brought and kept on the table by the nursing student. Without even checking for the details on the blood bag she simply passed on responsibility of the transfusion to her amateur/new junior colleague. Moreover, she did not follow up the patient and failed to monitor the patient.

Hence, this complaint was filed, seeking the following reliefs:

- ₹5 lakhs towards re-imbursement of medical and other expenses;
- ₹15 lakhs towards loss of earnings of husband Desraj, since he will now be unable to earn as he will have to attend to his wife forever (@ ₹5,000/- per month for 25 years, life expectancy being 60 years).
- ₹9 lakhs towards loss of earnings of Suman, as she will also be unable to work for her entire life. (@ ₹2,500/- per month for 30 years, life expectancy being 60 years).
- ₹54 lakhs towards minimum expected expenditure to be incurred on medicines for an entire lifetime @ ₹500/- per day for 30 years as the life expectancy is 60 years.
- ₹2 lakh each as token damages for each of the children to compensate them for the physical and emotional loss of mother's love and care.
- ₹3 lakhs each as punitive damages against each of the guilty doctors, OP Nos. 2, 3 and 4 as token punishment for their medical negligence.

Coming to the quantum of compensation, It is evident that a sum of ₹50,000/- vide cheque no. 391290 dated 10.02.2011, as monetary compensation, was given by the Office of the Deputy Commissioner, UT, Chandigarh to the complainants. Expenditure of ₹8,434/- incurred on the treatment of complainant no. 1, was also reimbursed by the OP no. 1-Hospital under the budget of Rogi Kalyan Smiti. In our considered view, this amount of compensation of ₹50,000/- is too meagre, to meet the ends of justice. Keeping in view the financial status of the complainants, who belong to a poor family, death of the foetus, loss of income of the complainant no. 2 (being a labourer) during the period of treatment of her wife, i.e., Mrs. Suman (being housewife), loss of income of Suman-complainant no. 1 during the period, she remained admitted in the hospital, the mental agony and physical harassment suffered by them due to the negligence of the Opposite Parties, we deem it appropriate to award a consolidated compensation of ₹4 lakhs to them (complainants) on all these counts. Besides this, we are of the considered opinion that it is the bounden duty of the OP no. 1-Hospital to bear all the expenses of the future treatment of complainant no. 1, if she required the same besides the amount already given to the complainants.

For the reasons recorded above, the complaint was allowed with costs. The Opposite Parties were jointly and severally directed to pay a sum of ₹4,00,000/- as compensation to the complainants. The Opposite parties were also directed to pay to the complainants ₹50,000/- as cost of litigation. Opposite Party no. 1 was also directed to bear all the expenses, which may be incurred on the future treatment of complainant no. 1, in any government hospital/health centre/dispensary etc.

This order be complied with, by the Opposite Parties within one month, from the date of receipt of a certified copy of the same, failing which, they shall be liable to pay the amount of ₹4 lakhs along with penal interest @ 12% p.a., to the complainants, from the date of filing of complaint, i.e., 21.01.2011, till its realization, besides costs of litigation.

Certified Copies of this order was ordered to be sent to the parties, free of charge. The file was consigned to Record Room, after completion.

Dated 01.03.2012 [JUSTICE SHAM SUNDER] PRESIDENT [NEENA SANDHU] MEMBER [JAGROOP SINGH MAHAL] MEMBER
Dr Rajiv Wadehra, medical superintendent of GMH and director, health and family welfare, Chandigarh, appeared in person before the commission following an order of September 27 that summoned him to explain why Suman had not been paid full amount as per the earlier orders and why he should not be sentenced to imprisonment for defying the orders. Dr Rajiv tendered an amount of ₹4,38,515 through cheque drawn on the treasury department, Chandigarh, in favour of Suman. He said the delay in payment was due to late approval (received on

October 9) by the UT finance department. Pankaj Chandgothia, counsel for Suman, said the commission had passed orders on March 1, 2012, directing GMH and its three doctors, Kirti Sood, Navdeep Kaur and Manpreet Kaur, to pay ₹4 lakh as compensation and ₹50,000 as legal costs. The payment was to be made within a month. The hospital was also directed to bear her treatment cost for rest of her life. Chandgothia said though GMH was held vicariously liable for the fault of its employees, it had only paid a sum of ₹1 lakh towards compensation and ₹12,500 towards legal costs.

HIGH COURT OF JUDICATURE AT ALLAHABAD ORDERS
DATED 9.10.2015
(Dr. Amit Verma vs. State of U.P. & another on 9 October, 2015)

Criminal case no. 1948/2015 (State v/s. Amit Verma and others) u/s 304-A, 336, 337, 338 IPC, crime no. C-11/2009, P.S. Nazeerabad, district Kanpur Nagar pending in the court of ACMM-II, Kanpur Nagar regarding death because of transfusion of blood of wrong blood group.

Application u/s 482 Cr.P.C. was filed for quashing the proceedings of criminal case no. 1948/2015 State v/s. Amit Verma Criminal case, crime no. C-11/2009 was registered after allowing of application u/s 156(3) CrPC. of the complainant Rizwan Khan. After completion of the investigation, police had submitted the charge-sheet against the applicant for the aforesaid offences, on the basis of which criminal case no. 1948/ 2015 was registered and preceded against him. After his appearance, the accused-applicant requested for discharge, and relied on case of 'Jacob Mathew v/s. State of Punjab'. After hearing his request for discharge was rejected by the trial court and charge for offences u/s 336, 337, 338, 304-A IPC were framed. Then applicant-accused moved application u/s 482 CrPC. for quashing the entire proceedings of the aforesaid case no. 1948/2015 pending against him.

Prosecution case in brief was that applicant Amit Verma and four others doctors, namely, Dr. Rajan Luthra, Dr. B.K. Gupta, Dr. J.P. Singh and Dr. Sanjay Gupta were carrying on their medical profession in Kanpur Medical Center, and Dr. P.K. Singh was in-charge of Blood-Bank of G.S.V.M. Medical College, Kanpur Nagar. On 06.11.2009 complainant's wife Yasmin Begam was admitted in Kanpur Medical Center, where her treatment started under the supervision of Dr. Rajan Luthra and Dr. B.K. Gupta. After sometime, they had asked complainant to arrange blood from Blood-Bank of G.S.V.M. College and gave a written a slip for bringing blood of O+ blood group.

On 07.11.2009 and 08.11.2009 blood brought by the complainant from G.S.V.M. Medical College Blood-Bank and was administered in the body of Yasmin Begam. On 08.11.2009 the bottles of blood brought by the complainant was handed over in said hospital and was administered to Yasmin Begam without properly testing and matching it with the blood of patient. When said blood was administered, the condition of patient started deteriorated suddenly. Then administration of blood was stopped, and on testing it was found that said blood was of 'B+' group instead of 'O+' group. Due to such administration of wrong group of blood, kidney and other organs of the body of the Yasmin Begam were damaged and died on 08.11.2009 at about 05:00 pm. in evening. For her death the doctors Rajan Luthra, Dr. B.K. Gupta, P.K. Singh and staff of Blood-Bank as well as Dr. Piyush Mishra, Dr. J.P. Singh and Dr. Sanjay Singh were held responsible because their negligence and administration of wrong blood without testing resulted in death of Yasmin Begam. Out of two bottles brought from the Medical College Blood-Bank, one bottle was administered and other bottle supply no. 26906 was not administered.

HIGH COURT in its order dated 09.10.2015 dismissed the application u/s 482 with the observations that the evidence collected during the investigation appears to be prima facie proof of medical evidence on the part of attending doctors, therefore the said proceedings before the trial court must continue to reach its logical conclusions. Therefore, the grounds mentioned in application for exercise of inherent jurisdiction for quashing the proceedings of the court below were not found sufficient.

STATE CONSUMER DISPUTES REDRESSAL COMMISSION, UP

C-1 Vikrant Khand 1 (Near Shaheed Path), Gomti Nagar
Lucknow-226010

Dr Pankaj Mehrotra vs Salim Ansari on 13 September, 2017

First Appeal No. A/2006/1211 (Arisen out of Order of District State
Commission)

Date 17.10.2017

JUDGMENT

Facts leading to the appeal no. 1203 of 2006, in short, are that the
respondent/complainant got his daughter Rani Faraz Jahan admitted
in the hospital of the appellants/OP no. 1 on the advice of the OP
no. 2 for her treatment on 11.9.2002 and had deposited ₹10,000.00 as
advance. The complainant's daughter was operated upon by the OP no.
2 and thereafter, as per the prescription, her treatment continued on the
advice of OP no. 1 & 2. For transfusion of blood the complainant from
time to time brought the blood for transfusion. On 13.9.2002, the OP no.
3 charged ₹1,600.00 for providing B+ blood. On the advice of doctors the
complainant again brought blood from the OP no. 3 on 23.9.2002 but
after transfusion of blood the condition of the complainant's daughter
became much worsen as the bleeding started from the anus side but the
OP no. 1 & 2 did not take it seriously. Again on 25.9.2002 a slip was given
for transfusion of blood whereupon the blood was brought from the OP
no. 3 and again there was transfusion of blood but the condition of his
daughter kept worsening. The complainant thereafter, found that A+
blood was transfused as there was a bottle with A+ blood group inscribed
on it. Because of the wrong transfusion of blood that the condition of the
complainant's daughter became very serious and she was discharged
from the hospital on 28.9.2002 to be taken to some other hospital. The
patient was taken to Hallet Hospital where he was informed that there
was no chance of survival of the patient because of wrong transfusion of
blood. Ultimately, she was taken to Kanpur Medical Centre where she
died on 29.9.2002. It was because of the wrong blood supply by the Blood
Bank and wrong transfusion of blood by the doctors in the hospital that
the complainant's daughter died. The complainant, thereafter, filed a
complaint case in the Forum below where the appellant and other OPs
filed their written statements. After hearing the parties the ld. Forum
below passed the impugned order on 18.4.2006 as under:-

"परिवाद स्वीकार किया जाता है, विपक्षीगण को आदेश दिया जाता है कि इस निर्णय के
दिनांक से दो माह के अन्दर विपक्षी सं0 1 रू 1,00,000/- (एक लाख) तथा विपक्षी सं0 2
रू 50,000/- (पचास हजार) व विपक्षी सं0 3 रू 1,50,000/- (डेढ़ लाख) परिवादी को उसकी
पुत्री की चिकित्सा एवं मृत्यु के लिए छतिपूर्ति परिवादी का भुगतान करें। निर्धारित समय में भुगतान

न करने पर विपक्षीगण द्वारा उक्त धनराशि पर 10 प्रतिशत वार्षिक साधारण ब्याज भी फोरम में वाद प्रस्तुत होने के दिनांक से देय होगा।"

"Feeling aggrieved with the impugned order, the appellant filed the appeal no. 1203 of 2006 mainly on the grounds that the Learned Forum has not considered the facts that the appellant has categorically denied that any wrong transfusion of blood was made and also the fact that if any wrong transfusion of blood is made then the patient could not survive such a long period of six days. The complainant had not made payment of ₹23,960.00 which was payable at the time of discharge and has filed the complaint to escape the payment. The patient was suffering from T.B. and she had died of Cardio Respiratory Arrest and not by the wrong transfusion of blood, hence, the impugned order is based on wrong appreciation of facts and evidence and is liable to be set aside."

It is interesting to note that according to the complainant the blood of wrong group was transfused from 23.9.2002 and there is the evidence on record to show that the blood A+ group was purchased on 25.9.2002 in the name of the patient Rani and hence, there is compelling reason to believe the statement of the complainant that the wrong blood group was transfused on 25.9.2002 and therefore, the worsening of the condition of the patient was due to this wrong transfusion of blood at least on 25.9.2002 positively and hence, the record of blood transfusion notes from 23.9.2002 are not provided by the appellant Hospital which is indicative of the fact that those records would have clarified the blood group which was transfused to the patient from 23.9.2002 onwards.

From the arguments of the ld. counsel for the appellant/OP no. 2 Dr. Pankaj Mehrotra, it transpires that the report of blood group was prepared by some other doctor of the hospital. Under the circumstances, the hospital authorities are also responsible for wrong transfusion of blood to the patient. It is argued by the ld. counsel for the appellants that there is no expert opinion to prove the point as to whether there was any wrong transfusion of blood to the complainant's daughter whereby she died and therefore, it cannot be said that there was wrong transfusion of the blood to the patient but we find that in a case like this, there is no need of expert opinion as only thing that is proved in the case is as to whether there was wrong transfusion of blood or not because wrong transfusion of blood itself is a very serious fatal mistake and in the instant case, from the discussions made above, it is proved that there was wrong transfusion of blood to the complainant's daughter whereby ultimately she dies in another hospital.

Therefore, there is serious deficiency in service firstly, on the part of the Blood Bank to supply blood of wrong group and then on the part of the hospital and Dr. Pankaj Mehrotra in getting the blood of wrong blood group transfused to the patient whereby she ultimately died. Therefore, the ld. Forum has passed a very reasoned order finding the appellants/OPs guilty of deficiency in service and therefore, there is no scope to interfere in the impugned order. Hence, all the appeals deserve to be dismissed.

No order as to costs. Certified copy of the judgment be provided to the parties in accordance with rules. Let a copy of this judgment be placed on the records of the Appeals no. 1211 of 2006 and 1160 of 2006.

IN THE HIGH COURT AT CALCUTTA
[A CONSTITUTIONAL WRIT JURISDICTION APPELLATE SIDE]
State of West Bengal & Ors vs. Dr. Subiman Saha and ANR on
18 February, 2019

Hon'ble Justice Dipankar Datta and Hon'ble Justice Bibek Chaudhuri

1. W.P.S.T. 176 of 2016 [State of West Bengal & ors. v/s Dr. Subiman Saha and anr.]
2. W.P.S.T. 177 of 2016 [State of West Bengal & ors. v/s Dr. Subiman Saha and anr.]

- These writ petitions, having a common genesis, involve the same parties. The same were naturally heard together and we propose to dispose it of by this common judgment and order.
- By an order dated June 19, 2000, the Principal Secretary to the Government of West Bengal, Labour Department placed Dr. Subimana Saha under suspension with immediate effect and until further orders, in contemplation of an inquiry against him for gross negligence of duty and misconduct. At the relevant time, Dr. Saha was posted as the Medical Officer, Blood Bank, ESI Hospital, Manicktola, Kolkata. A charge-sheet dated August 25, 2000 followed soon thereafter. The articles of charge framed against him, read as follows:
- That Dr. Subiman Saha, Ex-M.O. Blood Bank, ESI Hospital, Maicktala, committed gross blunder in detecting blood group of the deceased patient. It is highly irregular and unbecoming on the part of a responsible physician like him.
- Consequent upon wrong determination of Blood Group and Rh factor of the patient Ku. Soma Porey by the said Dr. Subiman Saha, an unusual delay in transfusion of blood was caused. As a result, the patient breathed her last on 14.6.2000. The said Dr. Subiman Saha committed serious misconductand created unnecessary harassment to the patient party.
- That Dr. Subiman Saha, committed gross negligence of duty in determining wrong blood group and Rh factor in respect of deceased patient. Such lapse of treatment of Dr. Subiman Saha acted irresponsibility and lack of devotion to duty as a public servant."
- The charge-sheet in its annexure-III listed the particular documents by which the charges framed against Dr. Saha were proposed to be sustained and annexure-IV contained the list of witnesses who were likely to adduce evidence on behalf of the prosecution. Dr. Saha replied to the charge-sheet on August 13, 2001. At the outset, he ventilated a grievance that despite his repeated prayers photo copies of the documents listed in annexure-III of the charge-sheet had not been furnished to him and, therefore, the reply was being

submitted by him without prejudice to his rights and contentions and reserving his right to submit further additional written defence. Certain portions of the reply which could be relevant for the purpose of decision on these writ petitions are quoted below: *"I also submit that, faulty determination of Rh. Type of Blood is a multifactorial technical error for which I cannot be held responsible solely. I submit that in the instant case the blood grouping was made correctly but due to multifactorial technical reasons and other aberrant technical parameters Rh. Typing of the Blood could have been fallacious. In that instant case while I was determining the blood grouping with the help at a glass slide only without microscope and even without Khan tube (for Coomb's Test), in absence of any technical assistant in a Blood Bank at 12 O' Clock in the midnight. In such situation, there are many possibilities of human error in the report regarding Rh. Typing without any wilful negligence on the part of the concern Doctor. I was not assisted by any technical personnel and Tube confirmation (Coomb's Test) could not be done due to non-availability of equipment like Microscope, Khan Tube, Coomb's reagent etc. during that very moment. I submit humbly that I cannot be held responsible for lack of such essential infrastructure which the blood bank in-charge could not provide in spite of our requests. In the article of charges it has been alleged that due to delay in transfusion of Blood, delay in treatment was caused, resulting unfortunate death of the patient. I also submit that since no post mortem examination was conducted by which it could be reasonably ascertained that the patient had died out of delayed blood transfusion. I am to submit further that the sex of the patient (Female, Aged 12 years), Marital Status (Unmarried), recoverable disease (Pubertal Menorrhagia), and considering her future possibility of pregnancy and so as to prevent the chance of haemolytic disease of the new-born: it was prudent on my behalf to give the diagnosis 'Rh' Negative When there is dilemma regarding clumping of R.B.Cs and to prevent future Immuno-sensitization, (As because immuno-incompatibility occurs when 'Rh' positive blood given to 'Rh' Negative person; but the Reverse is not True) it is justified to label the patient 'Rh' Negative. Under the circumstances the allegation of lack of sense of responsibility and devotion to duty and wilful disregard of medical ethics cannot and does not arise at all".*

The inquiring authority submitted his (undated) report of inquiry holding Dr. Saha guilty of article of charge III only. Articles of charge I and II were held not to have been proved. The Inquiring Authority held that Dr. Saha was guilty of committing serious mistake in determining the Rh. Factor in the blood of the patient. It was observed by the I.A. that this error ultimately led to the death of the patient. Dr. Saha moved the tribunal for the first time by presenting O.A. 1122 of 2002. In such application, he prayed for setting aside/quashing of the charge-sheet, the inquiry proceedings and the show-cause notice proposing punishment dated July 4, 2002.

The tribunal disposed of the application recording that the final order must be passed after considering the reply and the additional reply submitted by Dr. Saha, within a period of six months, whereupon copy of the order must be served on Dr. Saha. Liberty of Dr. Saha to pursue his statutory right of appeal was reserved. The concluding paragraph of the order records that the learned advocate for Dr. Saha had prayed for liberty to file the additional reply, if the same had not been filed before the disciplinary authority on any earlier occasion. Such prayer was granted and two months' time was given to Dr. Saha to file his reply without fail.

Aggrieved by the orders dated July 9, 2012 and June 6, 2013 allowing O.A. 581 of 2011 and dismissing R.A. 9 of 2012 respectively, the State challenged the same in an application under Article 227 of the Constitution before this Court, dated April 11, 2014. Such application was registered as COST 6 of 2014. It was listed for consideration before a Division Bench presided over by Hon'ble Jayanta Kumar Biswas, J. (as His Lordship then was) (hereafter the 1st DB) on August 29, 2014. The order passed on such application on August 29, 2014 is quoted below:

"Mr. Banerjee appearing for the State has submitted that he has received instructions to withdraw the COST with liberty to file an appropriate WPST against the same order of the West Bengal Administrative Tribunal. Mr. Chowdhury appearing for the first respondent has submitted that the State has partly complied with the order of the Tribunal. Correctness of this submission has been disputed by Mr. Banerjee. We are of the opinion that the prayer for withdrawal should be allowed. Hence we allow the prayer. The COST is dismissed. No costs. Certified xerox."

The aforesaid order by which COST 6 of 2014 was dismissed as withdrawn and no liberty was granted, as prayed for, to present a fresh application, did not result in any immediate action on behalf of the State and its officers to question it. More than eight months after the order dated August 29, 2014 was passed, the State presented WPST 101 of 2015 on April 6, 2015, being a writ petition under Article 226 of the Constitution, challenging the orders dated July 9, 2012 and June 6, 2013 (which were earlier challenged in COST 6 of 2014, together). WPST 101 of 2015 was considered by another Division Bench presided over by Hon'ble Nishita Mhatre, J. (as Her Ladyship then was) (hereafter the 2nd DB) and the order dated August 11, 2016 passed thereon is set out below:

"The learned Counsel Mr. Dutta, appearing for the petitioners/State, seeks leave to withdraw this petition and to file three separate petitions challenging the orders, which have been impugned in this petition. The petition is allowed to be withdrawn with liberty as prayed for subject to the question of maintainability of the writ petitions to be filed being considered at the stage of admission.

High Court passed that Dr. Saha having attained the age of superannuation during the pendency of proceedings before this Court, the State is entitled to proceed against him in terms of Rule 8 of the West Bengal Services (Death-cum-Retirement Benefit) Rules, 1971 (hereafter the DCRB Rules) and leave may, accordingly, be granted.

High Court further stated that the bruises and scars that an order of suspension, continued for unduly long period of time, brings about is, at times, more punishing than major penalties like reduction in rank or pay. It is because of these that the Supreme Court in a catena of decisions has deprecated continuance of suspension for unduly long period. The Bench felt that Dr. Saha having spent an inglorious life for all the time he was under suspension, it is sufficient admonition for him to have committed the lapse of determining the Rh factor erroneously. Justice would be sub-served, if the matter is allowed to rest now.

For the reasons aforesaid, WPST 176 of 2016 and WPST 177 of 2017 were dismissed both on the ground of maintainability as well as merits. Bench further ordered that whatever service and terminal benefits are outstanding shall be released in favour of Dr. Saha by the petitioners as early as possible, but not later than four months of receipt of a copy of this judgment and order. Bench observed that this much Dr. Saha was entitled to without even filing a fresh original application, for the ordeal he had faced in this century.

IN THE SUPREME COURT OF INDIA
CRIMINAL APPELLATE JURISDICTION
(Anjana Agnihotri vs. The State of Haryana on 6 February, 2020)

CRIMINAL APPEAL NO. 770/ 2009

ORDER

DEEPAK GUPTA .....J   HEMANT GUPTA.....

This Appeal is directed against judgment dated 23.04.2008 of the Punjab & Haryana High Court whereby the High Court upheld the order of Additional Sessions Judge dated 24.09.2004 by which the order dated 30.11.2000 of the learned Sub-Divisional Judicial Magistrate, Dabwali discharging the appellants for having committed offences under Section 304A IPC, 1860 and Section 18-C/27-B of the Drugs & Cosmetics Act, 1940, was set aside.

The prosecution story is that Santosh Rani (deceased) was admitted to the Agnihotri Hospital run by the appellants herein. On 15.11.1998 at about 5.00 a.m. Santosh Rani was expecting a child and she was advised caesarean operation. Such operation was conducted at about 8.00 a.m. and a male child was born. After the birth of the child the doctors felt that blood was required to be given to Santosh Rani. Thereafter, her husband Nand Lal and brother Bhajan Lal offered to give blood and this blood was taken and transfused to Santosh Rani at about 2.30 p.m. At about 2.00 a.m. the next morning Santosh Rani expired. Thereafter, Mulkh Raj, brother of the husband of the deceased filed an FIR with the police. It is important to note that in the FIR it is stated that in the hospital the blood of Nand Lal and Bhajan Lal was taken by the dispenser and Dr. Agnihotri of the hospital (without holding any blood bank License). It is further stated that these two persons tested the blood and transfused it to Santosh Rani and oxygen was also administered.

The main allegation against the appellants in the case is that they did not attend to Santosh Rani from 2.30 p.m. to 2.00 a.m. The Trial Court on the application of the accused discharged them relying upon the judgment of this Court in Jacob Mathew vs. State of Punjab & Anr. (2005) 6 SCC 1 case. The Additional Sessions Judge set aside the order of discharge and the order of Additional Sessions Judge in revision were upheld by the High Court. In Jacob Mathew's Case this Court clearly held that in criminal law medical professionals are placed on a pedestal different from ordinary mortals. It was further held that to prosecute the medical professionals for negligence under criminal law, something more than mere negligence had to be proved. Medical professionals deal with patients and they are expected to take the best decisions in the circumstances of the case. Sometimes, the decision may not be correct, and that would not mean that the medical professional is guilty of criminal negligence. Such a medical profession may be liable to pay damages but unless negligence of a high order is shown the medical professionals should not be dragged into criminal proceedings. That is why in Jacob Mathew's case this Court held that in case of criminal negligence against a medical professional it must be shown that the accused did something or failed to do something in the given facts and circumstances of the case which no medical professional in his ordinary senses and prudence would have done or failed to do. Therefore, this Court also directed in such cases an independent opinion of a medical professional should be obtained in this regard. This Court had made reference to the following observations in Jacob Mathew's case. While concluding the judgment this Court gave certain guidelines. This Court only refer to Para 48(7) which was relevant is as under:

"To prosecute a medical professional for negligence under criminal law it must be shown that the accused did something or failed to do something which in the given facts and circumstances no medical professional in his ordinary senses and prudence would have done or failed to do. The hazard taken by the accused doctor should be of such a nature that the injury which resulted was most likely imminent." Further this Court held in para 52 as under: "The investigating officer should, before proceeding against the doctor accused of rash or negligent act or omission, obtain an independent and competent medical opinion preferably from a doctor in government service, qualified in that branch of medical practice who can normally be expected to give an impartial and unbiased opinion applying the Bolam test to the facts collected in the investigation." In the present case the appellants failed to obtain any opinion of an independent doctor. The post-mortem report does not show that the death of Santosh Rani had occurred due to the transfusion of blood. The only negligence that could be attributed to the accused is that they carried out the blood transfusion in violation of some instructions issued by the Chief Medical Officer that blood should be obtained from a licensed blood bank and that no direct blood transfusion from the donor to the patient should be done. The Supreme Court therefore was of the opinion that even if this is true, the negligence is not such as to fall within the ambit of Jacob Mathew's case.

In view of the above, the judgment of the High Court was set aside and the order of the trial court was restored and discharged the appellants. The Appeal was accordingly allowed.

MADHYA PRADESH HIGH COURT BENCH AT GWALIOR

Hariom Sharma vs The State of Madhya Pradesh on 6 July, 2021

W.P. No. 11460/2021

Judge: Sushrut Arvind Dharmadhikari

Brief facts leading to filing of this case are that on 13.06.2021, the petitioner admitted his son aged about 2 years in J.A. Hospital, Gwalior, where he was diagnosed with jaundice. On 14.06.2021, one unit blood of B+ blood group was transfused to him, due to deficiency of blood in his body. Thereafter, on 15.06.2021, the son of the petitioner was admitted in the hospital of respondent no. 5, where he was tested COVID-19 positive on which the doctors were asked for transfusion of one unit blood and one unit plasma. On the same day, one unit blood and one unit plasma was transfused to the petitioner's son. After the blood and plasma was transfused, suddenly the son of the petitioner became serious and red spots were raised on his body. Thereafter, it was found that blood of wrong blood Group was transfused to his son by respondents no. 5 and 6. On the basis of the aforesaid, a complainant was made to the Superintendent of Police, Gwalior and also at Police Station Padav, District Gwalior but no action whatsoever has been taken thereupon. As such, the instant petition has been filed.

Per contra learned Government Advocate for the respondents/ State contends that the relief prayed in this petition cannot be granted to the petitioner in view of the fact that petitioner is having an alternative efficacious remedy of filing complaint before the Magistrate under section 156(3) of the Cr.P.C. He further submits that it is well settled that disputed questions of fact cannot be looked into by this Court in Article 226 of the Constitution of India. As such, the present petition is liable to dismissed at the threshold.

In view of the legal conspectus on the point in issue, as cited above, since the petitioner has rushed to this Court without availing the alternative efficacious remedy as envisaged under the Cr.P.C., this writ petition cannot be entertained and is, accordingly, dismissed.

So far as medical negligence against respondents no. 5 and 6 is concerned, the petitioner is free to avail alternative remedy as available under the law. However, if the petitioner approaches the Magistrate concerned under the provisions of the Code of Criminal Procedure, the Magistrate concerned shall proceed in accordance with law including the precedents enumerated hereinabove.

PUNJAB-HARYANA HIGH COURT
(Baldev Singh Romana vs. State of Punjab on 14 February, 2022)

CRM-M-41584-2020 (O&M)   Date of Decision: 14.2.2022

CORAM: HON'BLE MR. JUSTICE GURVINDER SINGH GILL

- The petitioner sought grant of regular bail in a case registered against him vide FIR No. 185 dated 10.10.2020 under Sections 269, 270, 307 IPC and Section 29 of the Drugs and Cosmetics Act, 1940 at Police Station Kotwali, District Bathinda.

- FIR in question was lodged by Civil Surgeon, Bathinda pursuant to an inquiry conducted by a three member Committee in the matter pertaining to transfusion of HIV positive blood to two patients. Report of the three member Committee constituted by Senior Medical Officer (SMO), Civil Hospital, Bathinda submitted its findings broadly to the following effect:

- That on 6.5.2020 Blood Bank, Civil Hospital, Bathinda, issued blood to be transfused to Rekha Rani who was getting treatment from Dr. Gurinder Kaur, Medical Specialist in Medical Ward. However, the said blood which had been taken from Blood Bag No. 2765 (HIV +ve) was infected blood. The blood had been issued by Richu Goyal, MLT (Medical Laboratory Technician) who was an out-sourced employee. The blood donor of the infected blood was Rajinder Kumar;

- That subsequently, on 3.10.2020, a minor girl, aged 7 years, namely Nimarpreet Kaur suffering from Thalassemia was also transfused infected blood donated by the same donor namely Rajinder Kumar. Even on the said occasion, the blood had been issued by Richu Goyal, MLT. During inquiry, it was held that the Blood Bank Incharge, Dr. Krishma Goyal, by not informing her superiors and keeping them in dark about the said facts was negligent and that in fact in May 2020 itself she knew that Rajinder Kumar donor is HIV positive. It was found that she had not even informed the patient and had played with the life of patient;

- That the senior-most MLT namely Shri Baldev Singh Romana (petitioner) was also under suspicion inasmuch as his relation with Dr. Krishma Goyal and Richu Goyal, MLT were not cordial. Though, Baldev Singh Romana stated before the Inquiry Committee that he did not know donor Rajinder Kumar and was not having his mobile phone but it was found that it is Baldev Singh Romana himself, who had called Rajinder Kumar to the Blood Bank for blood donation, while being aware that Rajinder Kumar is HIV positive. It was found that Baldev Singh Romana had made a call to Rajinder Kumar from his mobile phone no. 94176-81770 on 1.10.2020 at 11:45 a.m.;

- That when the infected blood was transfused to minor Nimarpreet Kaur, then Baldev Singh Romana went to the Children Ward and all of a sudden took the blood bag from nurse Kuldeep Kaur informing her that the same was HIV positive. He got the blood tested without any authorization from superiors and himself went to the office of SMO with the blood report and blood bag and informed him that HIV positive blood had been transfused. It was found that Baldev Singh Romana had also committed a wrong by not timely informing his superiors about the transfusion of infected blood and in case he had done so, the horrifying incident could have been avoided; and

- That it was also reported that there was some irregularity in purchase of HIV kits as the Test Kits had been purchased from outside and regarding which it was recommended that a separate inquiry be conducted.

- The learned counsel for the petitioner has submitted that the petitioner has no role whatsoever in the matter in hand and that it was the responsibility of Richu Goyal, MLT to ensure that the blood issued to the patient for transfusion is not HIV positive. It has been submitted that the infected blood as well as other blood was stored and kept separately and in these circumstances, it is Richu Goyal, MLT who was extremely negligent in her conduct leading to transfusion of HIV positive blood to two patients. The learned counsel has submitted that the main accused i.e. Richu Goyal, MLT who was responsible for the issuance of the blood has already been granted interim bail by this Court vide order dated 24.3.2021 passed in CRM-M-43650-2020.

- On the other hand, the learned State counsel has submitted that the complicity of the petitioner is clearly evident in as much as it is he himself who had called Rajinder Kumar to donate the blood though he was fully aware that he was HIV positive. He has submitted that although he stated falsely before the Inquiry Committee that he did not know Rajinder Kumar but the call details reflect that it is he who had called Rajinder Kumar by making a phone call from his own mobile phone. It has been submitted that it was for the purpose of settling some personal scores with Dr. Krishma Goyal and Richu Goyal that the petitioner intentionally got infected blood donated and transfused so that the persons who are incharge of the Blood Bank particularly Dr. Krishma Goyal and Richu Goyal are held responsible. The learned State counsel has, however, informed that the petitioner as on date has been behind bars since the last 1 year and 4 months and that trial has not commenced so far. The Court considered rival submissions addressed by the parties and observed as under. "It is indeed an unfortunate incident where two patients have been transfused with blood which was HIV positive. However, the question as to whether the same was done intentionally or was done on account of negligence is a question which would be debatable and can only be decided after evidence is recorded by the trial Court. In any case, the petitioner has been behind bars for a substantial period of about 1 year and 4 months and is not stated to be involved in any other case. Conclusion of trial is likely to consume time as the trial has not commenced so far.

- The petition, as such, was accepted and the petitioner was ordered to be released on regular bail on his furnishing bail bonds/surety bonds to the satisfaction of learned trial Court/Chief Judicial Magistrate/Duty Magistrate concerned.

THE HIGH COURT OF MADHYA PRADESH
(Criminal Revision No. 3152/2021)
(Naresh Kumar Gupta vs. State of M.P. and others Gwalior,
Dated: 21/02/2022)

1. This application under Section 482 of Cr.P.C. was filed against the order dated 12/10/2021 passed by Additional Sessions Judge, Gwalior in ST no. 256/2012, by which the application filed by the applicant under Section 193 of Cr.P.C. for taking cognizance against respondents no. 2 and 3 was rejected.

2. The necessary facts for disposal of the present application in short are that an adulterated plasma was supplied by the accused persons who are facing trial. An application under Section 193 of Cr.P.C. was filed for taking cognizance against respondents no. 2 and 3 on the allegations that the brother of the applicant namely, Manoj Gupta was admitted in R.J.N. Spectra (Apollo) Hospital for treatment of COVID-19. The family members of the patient provided plasma to the doctors as the condition of the patient Manoj Gupta was serious and as per the protocol for treating the COVID-19 virus, transfusion of plasma was one of the treatment. It is alleged that when the doctors were transfusing plasma, they found that the condition of the patient was deteriorating, therefore, transfusion of plasma was stopped and patient Manoj Gupta was shifted to ventilator. It is alleged that after first unit of plasma was given to patient Manoj Gupta, the doctors demanded for additional plasma and when the applicant requested to respondents no. 2 and 3 that since they are outsiders, therefore, they are not in a position to make arrangement, then it is alleged that respondent no. 3 directed to contact his employee Jagdish Bhadkariya, who gave the mobile number of co-accused Mahesh Mourya. He in his turn, arranged for talks with one Ajay Tyagi, who provided plasma for a consideration of ₹18,000/-. It is alleged that when the doctors started transfusing plasma, they found reaction, accordingly transfusion was stopped and the patient was shifted to ventilator. It is alleged that the Doctors had started transfusing plasma without verifying the plasma bag as well as without cross matching with the blood of the patient Manoj Gupta and, therefore, they are also liable to be prosecuted under Sections 304, 420, 465, 467, 468, 471, 120-B of IPC. The Trial Court by the impugned order has rejected the application on the ground that an action can be taken against the respondents under Section 319 of Cr.P.C. and at this stage, there is no good reason for taking cognizance against respondents no. 2 and 3.

3. The important aspect of the matter is that during the first wave of COVID-19 pandemic the patient Manoj Gupta was admitted in

the hospital, as he was suffering from COVID-19 virus. There was a rush of patients in the hospitals. Every efforts were being made by the doctors to save the patients. Since transfusion of plasma was one of the protocol for treating the COVID-19 patients, therefore, it cannot be said that as respondents no. 2 and 3 had asked for further unit of plasma for transfusing the same to the patient Manoj Gupta, therefore they had committed any medical negligence. The plasma was arranged by the family members of Manoj Gupta by purchasing the same from Ajay Tyagi. The doctors started transfusing the plasma, but as soon as they realized that the plasma had reacted, they stopped transfusing plasma and returned the same to the family members of the patient. Thus, it was clear that after the transfusion of plasma started, there was no medical negligence on the part of the doctors and as soon as they realized that the plasma which has been arranged by the family members of the patient has resulted in reaction, the transfusion was stopped. The only allegation made against respondents no. 2 and 3 is that before transfusing the plasma, the plasma bag was not seen and without verifying the report of the cross match pasted on the plasma bag, the doctors started giving plasma treatment to the patient Manoj Gupta.

4. High Court directed that whenever a complaint was received against a doctor or hospital by the Consumer Fora (whether District, State or National) or by the criminal court then before issuing notice to the doctor or hospital against whom the complaint was made the Consumer Forum or the criminal court should first refer the matter to a competent doctor or committee of doctors, specialized in the field relating to which the medical negligence is attributed, and only after that doctor or committee reports that there is a prima facie case of medical negligence should notice be then issued to the doctor/hospital concerned. This is necessary to avoid harassment to doctors who may not be ultimately found to be negligent. The High Court further warn the police officials not to arrest or harass doctors unless the facts clearly come within the parameters laid down in Jacob Mathew case [(2005) 6 SCC 1 : 2005 SCC (Cri) 1369], otherwise the policemen will themselves have to face legal action.

High Court viewed that the facts of the case at hand have to be examined in the light of the aforesaid principle of law with a view to find out as to whether the appellant, a doctor by profession and who treated Respondent 1 and performed surgery on her could be held negligent in performing the general surgery of her gall bladder on 8-8-1996. Thus, unless and until the committee constituted as per the directions given by the Supreme Court in the case of Jacob Mathew gives its report about the medical negligence of the doctors, the doctors should not be prosecuted.

5. In the present case, the applicant has not filed any report of the committee. It is his contention that on the instructions given by respondents no. 2 and 3 he had arranged plasma from Ajay Tyagi, as he had contacted one Jagdish Bhadkariya, who in his turn gave him the mobile number of Mahesh Mourya and Mahesh Mourya in his turn, arranged the talks of the family members of the patient Manoj Gupta with Ajay Tyagi. This Court cannot lose sight of the fact that the hospitals were overburdened in treating the patients in the first wave of COVID-19 pandemic. The situation was horrible and the patients were in need of immediate treatment. It is not in dispute that every plasma bag contains the cross match report. Whether the doctors had sufficient time to send the plasma to the laboratory for re-examination of plasma including cross matching or not, cannot be adjudicated by the Court and in absence of any report by the Medical Board constituted as per the guidelines laid down by the Supreme Court in the case of Jacob Mathew High Court was of the considered opinion that the Trial Court did not commit any mistake in rejecting the application filed by the applicant under Section 193 of Cr.P.C.

6. Accordingly, the order dated 12/10/2021 passed by Additional Sessions Judge, Gwalior in ST no. 256/2012 was affirmed, although on different grounds. The application under Section 482 therefore, was dismissed.

NATIONAL CONSUMER DISPUTES REDRESSAL COMMISSION
NEW DELHI

(M/S. Samad Hospital vs. S. Muhammed Basheer decided on
25 May, 2022)

FIRST APPEAL NO. 172 OF 2012 (Against the Order dated 09/01/2012 in
Complaint No. 27/2003 of the State Commission Kerala)

BEFORE: HON'BLE MR. JUSTICE R.K. AGRAWAL, PRESIDENT
HON'BLE DR. S.M. KANTIKAR, MEMBER

Dated: 25 May 2022

ORDER

- The married couple, A. K. Nazeer and his wife Sajeena
  were undergoing infertility treatment at Samad Hospital,
  Thiruvananthapuram (hereinafter referred to as the 'Opposite Party
  No. 1'). The abdominal Ultrasonography (USG) scan revealed fibroid
  uterus and advised laparoscopic removal of the fibroids. Sajeena
  (hereinafter referred to as the 'patient') underwent laparoscopic
  surgery on 01.08.02 and she was shifted to the post-operative ward.
  In the evening at 7.30 PM, Dr. Sathi M. Pillai (hereinafter referred to
  as the 'Opposite Party No. 2') asked for blood transfusion. The blood
  transfusion was started at 8.30 p.m., but immediately she developed
  blood transfusion reactions and complications. It was alleged
  to have happened due to mismatched blood by transfusion. It is
  alleged that one staff of Cosmopolitan Hospital disclosed to the 2nd
  Complainant and his brother Ashraf about the mistake committed
  at Samad Hospital by giving B+ve blood instead of O+ve blood.
  The Complainants have also written in their written complaint
  that mismatched blood was given to the patient Sajeena at the first
  Opposite Party Hospital. It was confirmed by Dr. Sahadulla, the
  Consultant Physician (hereinafter referred to as the 'Opposite Party
  No. 4') at KIMS Hospital, Thiruvananthapuram. Being aggrieved
  by the alleged negligence, during blood transfusion and further
  treatment, the Complainants filed the Consumer Complaint before
  the State Commission, Kerala and prayed for compensation of
  ₹45 lakh with interest + ₹4.5 lakh towards medical expenditure and
  ₹50,000/- as costs.
- The Opposite Parties Nos. 1 and 2, in their written versions, denied
  the mismatched blood transfusion to the patient Sajeena. It was
  submitted that the patient developed complications which were
  beyond their control and expectation. The complications were
  promptly treated but the patient developed DIC (Disseminated Intra
  Vascular Coagulation), a very serious condition. The doctors took
  expert consultation of Dr. R. K. Prabhu from the Taluk Hospital and

the patient was referred to a higher centre immediately for better management.

- The State Commission partly allowed the Complaint and directed the Opposite Parties Nos. 1 and 2 to pay a total compensation of ₹9,33,000/- to the Complainants Nos. 2 to 6 with cost of ₹15,000/-.
- Being aggrieved, the Appellants (Hospital and the Opposite Party No. 2) filed this First Appeal.

The main questions before the Forum are:

- Whether wrong blood was transfused, if yes- then whether hospital or the blood bank is liable?
- Whether it was a transfusion reaction or DIC?

Admittedly, the surgery was uneventful, but within half an hour of the initiation of the transfusion, the patient suffered shivering and diagnosed it as a transfusion reaction. It is pertinent to note that the witness Dr. Valentina deposed that the transfusion blood of B+ve group whereas the patient was O+ve. From the evidence of Dr. Valentina and her notes in the case sheet (B6), it was a case of transfusion reaction due to mismatch blood resulting into DIC + ARF + severe bleeding.

The Hon'ble Supreme Court in the case of Postgraduate Institute of Medial Education and Research Chandigarh vs. Jaspal Singh & Others held that mismatch in transfusion of blood resulting in death of the patient after 40 days, a case of medical negligence. In the instant case wrong blood transfusion to Sajeena was an error which no hospital/ doctor exercising ordinary care would have made. Such an error is not an error of professional judgment but in the very nature of things a sure instance of medical negligence and the hospital's breach of duty contributed to her death. Thus, we have no hesitation to hold the Opposite Party No. 1 and 2 liable for deficiency in service and the medical negligence.

Compensation:

Before fixing the quantum of compensation Forum looked into several issues. The Complaint was filed by 6 complainants. The patient Sajeena and her husband A. K. Nazeer were undergoing treatment for infertility at Samad Hospital, therefore A. K. Nazeer (Complainant No. 1) was the most aggrieved party. He unfortunately died in a road accident during the pendency of the complaint before the State Commission. Accordingly, his name was deleted and the parents of deceased Sajeena are Complainants Nos. 2 and 3 whereas Complainant No. 4 to 6 are the two sisters and brother of Sajeena. The parent's most stressful event in their life and cause for a major emotional crisis was that they lost their 28 years married daughter due to medical negligence and son-in-law in road accident. In our view, the State Commission erred in quantifying the amount ₹9,33,000/- as a compensation, but the complainants deserve for enhanced compensation. The Complainants stated that the deceased was earning ₹15000/- per month, but nothing is on record to prove her earnings. Therefore, in the ends of justice putting reliance upon the recent judgment of Hon'ble Supreme Court in Arun Kumar Manglik v Chirayu Health & Medicare Pvt. Ltd. and in Lata Wadhwa v State of Bihar, we allow a lump sum compensation of ₹20 lakh to the parents of the deceased Sajeena.

Based on the foregoing discussion, the Appeal was dismissed with modification to the Order of the State Commission. The Appellants shall jointly and severally pay ₹20 lakh as a compensation and ₹1 lakh towards the cost of litigation within 6 weeks from today to the parents of deceased Sajeena. Any delay beyond 6 weeks, shall attract interest @ 7% per annum till its realization.

Glossary

Absorption: The removal of antibodies from serum/plasma through the addition of red blood cells (RBCs) having corresponding antigen.

Adsorption: The uptake of antibody onto the specific receptors on the RBC surface under optimal conditions, therefore, removing the antibody from the serum.

Ambient temperature: Means atmospheric temperature of the immediate surroundings.

Amplitude of the agitation: Means side-to-side movement of the trays in a platelet agitator. The amplitude is expected to be within the range of 3.6–4.0 cm.

Apheresis: Means the process by which blood drawn from a donor, after separating plasma or platelets or leukocytes, is retransfused simultaneously into the said donor.

ART: Antiretroviral therapy.

Atypical antibody: An antibody which occurs as irregular a feature in the serum of some individual, whose red cells lack the corresponding antigen.

Autoantibody: An atypical antibody that sensitizes or agglutinates own red cells.

Autologous blood: The blood drawn from the patient/recipient for retransfusion into him/her later on.

Blood: Means and includes whole human blood, drawn from a donor and mixed with an anticoagulant.

Blood center: Means a place or organization or unit or institution or other arrangements made by such organization, unit or institution for carrying out all or any of the operations for collection, to be returned for apheresis, storage, processing, and distribution of blood drawn from donors and/or for preparation, storage, and distribution of blood components.

Blood cold chain: Means continuous maintenance of mandatory storage conditions (e.g., 2–6°C for whole human blood) from the point of collection/preparation to the point of use of blood and its components.

Blood component: A drug prepared, derived, or separated from a unit of blood drawn from a donor, e.g., red cells, platelet concentrates, or fresh frozen plasma, etc.

Biomedical waste: Waste generated during the diagnosis, treatment or immunization of human beings or animals or in research activities pertaining thereto or in the production and testing biological products.

Blood product: Means a drug manufactured or obtained from pooled plasma of blood by fractionation, drawn from the donors.

Closed system: A system, the contents of which are not exposed to air or outside elements during preparation and separation of components.

Crossmatched blood: Donor's whole blood or its components matched with the blood of the recipient.

Defrost cycle: Process of removing of excess ice from plasma freezer cabinets without change in the temperature of the freezer. Whenever, such frost or ice builds up in the plasma freezer cabinets it requires to be removed to avoid excessive running of the compressor. Modern freezers have an automatic defrost cycle. The temperature of the cabinet should not rise during the defrost cycle.

Document: Written or electronically generated information and work instructions. Examples of documents include standard operating procedures (SOPs), procedures, forms, and quality manuals.

Donor: Means a person who voluntarily donates blood after he has been declared medically fit after medical examination, for donating blood, on fulfilling the criteria given hereafter, without accepting in return, any consideration in cash or kind from any source, but does not include a professional or paid donor.

Equipment: A durable item, instrument or device used in a process or procedure.

Eluate: A fluid medium containing the antibodies that have been deliberately removed from RBCs, allowing for antibody identification.

Elution: The removal of antibody from the RBC surface. Total elution removes the antibody coating the RBCs and destroys the antigens to which they were attached. Partial elution removes the antibody, but allows the antigen to remain intact.

Erythrocytapheresis: It is a collection of RBCs by automated apheresis.

FIFO policy: First-in-first-out policy.

Graft-versus-host disease (GvHD): Transfusion-associated GvHD is a complication of blood component therapy or bone marrow transplantation. It occurs if donor-functional lymphocytes engraft and multiply in a severely immuno-deficient recipient. These engrafted donor cells react against the foreign tissue of the host.

Hemovigilance: Hemovigilance is asset of surveillance procedures covering the whole transfusion chain from collection of blood and its components to the follow-up of its recipient intended to collect and assess information on unexpected or undesirable effects resulting from the therapeutic use of labile blood components and to prevent their occurrence and recurrence. It is an important tool for improving safe blood transfusion practices.

Labeling: Information required or selected to accompany a unit of blood, component, tissue, derivative, or sample, which may include content, identification, and description of process, storage requirements, expiration date, cautionary statements, or indications for use.

Incomplete antibody: Any antibody which sensitizes red cells suspended in saline but fails to agglutinate them. These antibodies react in albumin/enzyme medium or with antihuman globulin (AHG) serum.

Major crossmatch: Test to determine compatibility between donor serum and patient's red cells.

Measurement: Set of operation having the object of determining a value or a quantity.

Minor crossmatch: Test to determine compatibility between patient's serum and donor red cells.

Mixed field agglutination reaction: A reaction wherein a few cells are agglutinated while many cells are unagglutinated.

Nucleic acid amplification testing (NAT): It is a molecular technique for screening donated blood to reduce the risk of transmission-transmitted infections in the recipients, thus providing an additional layer of blood safety. NAT is highly sensitive and specific for viral nucleic acids, narrows the window period of human immunodeficiency virus (HIV), hepatitis B virus (HBV), and hepatitis C virus (HCV) infections. It is an optional test.

PLHA: Patients living with HIV/AIDS.

Plasmapheresis: It is the procedure in which the whole blood is withdrawn from donor/patient, prevented from coagulation immediately after withdrawal, separated into plasma and cellular constituents either by centrifugation or sedimentation with returning back of the cellular constituents.

Procedure: A series of tasks usually performed by one person according to instructions.

Process control: The efforts to standardize and control processes to produce predictable output, meet standards, and minimize variation.

Prozone phenomenon: Negative reaction of antibody in low dilution and positive reaction in higher dilution of the same antibody.

Processed blood: Blood which has been processed into components. Generally refers to the red cell component. The essential tests may or may not have been done.

Professional donor: Means a person who donates blood for a valuable consideration, in cash or kind, from any source, on behalf of the recipient-patient and includes a paid donor or a commercial donor.

Proficiency testing: The structured evaluation of laboratory methods assesses the suitability of processes, procedures, equipment, materials, and personnel.

Quality assurance: As part of the overall quality management program, the range of activities and systems that provide confidence within the organization and for the authorities that all quality requirements are met.

Quality control: A component of quality management, these are tests put in place to ensure that processes, procedures, and products meet the quality requirements.

Quality indicators: Measurable aspects of process outcomes that indicate condition or direction of performance over a while and progress toward stated quality goals or objectives.

Quarantine: Temporary storage in isolation. For example, unprocessed/untested blood is kept in isolation (not accessible for use) until all essential processes/tests are completed.

Reference standards: Reference standards define how or within what parameters an activity shall be performed and are most detailed than management system requirements.

Rouleaux formation: A form of pseudoagglutination in which the red cells look like pile of coins.

Replacement donor: Means a donor who is a family friend or a relative of the patient/recipient.

Standard operating procedure: Written instructions for the performance of a specific procedure.

Sterility: Freedom from the presence of viable micro-organisms.

Stroke: Number of times the tray of the platelet agitator moves from side to side per minute; 65–75 strokes per minute are considered adequate.

Screening: Preliminary testing.

Sensitivity: Probability that the test result will be reactive in an infected individual.

Serum: Fluid portion of clotted blood.

Specificity: Special affinity between an antigen and its corresponding antibody.

Therapeutic phlebotomy: The collection of blood from patients in order to improve their health.

Traceability: Traceability is the ability to trace each individual unit of blood or blood component derived thereof from the donor to its final destination, whether this is a recipient, a manufacturer of medicinal products or disposal, and vice versa.

Unit: A container of blood or one of its components in a suitable volume of anticoagulant obtained from a blood collection from one donor.

Validation: Confirmation and provision of objective evidence that the requirements for a specific intended use or application have been fulfilled. It is a part of quality assurance system that evaluates in advance the steps involved in operational procedures or product preparation to ensure quality, effectiveness, and reliability.

Vasovagal syncope: Syncope resulting from hypotension caused by emotional stress, pain, acute blood loss, fear, or rapid rising from recumbent position.

Wharton's jelly: Mucoid connective tissues that make the matrix of the umbilical cord.

"30-minute rule": General rule in the blood center stating that a maximum time of 30 minutes is allowed for a blood or its component issued from the blood center to a ward to be returned.

Bibliography

1. Anchinmane VT, Sankhe SV. Blood transfusion audit in tertiary care hospital blood bank. Int J Pharm Sci Rev Res. 2022;74(2):129-32.
2. Bharucha Z, Chauhan DM. Introduction to Transfusion Medicine, 1st edition. Mumbai: DK Publishers; 1990.
3. Bisht A, Singh S, Marwaha N. Hemovigilance program-India. Asian J Transfus Sci. 2013;7(1):73-4.
4. Blaney KD, Howard PR. Basic & Applied Concepts of Blood Banking and Transfusion Practices, 3rd edition. St. Louis, MI: Elsevier; 2013.
5. Blood Collection: Routine Venepuncture and Specimen Handling. [online] Available from http://library.med.utah.edu/WebPath/TUTORIAL/PHLEB/PHLEB.html. [Last accessed March, 2023].
6. Chavan SK, Patil G, Rajopadhye P. Adverse blood transfusion reactions at tertiary care hospital. Int J Res Med Sci. 2016;4(6):2402-7.
7. Chitnis V, Chitnis S, Patil S, Chitnis D. Treatment of discarded blood units: disinfection with hypochlorite/formalin versus steam sterilization. Indian J Med Microbiol. 2003;21(4):265-7.
8. Chitnis V, Vaidya K, Chitnis DS. Biomedical waste in laboratory medicine: audit and management. Indian J Med Microbiol. 2005;23(1):6-13.
9. Drugs and Cosmetic Act 1940 and Rules 1945.
10. Godkar PB. Textbook of Medical Laboratory Technology, 2nd edition, New Delhi: Bhalani Publishing House; 2003.
11. Guidelines for Quality Assurance Programmes for Blood Transfusion Services. Geneva: World Health Organization; 1993.
12. Guidelines for Setting up Blood Storage Centers. New Delhi: NACO, Ministry of Health and Family Welfare, Government of India; 2007.
13. Harmening DM. Modern Blood Banking and Transfusion Practices, 5th edition. Philadelphia: F.A. Davis; 2005.
14. Hindawi S. Systems for accreditation in blood transfusion services. ISBT Science Series. 2009;4:14-7.
15. Hoffbrand AV, Catovsky D, Tuddenham EGD, Green AR. Postgraduate Haematology, 6th edition. New Jersey: Wiley; 2011.
16. Joint Working Party of the Transfusion and Clinical Haematology Task Forces of the British Committee for Standards in Haematology. Guidelines for the clinical use of blood cell separators. Clin Lab Haematol. 1998;20:265-78.
17. Kumar A, Sharma S, Ingole N, Gangane N. An audit of blood bank services. J Edu Health Promot. 2014;3:11.
18. Makroo RN. Practice of Safe Blood Transfusion: Compendium of Transfusion Medicine, 2nd edition. Career Publication; 2009.
19. Manual on the Management, Maintenance and Use of Blood Cold Chain Equipment. Geneva: WHO; 2005.
20. Model Standard Operating Procedures for Blood Transfusion Service. New Delhi: WHO; 2002.

21. National Standards for blood centres and Blood transfusion services 2nd Edition, 2023: NBTC (National Blood Transfusion Council), Ministry of Health and Family Welfare, Govt. of India.

22. National Guidebook on Blood Donor Motivation, 2nd edition, 2003, Ministry of Health and Family Welfare, National AIDS Control Organisation, Government of India.

23. Roback J, Combs MR, Grossman B, Hillyer C. Technical Manual, 16th edition. Arlington, VA: American Association of Blood Banks; 2008.

24. Screening Donated Blood for Transfusion-Transmissible Infections: Recommendations. Geneva: World Health Organization; 2010.

25. Sehgal S, Prakhya LJ. Evaluation of bacterial contamination of blood components in a tertiary care centre. Bangladesh J Med Sci. 2022;21(1): 213-5.

26. Sen S, Gupta P, Sinha S, Bhambani P. Haemovigilance and transfusion safety: a review. Sch J App Med Sci. 2014;2(1A):85-90.

27. Standards for Blood Banks and Blood Transfusion Services. New Delhi: NACO, Ministry of Health and Family Welfare, Government of India; 2007.

28. Technical Resource Manual for Hospital Transfusion Services, BC Provincial Blood Coordinating Office, 2nd edition, 2005.

29. The Blood Cold Chain: Guide to the Selection & Procurement of Equipment and Accessories. Geneva: World Health Organization; 2002.

30. The User Manuals of Blood Bag Monitor & Tube Sealer. Terumo Penpol Pvt Limited.

31. Transfusion Medicine Technical Manual, 1991, Directorate General of Health Services, Ministry of Health and Family Welfare, Govt. of India.

32. Transfusion Medicine Technical Manual 3rd edition, 2022, (Technical support by WHO) Directorate of Health Services, Ministry of Health and Family Welfare, Govt. of India.

33. World Health Organization. Blood Transfusion Safety Team. (2001). The Clinical Use of Blood: Handbook. Geneva: WHO; 2001. [online] Available from https://apps.who.int/iris/handle/10665/42396 [Last accessed April, 2023].

34. Zammit V. (2004). A comparative study between antiglobulin crossmatch and type and screen procedures for compatibility testing. [online] Available from https://www.semanticscholar.org/paper/A-comparative-study-between-antiglobulin-crossmatch-Zammit/e7e9953b59b489f8953fb71d-10cc2560a5941063 [Last accessed April, 2023].

Index

Page numbers followed by *f* refer to figure, *fc* refer to flowchart, and *t* refer to table.